Three-dimensional Echocardiography

Thomas Buck
Andreas Franke
Mark J. Monaghan (Eds.)

Three-dimensional Echocardiography

Second fully revised edition

With 877 figures and 518 videos

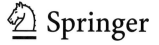 Springer

Editors
Prof. Dr. Thomas Buck
Klinikum Westfalen
Dortmund
Germany

Dr. Mark J. Monaghan
King's College Hospital
London
UK

Prof. Dr. Andreas Franke
Klinikum Siloah
Hannover
Germany

You can also find all video material for this book at:
http://www.springermedizin.de/vzb-echocardiography

ISBN-13 978-3-642-36798-4
DOI 10.1007/978-3-642-36799-1

ISBN 978-3-642-36799-1 (eBook)

Library of Congress Control Number: 2014932999

Springer Medizin
© Springer-Verlag Berlin Heidelberg 2011, 2015

Planning: Hinrich Küster, Heidelberg
Project Management: Kerstin Barton, Heidelberg
Copy Editing: Dr. Mary Gossen, Dietzenbach
Project Coordinator: Barbara Karg, Heidelberg
Cover Design: deblik Berlin
Cover Image: © Springer-Verlag (Prof. Buck)
Production: Fotosatz-Service Köhler GmbH – Reinhold Schöberl, Würzburg

Printed on acid-free paper

Springer Medizin is brand of Springer
Springer is part of Springer Science+Business Media (www.springer.com)

Preface

Real-time three-dimensional (3D) echocardiography, which became commercially available in 2002, is the most recent, major advancement in echocardiography. Providing direct viewing of 3D cardiac surfaces during live scanning, it adds fundamentally new information to the echocardiographic assessment of heart diseases, and it has already significantly changed echocardiographic diagnoses. Although echocardiographic examiners are used to interpreting cross-sectional images, conventional two-dimensional (2D) echocardiography requires mental 3D reconstruction of cardiac structures. This is prone to error and can be difficult to communicate. Real-time 3D echocardiography, in contrast, provides direct, anatomically realistic visualization of 3D structures, such as an en face view from the left atrium to the mitral valve or the direct view of a multifenestrated atrial septum. Beyond this, real-time 3D echocardiography allows for the first time accurate quantitative assessment of structures, volumes and spatial relationships without any geometric assumptions. Therefore, this gives the technique a unique advantage over conventional 2D echocardiography.

However, the practical application and data analysis of real-time 3D echocardiography has been shown to substantially differ from conventional 2D echocardiography. While in 2D echocardiography, the image information is all obtained from a 2D sector view that is manually optimized to present the best image information, real-time 3D datasets facilitate unlimited viewing from all directions of the dataset and unlimited viewing perspectives of structures within the dataset. This freedom of unlimited 3D visual assessment, however, requires knowledge and experience about how to live scan, acquire, and analyze volumetric datasets.

EyeCatcher

Practical application and data analysis of real-time 3D echocardiography differs substantially from conventional 2D echocardiography.

This book is both an illustrated textbook and a practical guide to real-time 3D echocardiography. It provides a comprehensive overview of this fascinating technology covering all clinically important aspects, including a substantial explanation of the basic principles of 3D technology, step-by-step introductions to basic aspects of clinical application, and detailed descriptions of specific applications in the broad spectrum of clinically important heart diseases. What also makes this book an invaluable companion, when working with real-time 3D echocardiography, is an in-depth review of the most recent literature which is provided in each chapter.

The book contains a large number of comprehensively illustrated clinical case examples, which demonstrate how real-time 3D modifies decision-making in echocardiographic practice. However, while focusing on real-time 3D echocardiography, the book does not claim to be a full textbook on either echocardiography or on cardiac diseases.

To illustrate the added benefit of 3D image information, most case examples also include conventional 2D image information for comparison. However, it is important to emphasize that the authors have aimed to highlight the complementary nature of the two techniques where, on the one hand, 3D visualization adds important diagnostic information to a standard 2D echocardiographic examination and, on the other hand, 2D cross-sectional information on structure and thickness of valves, walls, and masses is indispensible for complete understanding of 3D datasets.

EyeCatcher

Real-time 3D echocardiography and conventional 2D echocardiography should be considered complementary modalities.

The authors of this book have all been intensely involved in interactive training courses on 3D echocardiography over the past years and have included their training experience as well as the most illustrative case examples into each chapter. Thus, this book serves as a valuable educational compendium to both individual learning experiences as well as expert-guided training courses.

Since a strong focus of the book is on practical application of real-time 3D echocardiography in daily clinical routine, its chapters and case examples are organized so as to provide valuable tips and tricks for both beginners and experts. In addition, because the heart and echocardiographic imaging are both dynamic and because dynamic information is critical for understanding, the majority of echocardiographic images within the book are accompanied by the full video sequences on the included DVD.

■ **2ⁿᵈ edition**

After a very successful 1ˢᵗ edition, with more than 1000 copies sold, this book presents the 2ⁿᵈ edition which is a full revision of the 1ˢᵗ edition, preserving the overall concept and structure of the book but adding a comprehensive update of all chapters with new illustrative cases, new recommendations from recent guidelines, and new important literature.

Since the 1ˢᵗ edition was published in 2011, the field of real-time 3D echocardiography has demonstrated marked progress with new 3D acquisition software solutions such as one-beat full volume and live 3D color-Doppler, new 3D analysis software solutions such as the heart model 3D volumetry and the 3D navigator, and, importantly, publication of several recommendations on the clinical application of real-time 3D echocardiography. Furthermore, the recent technical advancements have resulted in real-time 3D echocardiography being used in new places in cardiac centers. For example, periinterventional guidance and monitoring in the catheterization lab has become and will continue to be the most rapidly progressing clinical application of real-time 3D echocardiography.

Thus, we believe that a 2ⁿᵈ edition of the book is timely and hope it will be as valuable to readers of various professions like sonographers, physicians, scientists, and students, as the first apparently was.

Thomas Buck
Andreas Franke
Mark J. Monaghan
June 2014

About the editors

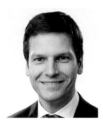

■ **Thomas Buck, MD, FACC, FESC**

Thomas Buck is Associate Professor of Medicine and Cardiology at the University Duisburg-Essen, Germany. Since 2014, he is Director of the Department of Cardiology of the Klinikum Westfalen in Dortmund, Germany. Prior to this at the University Hospital Essen, he held the position of Director of Echocardiography Laboratories as well as the appointments of Chief Consultant and Assistant Director of the Department of Cardiology at the West German Heart Center. Since the beginning of his academic career in 1992, 3D echocardiography has been a major field of his scientific interest. One of his primary clinical areas of expertise is the management of heart valve disease patients, where his early scientific work was stimulated while working as a Research Fellow at Massachusetts General Hospital, Boston, USA. As one of his official assignments, he was the Chair of the German Working Group of Echocardiography from 2005–2011. In addition to a considerable number of scientific articles and clinical guidelines, his work includes several teaching book contributions and international patents in the field of echocardiography. Since the introduction of real-time 3D echocardiography into clinical practice, he has regularly organized national and international training courses as an expert trainer.

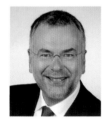

■ **Andreas Franke, MD, FESC**

Andreas Franke is Associate Professor of Medicine and Cardiology and Director of the Department of Cardiology, Angiology and Intensive Care Medicine of the Klinikum Siloah in Hannover, Germany. During his clinical and academic career starting in 1988 at the RWTH Technical University Aachen, Germany, echocardiography and congenital heart disease in adults have been his main fields of scientific interest and work. His primary clinical areas of expertise besides non-invasive cardiac imaging are the interventional therapy of coronary artery disease and the management of valvular disease. Since the early 1990s, he has been involved in further development of 3D echocardiography and has published numerous clinical studies on the topic. Between 1998 and 2001, he was a nucleus member of the Working Group on Echocardiography of the ESC as an organizer of the subgroup 3D echocardiography. Over the last 15 years, he also contributed to several textbooks and atlases on echocardiography. Moreover, since 2003 he regularly organizes national real-time 3D echocardiographic training courses as an expert trainer.

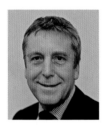

■ **Mark J. Monaghan PhD, FRCP(Hon), FACC, FESC**

Mark J. Monaghan is a Professor of Echocardiography, Director of Non-Invasive Cardiology and Associate Medical Director at King's College Hospital, London UK. He has worked in the field of echocardiography for over 25 years and has published extensively on the subject, especially on the use of 3D. In addition, he holds two international patents on echocardiographic technology and lectures widely at international meetings and cardiology conferences throughout the world. He runs several teaching courses and workshops on 3D echocardiography every year and has contributed to and co-edited several textbooks. Professor Monaghan has been a board member of the European Association of Echocardiography and is a past President of the British Society of Echocardiography.

Content

List of authors

Adhya, Shaumik, BSc MBBS MRCP CCDS
Consultant Cardiologist
Medway Maritime Hospital
Gillingham, Kent, UK

de Agustin, José Alberto
Senior Staff
Universidad Complutense de Madrid
Hospital Clínico San Carlos
Madrid, Spain

von Bardeleben, Stephan, MD
Director, Echocardiography
2nd Medical Clinic, Department of Cardiology
University Medical Center Mainz
Mainz, Germany

Buck, Thomas, MD, FACC, FESC
Associate Professor of Medicine
Director, Department of Cardiology
Klinikum Westfalen
Dortmund, Germany

Franke, Andreas, MD, FESC
Associate Professor of Medicine
Director, Department of Cardiology, Angiology
and Intensive Care Medicine
Klinikum Siloah
Hannover, Germany

Kisslo, Joseph, MD
Professor of Medicine
Duke University Medical Center
Durham, NC, USA

Kühl, Harald P., MD
Associate Professor of Medicine
Director, Department of Cardiology and Intensive Care
Medicine
Klinikum Harlaching
München, Germany

McGhie, Jackie
Chief sonographer
Department of Cardiology
The Thoraxcenter
Erasmus University Medical Center
Rotterdam, the Netherlands

Meijboom, Folkert J., MD, PhD, FESC
GUCH & pediatric cardiologist
Department of Pediatrics and Cardiology
University Medical Center Utrecht
Utrecht, the Netherlands

Miller, Owen I, FRACP, FCSANZ, FRCPCH
Head of Service, Clinical Lead
Paediatric and Fetal Cardiology
Evelina London Children's Hospital
London, UK

Monaghan, Mark J., PhD, FRCP (Hon), FACC, FESC
Professor of Echocardiography
Director of Noninvasive Cardiology
and Associate Medical Director
King's College Hospital, Denmark Hill
London, UK

Plicht, Björn, MD
Senior Cardiologist
Department of Cardiology
Klinikum Westfalen
Dortmund, Germany

Roelandt, Jos R.T.C., MD, PhD, FESC
Professor of Cardiology
Emeritus Chairman Thoraxcenter
Erasmus University Medical Center
Rotterdam, the Netherlands

Simpson, John
Professor of Paediatric and Fetal Cardiology
Director of Paediatroc Echocardiography
Evelina London Children's Hospital
Guy's and St Thomas' NHS Foundation Trust
London, UK

Thiele, Karl E., ME
Principal Scientist
Philips Healthcare
Andover, MA, USA

van der Zwaan, Dr. Heleen
Cardiology Resident
Department of Cardiology
The Thoraxcenter
Erasmus University Medical Center
Rotterdam, the Netherlands

Zamorano, José L., MD, FESC
Professor of Medicine
Director, Department of Cardiology
University Hospital Ramón y Cajal
Madrid, Spain

Three-dimensional echocardiography: lessons in overcoming time and space

Jos R.T.C. Roelandt, Joseph Kisslo

T. Buck et al. (Hrsg.), *Three-dimensional Echocardiography*,
DOI 10.1007/978-3-642-36799-1_1, © Springer-Verlag Berlin Heidelberg 2014

A more intelligible display of complex cardiac pathology and the need for more accurate left ventricular (LV) function assessment prompted investigators to develop three-dimensional (3D) echocardiography immediately after the introduction of two-dimensional (2D) echocardiography in the early 1970s. Indeed, the objective display of cardiac structures in their correct relationship to each other and avoiding assumptions about LV cavity geometry would greatly improve diagnostic accuracy. Several directions have been followed, but 3D echocardiography has followed two merging lines of development. One line is trying to make ultrasound systems work faster and faster, despite the limitations imposed by the fixed velocity of ultrasound in tissue. The second technical line is the attempt to provide meaningful images of the data acquired.

> Three-dimensional display of cardiac structures would greatly improve diagnostic accuracy.

1.1   Reconstruction techniques

The initial approach to 3D echocardiography was the offline reconstruction of a dataset using an external coordinate system or position locator (mechanical, acoustic, electromagnetic, or optical) linked to the transducer to continuously measure the spatial position of each individual image during freehand scanning (◘ Fig. 1.1, ► Techniques for 3D image acquisition) [1][2][3][4]. End-respiratory ECG-triggered 2D echocardiographic images were captured in end-diastole and end-systole using an intersectional line or a standard image plane as a reference for the position and orientation of all other recorded imaging planes [5]. LV endocardial cavity contours were manually traced to produce end-diastolic and end-systolic wireframe or surface-rendered reconstructions of the cavity by a computer (◘ Fig. 1.2).

> Techniques of 3D image acquisition
>   A. Reconstruction techniques
>   1. External reference systems (nonsystematic image acquisition by freehand scanning)
>   – Mechanical arm [1]
>   – Acoustic (spark gap) locator [2]
>   – Optical sensor [3]
>   – Electromagnetic sensor [4]
>   2. Internal reference systems (systematic image acquisition by predetermined transducer motion)
>   – Linear scanning [11][12]
>   – Fan-like scanning [13]
>   – Rotational scanning (stepwise or continuous) [14][15][16]
>   B. Volumetric real-time techniques
>   1. Real-time 3D volume acquisition (with sparse matrix array transducers) [17]
>   2. Real-time 3D imaging (with fully sampled matrix array transducers and micro-beamforming)

Subsequently, volumes were calculated using the summation of wedges method [6]. Freehand scanning had the advantage that it could be applied to most patients, because images could be obtained from several precordial windows. Unfortunately, not only was the whole procedure tedious and time consuming, but the display was static.

Consequently, this approach was not clinically used. However, research studies proved that quantification of cavity volumes and, more importantly, those of distorted aneurysmal ventricles and myocardial mass by 3D echocardiography was more accurate and reproducible than by 2D echocardiography [7][8][9][10].

In the late 1980s, data processing algorithms became available for direct conversion of basic images from a polar to a Cartesian coordinate system together with mathematical interpolation schemes and smoothing algorithms to fill the gaps between the images. These developments were used in the next generation of 3D echocardiographic techniques [18] which were based on an internal coordinate system, allowing a continuum of 2D echocardiographic images to be captured by stepwise transducer motion (linear, fan-like, or rotational) together with temporal information (► Techniques for 3D image acquisition). A diagram of the various modes of transthoracic and transesophageal image acquisition is shown in ◘ Fig. 1.3. Volumetric datasets which contained tissue grey scale information could now be constructed and sliced in any desired cross-section (anyplane, paraplane) resembling conventional 2D images [14][15].

1.1.1   The linear scanning approach

This was the earliest approach to dynamic 3D echocardiography and was based on 3D concepts used in MR and CT imaging. These were applied to ultrasound imaging by researchers at TomTec, who developed the Echo-CT in 1990 (TomTec Imaging Systems GmbH, Munich, Germany) [11][12]. They built a tomographic transesophageal transducer assembly known as »the lobster tail« for acquiring parallel, equidistantly spaced 2D images (◘ Fig. 1.4). The distal part consisted of multiple semicircular plastic segments, which were mechanically straightened after the assembly was advanced into the esophagus.

The transducer was mounted on a sliding carriage housed in this distal part and was moved in equal steps by a computer-controlled stepper motor which was moved using logic that considered heart rate and respiration phase. A water-filled balloon was used to ensure stable contact with the esophageal wall. The images were directly transferred to a workstation (Echo-View, TomTec Imaging Systems) and digitally converted into a prismatic shaped dataset. This transducer assembly was also utilized precordially in children and good results were reported [19].

The Echo-CT system remained a research tool and did not enter into practical clinical use because of difficulties with intraesophageal probe introduction, prolonged examination time under sedation, poor patient acceptance, and limited image quality. However, the method further stimulated interest in 3D echocardiography. The linear acquisition and reconstruction software was also used for ECG-gated 3D reconstruction of coronary artery segments from intracoronary ultrasound images

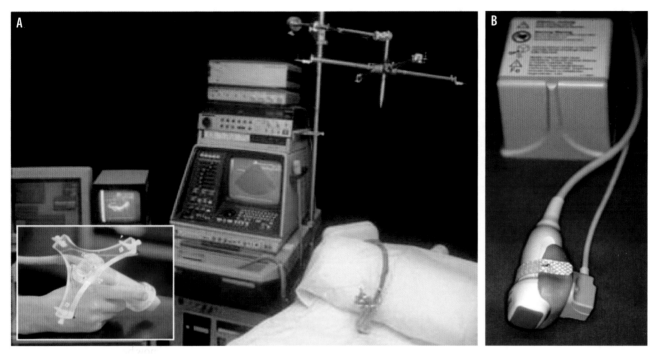

Fig. 1.1 A Setup for image acquisition using an acoustic spark gap device with three spark gap (sound) emitters. The insert shows a prototype which was marketed by TomTec GmbH in 1996 and could be fitted to most commercially available ultrasound transducers. When attached to a transducer, it permits unrestricted precordial freehand scanning and the continuous registration of the position and orientation of the transducer and its imaging plane by a stationary overhead external coordinate system, composed of a set of fixed microphone receiver arrays. From the travel time to each of these microphones, the x, y, and z coordinates and the spatial location of the transducer are calculated (courtesy of A.S. Gopal). **B** Electromagnetic sensor for unrestricted freehand image acquisition. A magnetic field is emitted by the rectangular magnetic box placed near the patient. A position sensor the size of a sugar cube is attached to the transducer and is connected via a microcomputer with the magnetic box; thus, the spatial position and orientation of the transducer and the image frame could be continuously measured

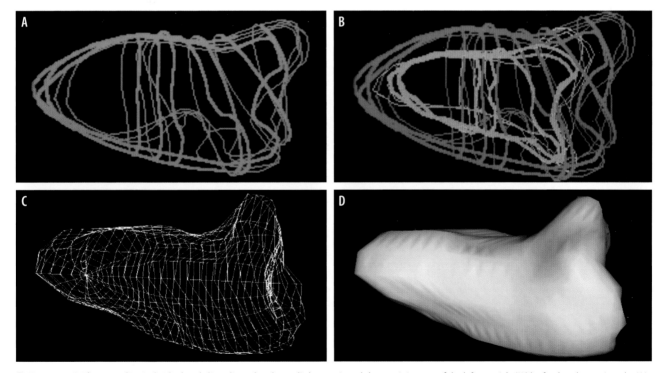

Fig. 1.2 A, B After recording individual end-diastolic and end-systolic long-axis and short-axis images of the left ventricle (*LV*) by freehand scanning, the LV contours are manually traced and saved with their spatial position and orientation (*blue* end-diastolic; *yellow* end-systolic contours) in the computer. These contours are used to create a wire-frame (**C**) or surface-rendered (**D**) reconstruction of the left ventricular cavity. From these reconstructions the end-diastolic and end-systolic volumes are calculated using a polyhedral surface reconstruction algorithm. Reprinted from [6]; Copyright American Society of Echocardiography

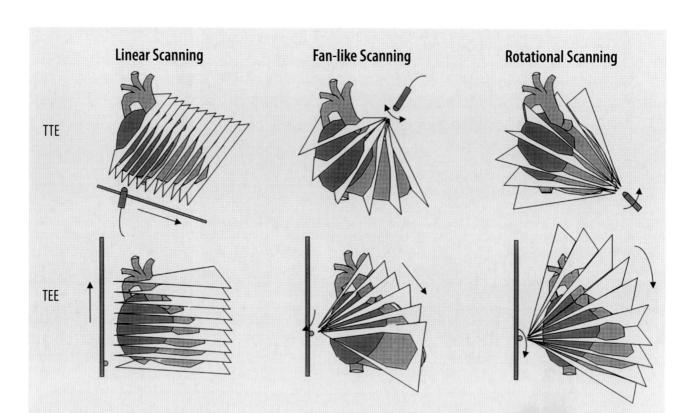

Fig. 1.3 Schematics showing various modes of data acquisition for 3D reconstruction with transthoracic (*TTE*) and transesophageal (*TEE*) approaches. With linear scanning, parallel cross-sectional images of the heart are acquired to create a prismatic dataset. Fan-like scanning allows a pyramidal dataset to be obtained and rotational scanning, where the transducer is rotated around the central axis of the imaging plane, provides a conical dataset

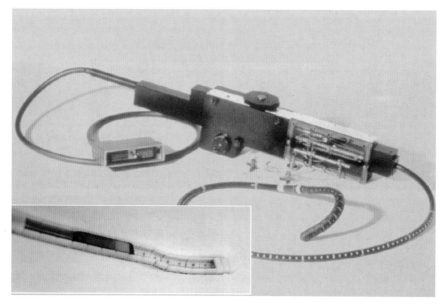

Fig. 1.4 The Echo-CT probe introduced in 1990. The insert shows the semicircular plastic segments (Bowden rings) which when straightened provide the sliding carriage for the linear and stepwise pull back of the transducer under computer control. Reproduced from [38]; Copyright Van Zuiden Communications BV

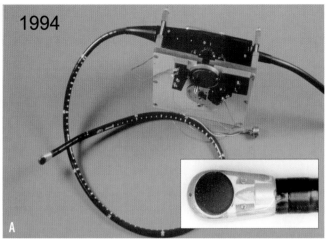
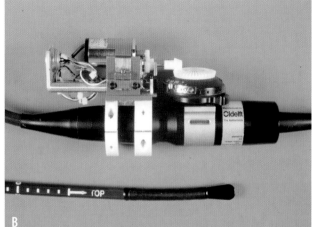
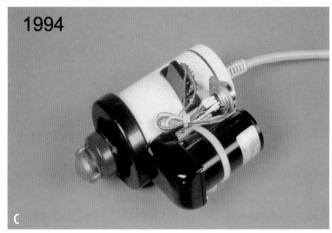
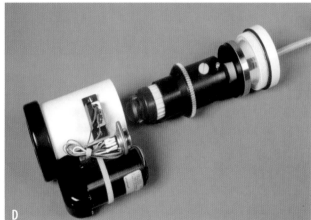

Fig. 1.5 Prototype wheel-work interfaces for rotational image acquisition built at the Thoraxcenter in 1994. **A** Using a transesophageal multiplane probe, the wheel-work device is attached to the control knob and turns the transducer using a stepper motor which is activated by a steering algorithm considering heart cycle variation and the respiratory phase. The multiplane phased array transducer is rotated in discrete adjustable increments through 180°. **B** This smaller wheel-work interface was more practical and used in most of the initial clinical studies. **C** Transducer assembly used at the Thoraxcenter in 1994 for precordial image acquisition. **D** A standard transducer is fixed with a cog wheel in a holder. A step motor is mounted on the holder and rotates the transducer via a wheel-work interface under control of the computer algorithm. The size and shape of the housing could be adapted to any standard precordial transducer. Reproduced from [14]; Copyright American Society of Echocardiography

and has remained the reference method for quantitative analysis of coronary artery disease and testing the effects of therapeutic coronary interventions [20].

> Early results with the transesophageal Echo-CT system further stimulated interest in 3D echocardiography.

1.1.2 The fan-like scanning approach

In this method, the transducer is placed over an acoustic window and moved in a fan-like arc at prescribed angles either manually or by a computer-controlled stepper motor (**Fig. 1.3**) [13][21]. The principles for temporal and spatial synchronization are similar to those for linear scanning. After image reconversion, pyramidal datasets are obtained. Initially, transesophageal probes were used to acquire equiangled short-axis [22] or longitudinal [23] cardiac cross-sections.

Because it was difficult to keep the probe stable in the esophagus during acquisition, investigators subsequently explored the precordial approach. In children, good results were obtained with subcostal scanning; however, in adults the results were suboptimal due to the limited arc over which the transducer could be tilted with good skin contact [24]. Overall, the fan-like scanning examination was rather tedious and the clinical success rate limited. The method was rapidly replaced by the rotational acquisition method.

1.1.3 The rotational scanning approach

In this method, the transducer is rotated in a semicircle around the central axis of the imaging plane (**Fig. 1.3**). In the early 1980s, researchers had already investigated the possibility of transthoracic manual transducer rotation for image acquisition to create LV cavity reconstructions [25]. However, stable image acquisition (axis alignment) and controlled rotation for obtaining more planes within the 180° rotation arc were problematic. Consequently, the use of external motorized stepper devices to rotate the transducer was explored mainly to produce static wire-

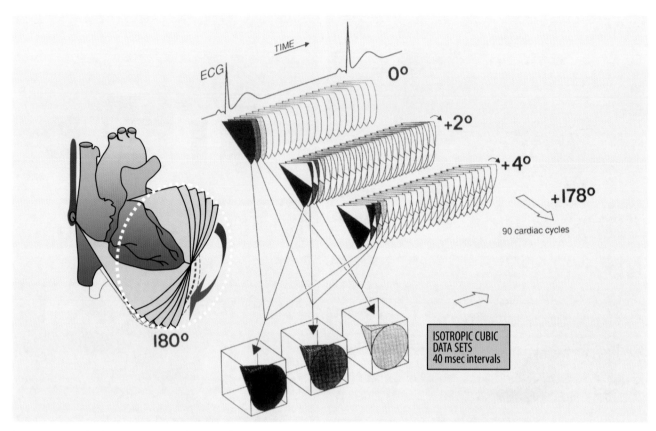

◻ **Fig. 1.6** Principle of 3D reconstruction of the heart from sequentially acquired images using the rotational scanning approach. At each scanning plane (starting from 0°) images of a complete heart cycle are sampled at 25 frames/s. The recorded images are digitized and stored on a computer. After recording 90 cardiac cycles at 2° intervals (to encompass a conical volume of 180°), the cross-sections are formatted according to their electrocardiographic phase and stored in a series of corresponding isotropic cubic datasets. Reproduced from [14]; Copyright American Society of Echocardiography

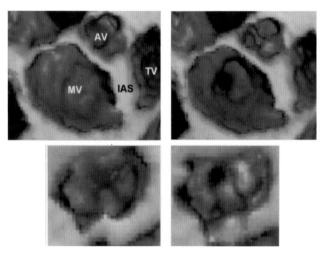

◻ **Fig. 1.7** Examples of the first dynamic volume-rendered 3D reconstructions of a patient with mitral valve stenosis recorded in April 1994. The mitral valve (*MV*) is seen from an atrial (surgical) perspective (*top*), and from within the left ventricle (*bottom*). During systole (*left*), the valve leaflets are closed, while the stenotic orifice of the valve is seen during diastole (*right*). *AV* aortic valve, *IAS* interatrial septum, *TV* tricuspid valve. Reproduced from [14]; Copyright American Society of Echocardiography

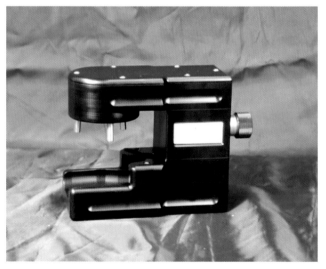

◻ **Fig. 1.8** Adapter that became commercially available in 1995 to rotate the control knob of a multiplane transesophageal transducer in discrete increments by a stepper motor under computer control for rotational image acquisition. Copyright TomTec Imaging Systems, Germany

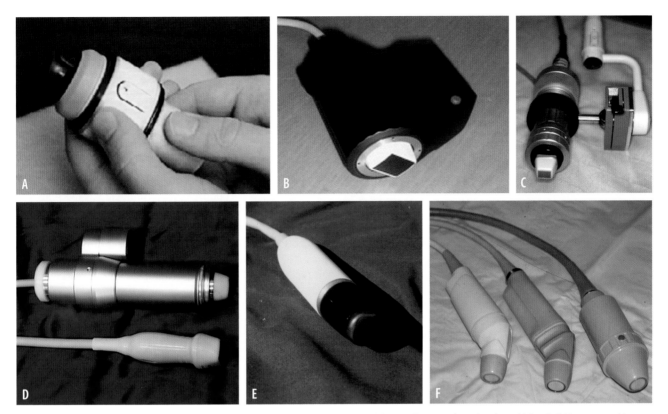

◘ Fig. 1.9 Precordial multiplane transducer assemblies for rotational image acquisition. **A** System for manual rotational acquisition. **B–D** Prototypes with external stepper motor devices for computer-controlled rotational image acquisition. Prototype with an internal step motor (**E**) and systems with an internal stepper motor which have been commercially available (**F**). Systems with an internally integrated motor allowed more stable image acquisition and, hence, better quality 3D reconstructions

frame or surface-rendered LV cavity reconstructions to measure LV volumes [26][27][28]. Manual rotation of a multiplane transesophageal transducer with increments of 18° had also been performed for static LV cavity reconstructions [29].

In early 1994, the steering logic algorithm which was developed for the linear scanning system (Echo-CT) was adapted to rotate the transducer by a stepper motor attached to the external control knob of a prototype transesophageal multiplane probe (Delft Instruments Medical Imaging B.V., Delft, The Netherlands; ◘ Fig. 1.5) [14][30].

The TomTec Echo-Scan software was used for image acquisition, processing, and volume rendering (◘ Fig. 1.6). This resulted in the first dynamic visualization of 3D volumetric reconstructions with a tissue grey scale resembling the actual anatomy of the heart and the display of any selected plane through the heart in cine loop format at 25 frames/s (◘ Fig. 1.7) [14]. Adaptors for rotational image acquisition using standard transesophageal probes soon became available (◘ Fig. 1.8), followed by systems with the stepper motor integrated into the probe handle.

At the same time, we also constructed a transducer assembly which could accommodate any commercially available standard transducer for precordial rotational image acquisition with an external stepper motor using the same steering logic and reconstruction software (◘ Fig. 1.5) [15]. The image quality of these reconstructions was good and transducer systems with an internally integrated stepper motor rapidly became commercially available (◘ Fig. 1.9) [15][31]. Nonetheless, despite the practical advantages,

the precordial system was not widely accepted because there were still too many artifacts due to the relatively long scanning time causing both displacement of the transducer and motion of the patient due to growing restlessness.

Because up to 65% of the referrals for echocardiographic examinations request evaluation of LV function, the possibility of precordial continuous rather than stepwise rotational acquisition was investigated in order to reduce acquisition and processing times for rapid LV volume measurement and perfusion studies. Thus, we constructed a transducer assembly with an internal, ultrafast rotating phased array transducer (160–480 rpm; ◘ Fig. 1.10) [16]. The rotational velocity set the number of independent volume datasets obtained during one heartbeat (e.g., at 480 rpm 16 volumes/s are obtained which means that 12 volumes are obtained at a heart rate of 80 bpm). This approach required the development of complex processing software. Clinical research studies confirmed the feasibility of this approach. Following the same idea, precordial scanning with a continuously rotating transducer to shorten acquisition time using eight planes for reconstruction and rapid LV volume measurement was later proposed by researchers at the Mayo Clinic [32].

The advantages of dynamic 3D imaging for analyzing complex pathomorphology and sectioning structures at various levels and angulations together with the en face visualization of pathology from any perspective were amply documented. It was also shown in many studies that the quantification of LV and right ventricular (RV) volumes and function is more accurate

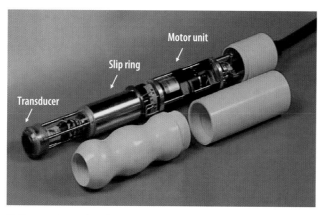

Fig. 1.10 Prototype of the continuously fast rotating ultrasound transducer assembly which has three major parts. The 64 element phased array transducer operating at 3 MHz. The slip ring device with 84 contacts allows ultrafast signal transfer from the ultrasound system to the rotating transducer and vice versa. The motor unit drives the phased array transducer at a rotational speed that ranges from 4–8 Hz

and more reproducible than with 2D echocardiography mainly by overcoming LV cavity foreshortening and avoiding the need of geometric assumptions. Because of these major clinical contributions, the transesophageal rotational approach for 3D reconstruction was rapidly implemented into clinical practice.

> The transesophageal rotational approach for 3D reconstruction was rapidly implemented into clinical practice.

1.2 Volumetric real-time (high-speed) scanning

Fundamental to understanding real-time 3D echocardiography (RT3DE) is to keep in mind that the machines must
- acquire and process vast amounts of ultrasound data (from every direction) and then
- display image(s) in real time.

Obviously, if data cannot be acquired and presented fast enough, rendering is not possible. In this section, the methods used for such high-speed scanning that allow for RT3DE imaging in all modern systems are presented.

All current 3D echocardiographic systems are based on volumetric real-time scanning principles and the history of the specific techniques stretch back nearly two decades from the inception of cardiac phased array scanning methods [33]. In RT3DE scanning, the ultrasound beam is electronically, rather than mechanically, moved throughout the scan volume. While faster than the mechanical methods described to this point, the development of real-time scanners is about making a beam move everywhere in a scan volume by overcoming timing limitations inherent to ultrasound scanning systems.

It is important to recall several very basic concepts. First, an ultrasound beam sent from a transducer (where electrical impulses are turned into ultrasonic waves transmitted into the body) requires that the ultrasound waves be reflected. Then the system

must wait for the returning signals, where ultrasound is converted into electrical impulses in the transducer and the images are then created in the scanning device – this all takes time. Second, ultrasound travels in the body at approximately 1540 m/s. In basic imaging, a receive sequence follows every transmit sequence in a regular pattern to write a line of data (1:1 receive:transmit). Third, together, this basic 1:1 writing of lines (in a 2D phased array imaging device) and beam movement result in approximately 256 lines of ultrasound data in every ultrasonic frame. Systems nominally write 30 frames/s. When color imaging is used, image lines are dropped so that lines representing spatial color data can be created. In short, a conventional 2D echocardiographic machine is at the limit of its technical capabilities.

Phased array scanners were used in the mid 1970s to overcome some of these physical limitations for electronically, rather than mechanically, moving the ultrasound beam throughout a 2D field of view. The prototype for such devices for cardiac scanning was the Duke University phased array system (version T1) [33]. By the mid 1980s, such phased array scanning devices had replaced all mechanically driven 2D systems.

A quantum leap forward in 3D echocardiography was achieved by extending the use of phased array devices, which used parallel processing techniques in combination with the development of multidimensional array transducers. This combination progressively allowed for the real-time acquisition, followed by volumetric rendering of pyramidal datasets from a fixed transthoracic transducer position. These advances obviated the need for ECG and respiratory gating and eliminated the movement registration artifacts of the early rotational scanners.

> A quantum leap forward in 3D echocardiography was achieved by the development of multidimensional array transducers.

The earliest steps using parallel processing schemes to achieve these goals were made with the original Duke T1 system in 1980. The profound effect of parallel processing can be easily seen in ◘ Fig. 1.11, showing a series of short-axis views from a patient with pericardial effusion. Actual scan lines are seen because there is no scan converter/image processing used. A 128 line scan using a traditional 1:1 receive:transmit scan sequence is shown in ◘ Fig. 1.11A. Here every received line is the consequence of a single transmitted line. In ◘ Fig. 1.11B, the system is dropped to a 24 line 1:1 receive:transmit scan sequence, where line density is obviously reduced and the image is unsatisfactory. Finally, ◘ Fig. 1.11C illustrates the results when a 4:1 receive:transmit sequence was employed (achieving four receive lines for every transmit line). Such multiple receive lines are collected nearly simultaneously and demonstrate the effect of such 4:1 parallel processing. The remarkable achievement here is that ◘ Fig. 1.11C resembles ◘ Fig. 1.11A, but was acquired in only a fraction of the time required by a traditional scanner. This meant it was possible to use the leftover lines to scan in multiple dimensions at the same time, or to use the leftover time to move the system at faster and faster frame rates.

The first simultaneous multidimensional scans were performed in 1986, again using the Duke University T1 scanner that employed a bow tie transducer array [34]. A long-axis image in a normal volunteer (slightly rotated to allow perspective) is shown

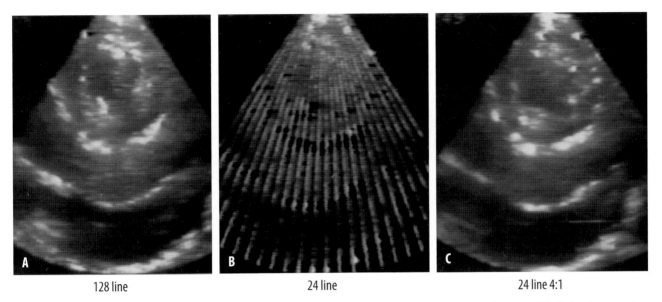

| 128 line | 24 line | 24 line 4:1 |

◻ **Fig. 1.11** Effects of parallel processing shown on the Duke T1 system in 1980. Serial short-axis images of a patient with a pericardial effusion demonstrating the possibilities with line parallel processing. The 24 line scan (**C**) is of similar quality to the 128 line scan (**A**), but it uses a 4:1 receive:transmit parallel process schema. This early work indicated real-time simultaneous imaging in multiple dimensions was possible. For details, see text

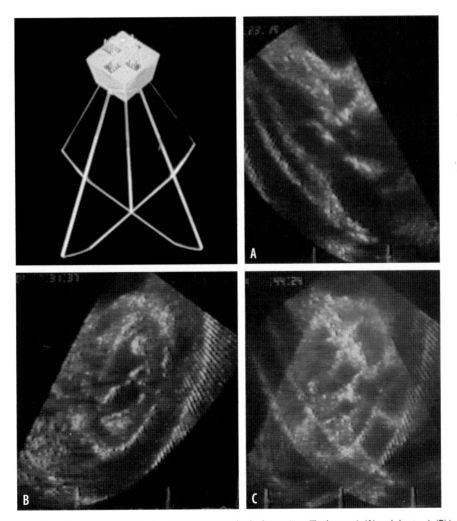

◻ **Fig. 1.12** Results from an early version of the Duke T1 system operating in multiple dimensions. The long-axis (**A**) and short-axis (**B**) images could be combined simultaneously into the two images (**C**) moving in real time. This demonstrated that simultaneous multidimensional imaging was accomplished. For details, see text

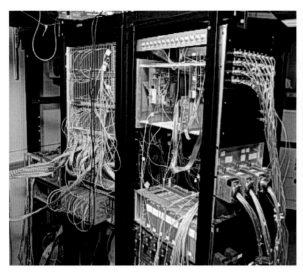
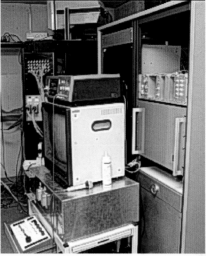
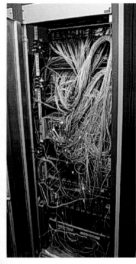

■ **Fig. 1.13** Pictures from the original real-time 3D imaging machine (Duke system T2). For details, see text

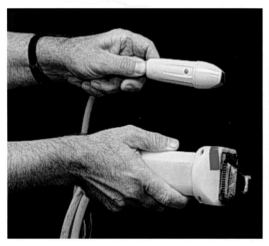
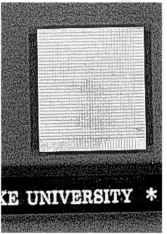

■ **Fig. 1.14** *Left* The original matrix transducer (*bottom*) of the Duke T1 system compared to a commercial transducer of the time (*top*). *Right* A picture of the matrix system is shown

in ■ Fig. 1.12A, while ■ Fig. 1.12B shows a short-axis view from the same individual that was achieved by simply electronically switching the scan plane by pressing a button. The paramount achievement is shown in ■ Fig. 1.12C, where the two orthogonal planes (called O-mode) are scanning at the same time. It then remained to scan in all dimensions simultaneously.

The first RT3DE system was developed at Duke University using the system shown in ■ Fig. 1.13. As can be seen, the system was so large that it was impossible to capture it in a single picture, while the complex circuitry goes without explanation. This is the first system in the world that could be used for RT3DE purposes. Called T2 (as a successor to T1), the system used a sparse matrix phased array transducer with 512 elements (■ Fig. 1.14) to scan a 60°×60° pyramidal volume [17].

This was a 16:1 parallel processed system and resulted in 17 pyramidal volumes/s at a depth of 16 cm. The original system displayed images that were not rendered, but rather comprised a simultaneous display of multiple planes within the pyramidal volume, usually two perpendicular long-axis views along with

one or more views orthogonal to the long-axis at selected depths (C-scans). A still frame from the first actual 3D scan ever performed in 1990 is illustrated in ■ Fig. 1.15. While not rendered, two separate ventricles were clearly observed in real time, particularly in the second C-scan on the top left.

> The first real-time 3D echocardiography system comprised a simultaneous display of multiple planes within a pyramidal volume.

A later version of the Duke System (T4) and commercial versions based on the Duke system are shown in ■ Fig. 1.16. The Volumetrics V360 (■ Fig. 1.16, right) was the first system available to produce real-time rendered images using these techniques. An example of a rendered image is shown in ■ Fig. 1.17 (bottom).

The latest version of the experimental Duke system is T5 and is shown in ■ Fig. 1.18. It uses 1000 channels, two simultaneous beams, each in 32:1 parallel process schema, that result in an 82° pyramidal volume and is capable of obtaining 40 or more

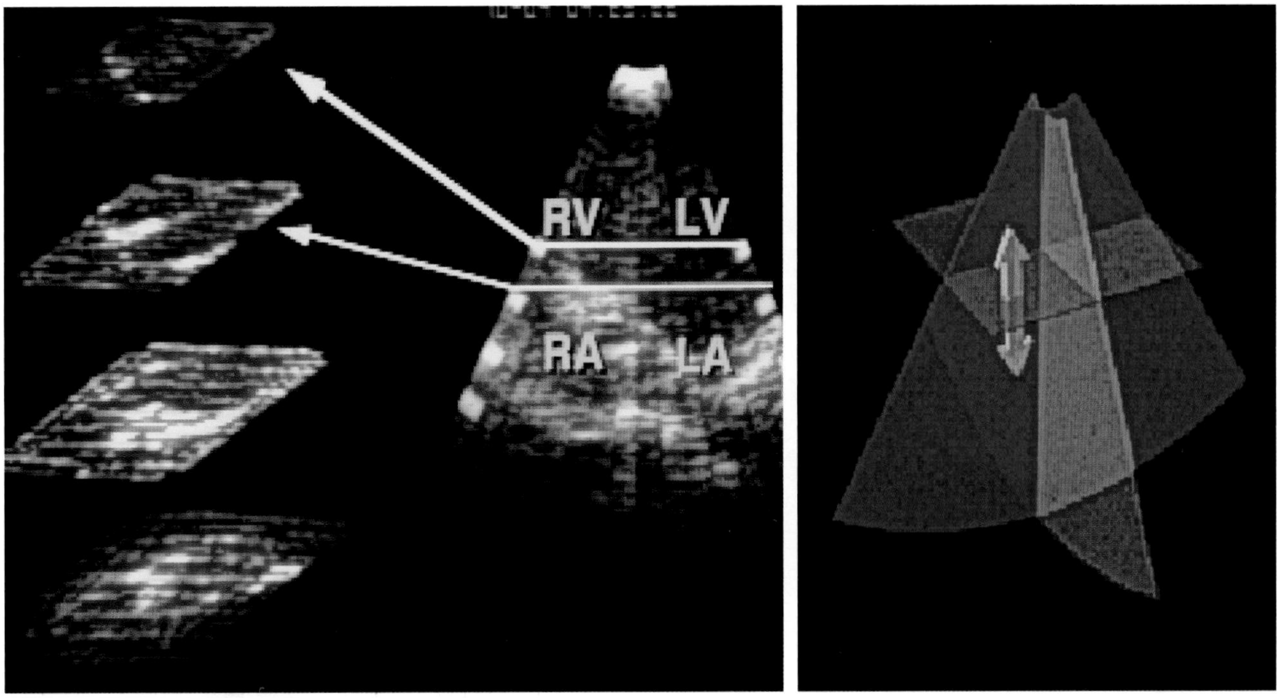
RV
LV
RA
LA

Fig. 1.15 A still frame image from the first real-time 3D image ever scanned (October 3, 1990). Four C-scans (*right*) are simultaneously acquired at different depths with the B-mode. The schematic shows how a C-scan is parallel to the skin surface, rather than perpendicular like a B-mode. *Left* The second C-mode image clearly shows a septum and two ventricles. *RV* right ventricle, *LV* left ventricle, *RA* right atrium, *LA* left atrium

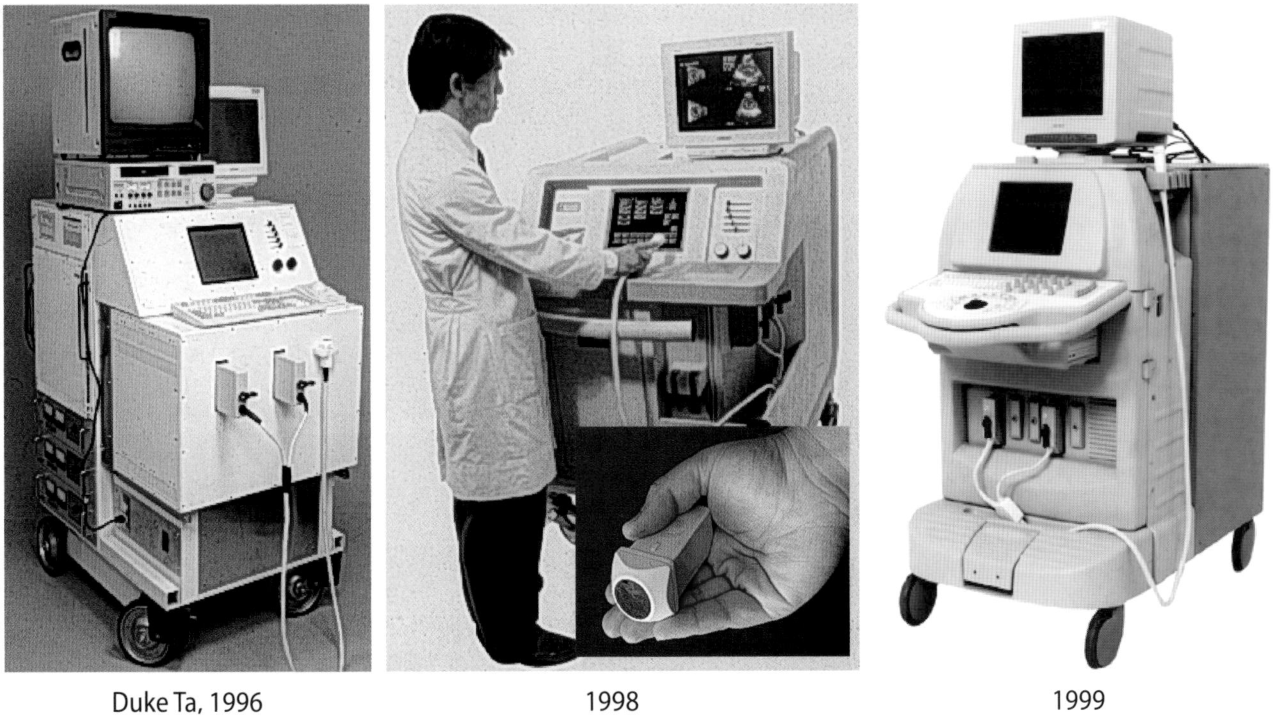
Duke Ta, 1996
1998
1999

Fig. 1.16 Later versions of the Duke RT3DE system (T4). *Left and middle* Two of the first commercially available RT3DE systems manufactured by Volumetrics, Inc. *Right* The first RT3DE system capable of rendering in real time (Volumetrics, Inc., Model V360)

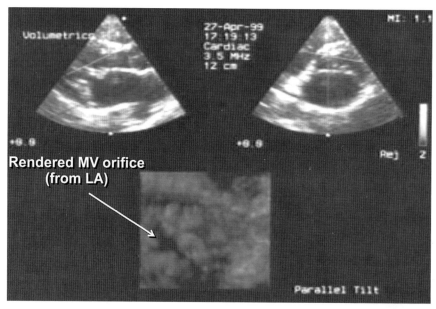

■ **Fig. 1.17** A still-frame image obtained from a Volumetrics Model V360 system. There are two intersecting B-modes (O-mode; *top*) and an early example of a real-time rendered image (*bottom*). *MV* mitral valve, *LA* left atrium

volumes/s in the 3D mode and almost 300 frames/s in the 2D mode. This system is capable of calculating data at the rate of 1.6 teraflops/s (calculations/s) and is about 40 times faster than current commercial systems. The transducer used in this experimental system is obviously large.

The T5 system creates paired diastolic and systolic, long-axis and short-axis images in 2D formats (■ Fig. 1.19); thus, multidimensional ultrasound data can be obtained in about 3 ms and is, thus, suited for the study of complex multidimensional LV movement. The system is currently being implemented with feature tracking capabilities to study complex movements of myocardial stress that are similar to what is generally understood as speckle tracking [35][36].

❯ RT3DE systems with matrix array and micro-beamforming technology were extremely fast and allowed real-time display of rendered images.

Another early real-time method was the surface rendering of LV cavities based on three equally spaced long-axis views simultaneously acquired with a matrix array transducer from the same heart beat (real-time tri-plane 3D echocardiography).

Later generations of RT3DE systems used a complex matrix array containing 3000 miniature elements. Each of these elements is electronically controlled by a micro-beamformer (▶ Chapter 2) incorporated into the transducer head to achieve multidirectional beam steering through a pyramidal volume of 30°×60° (■ Fig. 1.20).

Powerful microelectronics process multiple data streams in the transducer and the cardiac structures are reconstructed and rendered in the ultrasound system. This process is extremely fast and allows the real-time display of the rendered images. To capture a dataset large enough to encompass the whole (dilated) LV from the apical transducer position, four or seven consecutive ECG-triggered real-time additional volumes of 20°×90° are acquired

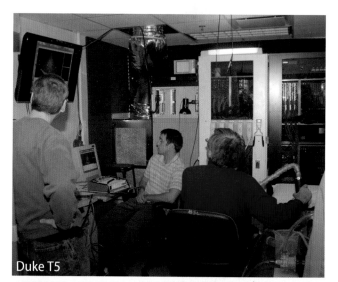

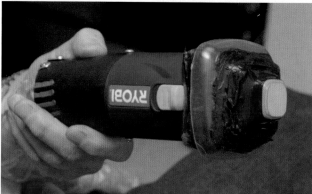

■ **Fig. 1.18** The latest generation experimental Duke RT3DE imaging system (known as T5). The system requires its own ventilation (ducting seen at the rear). The transducer housing is from a commercially available electric bench tool, whereby the original electronic contents have been replaced by the transducer and wiring (*bottom*)

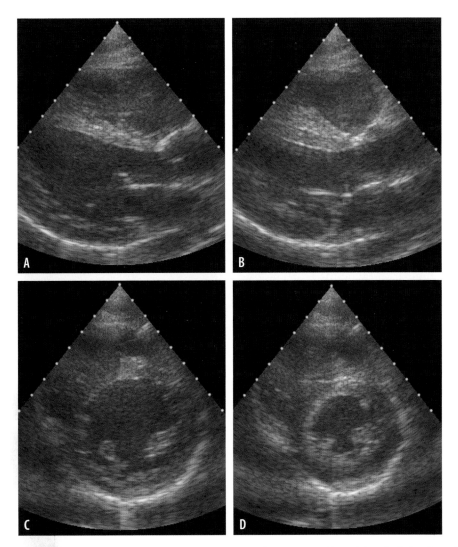

◨ **Fig. 1.19** Still frames (in 2D) from the Duke T5 system that took only 3 ms to create. The acquisition of paired diastolic (*left*) and systolic (*right*) long-axis (*top*) and short-axis (*bottom*) multidimensional images makes it possible to image rapid and detailed components of ventricular mechanics. For details, see text

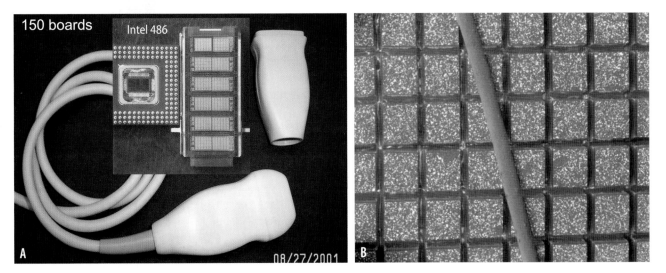

◨ **Fig. 1.20** Matrix transducer for real-time volumetric data acquisition introduced by Philips Medical Systems (Andover, USA) in 2001. **A** Much of the beam steering and reception processing is performed in the probe, which contains the equivalent of 150 Intel 486 printboards compressed into an ergonomic housing. **B** A microscopic view shows the miniature crystals of the matrix array in the transducer for RT3DE image acquisition together with a human hair to appreciate their size. Copyright Philips Medical Systems

during held respiration and electronically »stitched« together into a composite pyramidal data set of 80°×90° or even larger. Real-time 3D color Doppler flow has been integrated in the volumetric images and allows the combined real-time display of the origin, direction, and size (volume) of jets and surrounding tissue data. For this type of real-time 3D color Doppler acquisition, seven consecutive ECG-triggered real-time volumes are needed.

Because of cost, size, and some technical limitations, the current commercial systems are only now beginning to approach the high-speed capabilities (high line density and high frame rate/volume rates) of the early Duke experimental systems. The ability of these commercial systems to render images is, nevertheless, excellent.

Developments in microelectronics are evolving rapidly and will further improve image quality. Real-time anyplane and para-plane cross-sectional planes for the accurate measurement of various dimensions and surface areas of defects and diseased valves and online assessment of the relationship, orientation, and motion of any structure and blood flow from different perspectives offer important diagnostic information.

The next major step was the introduction of broadband (1–5 MHz) monocrystal transducers (■ Fig. 1.21). The electro-mechanical efficiency of these monocrystals is 80–100% better than that of the currently used piezoelectric crystals, thus, making them twice as sensitive. This results in not only better penetration and resolution, but also a better signal-to-noise ratio. These transducers allow high-resolution harmonic imaging with improved cavity delineation. They also offer advantages when left heart contrast agents are needed in patients with less than optimal image quality as the tissue/contrast echo separation is better. Because of their higher efficiency, smaller matrix transducers with good performance can be constructed.

Clinical results with the transthoracic pediatric monocrystal matrix array transducer showed that the image quality and the resolution are excellent and competitive with magnetic resonance imaging (MRI). An advantage over MRI in infants and small children is that no sedation is needed during the examination.

The efficiency of the monocrystal matrix array transducers and miniaturization have also rapidly led to the introduction of transesophageal RT3DE. Earlier prototypes using conventional piezoelectric crystals were built by researchers at Duke University (■ Fig. 1.22). Early data on intracardiac RT3DE for guiding interventional procedures were reported in 2002 (■ Fig. 1.23) [37].

1.3   High speed imaging

Readers of the preceding pages of this chapter will recognize the creativity of the engineering and medical scientists who established the methodologies for 3D imaging. Most of these approaches still form the structural basics of current day devices. The most important thing to realize is that techniques (such as parallel processing) overcome the physical limitations induced by the limited speed of sound in tissue. Without these early advances, simultaneous imaging with multiple lines in multiple

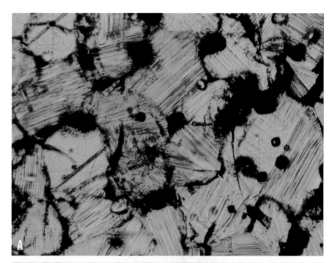

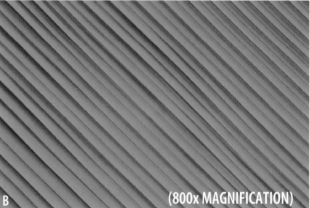

■ **Fig. 1.21** Piezoelectric ceramics (PZT) are used in conventional transducers. **A** The picture shows the randomly oriented multicrystalline grains in a transducer. **B** The almost perfect arrangement in a monocrystal transducer at the atomic level is shown. Thus, transducers that are smaller, being much more efficient with greater bandwidth, sensitivity, and image resolution, can be produced. Copyright Philips Medical Systems

directions (space), while still capturing detailed cardiac motion (time) would not be possible. Imaging of the heart presents unique problems compared to other bodily organs because it is in constant motion.

All users need to look beyond simple transmit and receive and into these more complex imaging principles in order to properly use 3D devices. Phased arrays allowed electronic steering of an ultrasound beam and opened the door for modern 2D machines in use worldwide. These led directly to RT3DE. The story of the system development is not only in new hardware or new computer technology. It is also dependent on new thoughts and ideas that create desired applications that drive system development.

One intriguing new field of exploration is using advanced capabilities for imaging in space and time to create images of cardiac micromechanical events. One such device capable of advanced exploration is the Duke T5, shown in ■ Fig. 1.18 and ■ Fig. 1.19 and described in the accompanying text. T5 is capable of producing B-mode images at rates of 400–600 frames/s with 32 to 1 parallel processing in receive as well as simultaneous transmission of multiple interrogating beams. The data storage computer scanner interfaces permit very high data transfer rates

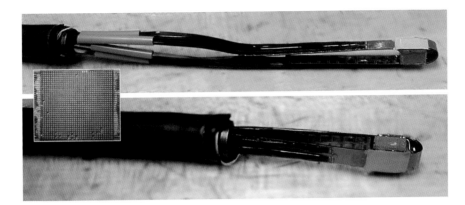

◘ Fig. 1.22 Prototype of the first transesophageal RT3DE probe developed at Duke University

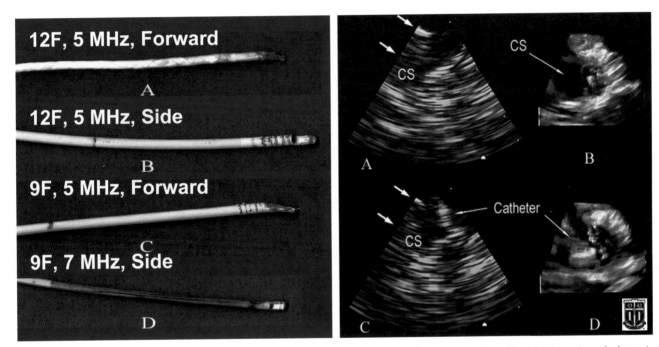

◘ Fig. 1.23 Intracardiac catheters with matrix arrays for real-time 3D imaging. Prototypes of 9F and 12F sizes operating at 5 and 7 MHz are shown for forward and side imaging. **A** A sector image of the left atrium together with the forward 3D view (**B**) without a catheter. **C, D** The same views with a catheter in place in an experimental animal. *CS* coronary sinus. Reproduced from [37]; Copyright John Wiley and Sons

and provide storage of real-time volumetric and high-speed B-mode images. Images acquired at high speed can then be played back at slower speeds, or frame by frame, to analyze and quantitate temporal micromechanical activity. Early results show a variety of ventricular wall and valve motions heretofore unseen in conventional B-mode or RT3DE images.

Current methods for display of such micromotions are not, however, well developed. One such motion detection scheme is based on subtraction of successive image frames to enhance the visualization of change. In this approach, targets that do not move disappear (shown in black), while slow moving targets are dim, and fast moving targets will appear brighter. A surprising finding during these studies was the visualization of a traveling brightness phenomenon in the interventricular septum (now called the *event* for current lack of a better name) late in the QRS complex. This event travels at 2–3 m/s and occurs near mitral valve closure.

Recent study of volunteers and patients with this high speed T5 system uses a 96 element, 3.5 MHz one-dimensional linear array and shows this event in the parasternal long axis of all individuals examined. An example of the regional change in brightness derived from a 22-year-old male volunteer in sinus rhythm is shown in ◘ Fig. 1.24. The brightness data from the difference images was detected from 5 segments of the interventricular septum (left panel). The brightness data (right panel) was then plotted as a function of time for each of these 5 segments, spaced 5 mm apart, together with the ECG (top line). Tracings are shown from the most basal segment (second line) to the more apical segment (bottom line). The slanted line identifies the onset time of the event in each of the segments and the slope of that line corresponds to the event velocity.

For reference, ◘ Fig. 1.25 shows a plot of the brightness variation from the difference images throughout one cardiac cycle. The event, aortic valve opening and closure, and mitral valve

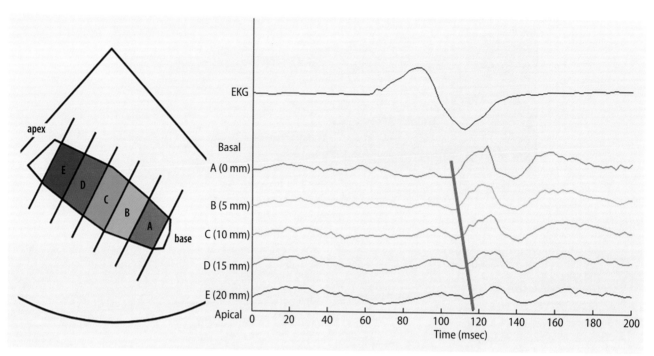

Fig. 1.24 Summed difference brightness across the septum. The top trace is the ECG. The remaining traces are displayed from most basal at top to most apical at bottom. The superimposed line indicates onset of the event in each window. (Courtesy of Cooper Moore and John Castellucci)

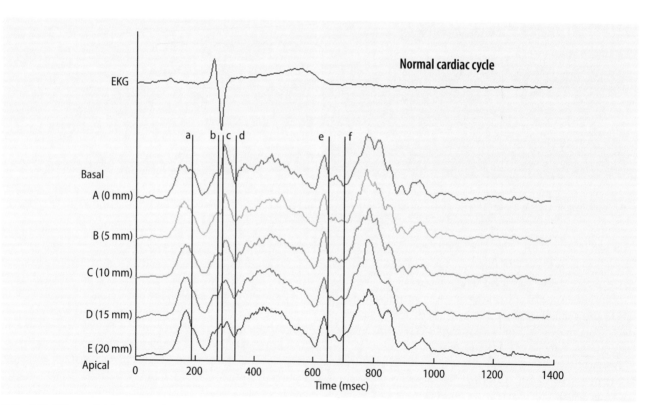

Fig. 1.25 Difference brightness in each window over the course of the cardiac cycle. Vertical lines (**A–F**) indicate mechanical events in the heart as observed in the original ultrasound image: end of A-wave (**A**), mitral valve closure (**B**), the event (**C**), aortic valve opening (**D**), aortic valve closure (**E**), and mitral valve opening (**F**). (Courtesy of Cooper Moore and John Castellucci)

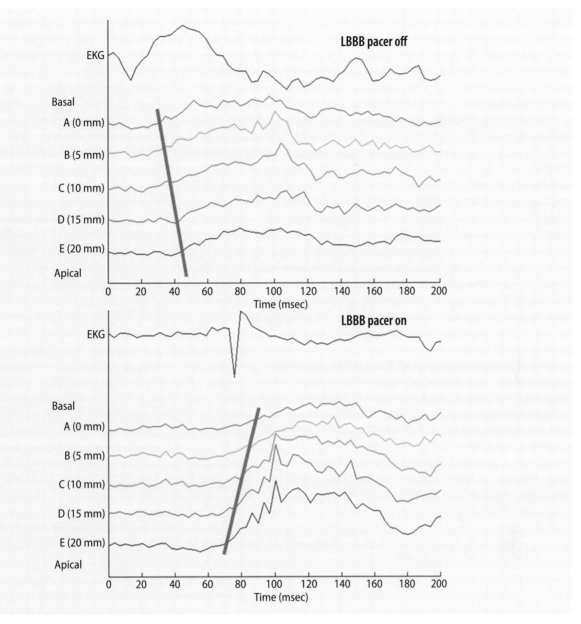

Fig. 1.26 Example traces from an 86-year-old woman with left bundle branch block (LBBB) and a biventriclular pacemaker. Images acquired with the pace-maker turned off (*top*) and images acquired during biventricular pacing (*bottom*). Note the change in slope of the superimposed line, indicating a change in direction of the event. For details, see text. (Courtesy of Cooper Moore and John Castellucci)

opening and closure are indicated. The timing of events was derived from the original B-mode sequences by counting frames. At the 400+ frame rates, valve closures can be resolved with ±2.5 ms accuracy. Aortic valve opening occurs in 10 ms, while closure occurs in about 13 ms. Mitral valve closure occurs over a 80–85 ms period.

The timing of the event indicates it can be associated with one, or more, of several hypothesized factors such as

- sequential tensing of the myocardium associated with the early onset of isometric contraction and mitral valve closure,
- direct or consequent relation to the electrical depolarization/repolarization cycle,
- cessation of coronary blood flow, etc.

Any of these events represent the potential for ultrasound to image cardiac microevents that reflect physiologic changes never thought possible with ultrasound.

Initial results exploring the physiologic changes behind this traveling event have first centered around its association with electrical events (either depolarization or repolarization) of the specialized conducting system in the septum. An early study included patients with intact atrioventricular conduction but with left bundle branch block (LBBB) and implanted biventricular pacemakers for cardiac resynchronization therapy (CRT). Images were obtained with the pacing device turned on/off.

In **Fig. 1.26**, the resultant brightness change traces from one of these patients, an 86-year-old woman with the right ventricular lead placed distal along the interventricular septum, is shown. In this patient, as in all with biventricular pacers, the electrical conduction was from the base towards the apex with the pacemaker turned off (top panel). The sequence of depolarization was always base to apex without pacing and the sequence of the event was the same (base to apex). When the pacers were turned on, the sequence of the event was reversed and travelled from apex to base. All paced leads were set to zero offset between the LV and RV leads (bottom panel).

The slanted line in ◘ Fig. 1.26 (top) connects the onset of the event with the pacer off (base to apex) and the slanted line in ◘ Fig. 1.26 (bottom) connects the onset of the event with the pacer on (apex to base). While presently uncertain as to the actual physiologic origin of the event, these findings do demonstrate that RT3DE and its high speed progeny of the original (such as the Duke T5) are capable of uncovering cardiac microevents in the 2–3 ms time range. Whether due to a traveling contractile wave (due to actual motion) or a change in acoustic impedance of septal tissue (thus brightness change without motion), such findings open new windows for cardiac imaging and the possibility of microtime domain imaging of electrical–mechanical coupling.

Such rapid spatial imaging speed was never thought possible with any technique and such findings have never been previously observed. Just as the first 2D echocardiography with electronic phased array systems and then related RT3DE systems were once thought impossible, these methods have proved clinically useful. It is likely that high speed microevent imaging in two and/or three dimensions may also become commonplace one day. In future years, look for even newer editions of this textbook to further demonstrate the evolution of high speed 2D and 3D imaging and development of its clinical possibilities.

1.4   The future is based on the past

Proven benefits of RT3DE compared with 2D echocardiography are the diagnosis of complex conditions and the more accurate and reproducible calculation of cavity volumes, LV ejection fraction, and myocardial mass, which are the most common requests for an echocardiographic study. RT3DE is less operator dependent than other echocardiographic examinations, and the results are comparable to MRI. Since RT3DE is more widely available and less expensive, it will become the technique of choice for these applications in daily practice, and its availability and versatility offers advantages in many clinical scenarios (e.g., interventions, intensive care units, emergencies). Unique are its diagnostic applications in newborns and small children (no sedation), and the intraoperative decision-making and guiding of interventional procedures with transesophageal RT3DE.

Newer, sensitive transducers and the rapid development of faster microprocessors will continually increase spatial and temporal resolution as well as the speed of quantitative analysis. However, the imaging rate is currently still too slow for accurate wall motion analysis.

Parametric analysis and imaging are now possible thanks to RT3DE and will further expand the diagnostic capabilities of echocardiography by providing diagnostic information that is currently beyond our clinical capabilities.

With more and more powerful imaging computers, we may expect that the holographic display of cardiac images will become a reality in the future. Virtual reality, the immersive environment created by ultrafast computers and RT3DE, will also become accessible. This will allow the cardiologist to interact with cardiac data and heralds a revolution in cardiac teaching, diagnosis, and treatment (e.g., remote robotic surgery assistance) via internet.

References

1. Dekker DL, Piziali RL, Dong E Jr (1974) A system for ultrasonically imaging the human heart in three dimensions. Comput Biomed Res7:544–553
2. Moritz WE, Shreve PL (1976) A microprocessor based spatial locating system for use with diagnostic ultrasound. Proc IEEE 64:966–974
3. Frangi AF, Niessen WJ, Viergever MA (2001) Three-dimensional modelling for functional analysis of cardiac images: a review. IEEE Trans Med Imaging 20: 2–5
4. Raab FH, Blood EB, Steiner TO, Jones HR (1979) Magnetic position and orientation tracking system. IEEE Trans Aerospace Electron Systems 15: 709–718
5. King DL, King DL Jr, Shao MYC (1990) Three-dimensional spatial registration and interactive display of position and orientation of real-time ultrasound images. J Ultrasound Med 9:525–532
6. Gopal AS, King DL, Katz J et al (1992) Three-dimensional echocardiographic volume computation by polyhedral surface reconstruction: in vitro validation and comparison to magnetic resonance imaging. J Am Soc Echocardiogr 5:115–124
7. King DL, Harrison MR, King DL Jr et al (1992) Improved reproducibility of left atrial and left ventricular measurements by guided three-dimensional echocardiography. J Am Coll Cardiol 20:1238–1245
8. Gopal AS, Keller AM, Rigling R et al (1993) Left ventricular volume and endocardial surface area by three-dimensional echocardiography: comparison with two-dimensional echocardiography and nuclear magnetic resonance imaging in normal subjects. J Am Coll Cardiol 22:258–270
9. Handschumacher MD, Lethor JP, Siu SC et al (1993) A new integrated system for three-dimensional echocardiographic reconstruction: development and validation for ventricular volume with application in human subjects. J Am Coll Cardiol 21:743–753
10. Siu SC, Rivera JM, Guerrero JL et al (1993) Three-dimensional echocardiography. In vivo validation for left ventricular volume and function. Circulation 88:1715–1723
11. Wollschläger H, Zeiher AM, Klein HP et al (1989) Transesophageal echo computer tomography: a new method for dynamic 3-D imaging of the heart. Circulation 80:II-569 (abstract)
12. Wollschläger H, Zeiher AM, Klein HP (1990) Transesophageal echo computer tomography (ECHO-CT): a new method for perspective views of the beating heart. Circulation 82(Suppl. 3):III-670 (abstract)
13. Kuroda T, Kinter TM, Seward JB et al (1991) Accuracy of three-dimensional volume measurement using biplane transesophageal echocardiographc probe: in vitro experiment. J Am Soc Echocardiogr 4:475–484
14. Roelandt JRTC, Ten Cate FJ, Vletter WB, Taams MA (1994) Ultrasonic dynamic three-dimensional visualization of the heart with a multiplane transesophageal imaging transducer. J Am Soc Echocardiogr 7:217–229
15. Roelandt JRTC, Salustri A, Mumm B, Vletter WB (1995) Precordial three-dimensional echocardiography with a rotational imaging probe: methods and initial clinical experience. Echocardiography 12:243–252
16. Djoa KK, Jong N de, van Egmond FC et al (2000) Real-time three-dimensional data acquisition with the fast rotating scanning unit. Ultrasound Med Biol 26:863–869
17. Von Ramm OT, Smith SW (1990) Real-time volumetric ultrasound imaging system. J Digit Imaging 3:261–266

18. Levoy M (1988) Display of surfaces from volume data. IEEE Comput Graphics Application 8: 29–39

19. Fulton DR, Marx GR, Pandian NG et al (1994) Dynamic three-dimensional echocardiographic imaging of congenital heart defects in infants and children by computer controlled tomographic parallel slicing using a single integrated ultrasound instrument. Echocardiography 11:155–164

20. Bruining N, von Birgelen C, Di Mario C et al (1995) Dynamic three-dimensional reconstruction of ICUS images based on an ECG-gated pull-back device. Computers in Cardiology 633–636

21. Nixon J, Saffer SI, Lipscomb K, Blomqvist CG (1983) Three-dimensional echoventriculography. Am Heart J 16:435–443

22. Belohlavek M, Foley DA, Gerber TC et al (1993) Three-dimensional ultrasound imaging of the atrial septum: normal and pathologic anatomy. J Am Coll Cardiol 22:1673–1678

23. Martin RW, Bashein G, Zimmer R, Sutherland J (1986) An endoscopic micromanipulator for multiplanar transesophageal imaging. Ultrasound Med Biol 12: 965–975

24. Delabays A, Pandian NG, Cao QL et al (1995) Transthoracic real-time three-dimensional echocardiography using a fan-like scanning approach for data acquisition. Echocardiography 12:49–59

25. Ghosh A, Nanda NC, Maurer G (1982) Three-dimensional reconstruction of echocardiographic images using the rotation method. Ultrasound Med Biol 6:655–661

26. Machle J, Bjoernstad K, Aakhus S et al (1994) Three-dimensional echocardiography for quantitative left ventricular wall motion analysis. Echocardiography 11:397–408

27. Buck T, Schön F, Baumgart D et al (1996) Tomographic left ventricular volume determination in presence of aneurysm by three-dimensional echocardiographic imaging. J Am Soc Echocardiogr 9:488–500

28. Mele D, Levine RA (2000) Quantitation of ventricular size and function: principles and accuracy of transthoracic rotational scanning. Echocardiography 17:749–755

29. Nanda NC, Pinheiro L, Sanyal R et al (1992) Multiplane transesophageal echocardiography imaging and three-dimensional reconstruction. Echocardiography 9:667–676

30. Roelandt JRTC, Thomson IR, Vletter WB et al (1992) Multiplane transesophageal echocardiography: latest evolution in an imaging revolution. J Am Soc Echocardiogr 5:361–367

31. Papavassiliou D, Doelling NR, Bowman MK et al (1998) Initial experience with an internally rotating transthoracic three-dimensional echocardiographic probe and image acquisition on a conventional echocardiogram machine. Echocardiography 15:369–376

32. Belohlavek M, Tanabe K, Japrapanichakul D et al (2001) Rapid three-dimensional echocardiography: clinically feasible alternative for precise and accurate measurement of left ventricular volumes. Circulation 103: 2882–2884

33. Kisslo J, von Ramm OT, Thursone FL (1976) Cardiac imaging using a phased-array ultrasound system II: Clinical technique and application. Circulation 53:262–267

34. Snyder JE, Kisslo JA, von Ramm OT (1986) Real-time orhtogonal mode scanning of the heart I. System design. J Am Coll Cardiol 7:1279–1285

35. Kuo J, Atkins BZ, Hutcheson KA, von Ramm OT (2005) Ultrasound in Med & Biol 31:203–211

36. Kuo J, von Ramm OT (2008) Three-dimensional motion measurements using feature tracking. IEE Transactions on Ultrasonics, Ferroelectrics and Frequency Control 55:800–810

37. Smith SW, Light ED, Idriss SF, Wolf PD (2002) Feasibility of real-time three- dimensional intracardiac echocardiography for guidance of interventional electrophysiology. PACE 25: 351–357

38. Roelandt JRTC (1998) Technical aspects: approaches, clinical procedure and display. In: Roelandt JRTC (ed) Three-dimensional echocardiography of the heart and coronary arteries. Van Zuiden Communications BV, Alphen a/d Rijn, The Netherlands

Basic principles
and practical application

Thomas Buck, Karl E. Thiele

T. Buck et al. (Hrsg.), *Three-dimensional Echocardiography*,
DOI 10.1007/978-3-642-36799-1_2, © Springer-Verlag Berlin Heidelberg 2014

Current real-time 3D echocardiography (RT3DE) evolved from original volumetric three-dimensional (3D) echocardiography. Original volumetric 3D echocardiography described the acquisition of 3D datasets in real time at a rate of about 15–20 3D datasets per second using sparse matrix array transducer technology [1][2][3][4], thus, eliminating time-consuming 3D reconstruction of two-dimensional (2D) image planes which were prone to interpolation artifacts (▶ Chapter 1) [5][6][7][8]. Such pyramid-shaped, volumetric 3D datasets, once acquired, could be further analyzed by cropping and slicing.

Recent developments in RT3DE, however, go beyond this by allowing 3D visualization of volume rendered images during live scanning, commonly called live 3D echocardiography [9]. Thus, current RT3DE can be used as an integral part of routine echocardiographic examinations allowing rapid change between 2D cross-sectional views and 3D visualization with the press of a button. Because RT3DE works differently in many regards compared to conventional 2D imaging, the following chapter provides a comprehensive overview of the fundamentals of current real-time 3D technology, including the basic principles of volume data acquisition and requirements of 3D probes, followed by a practical introduction to 3D data acquisition and analysis. The wide spectrum of clinical indications for 3D examination will be covered in the subsequent chapters on special applications and clinical questions.

> Today, RT3DE can be used as an integral part of routine echocardiographic examinations.

2.1 How real-time 3D ultrasound works

Karl E. Thiele

Three-dimensional ultrasound can be challenging for clinicians to interpret. It is also challenging for ultrasound engineers to design. No other ultrasound mode has more limitations and more need for improved frame rates, resolution, image quality, and volume size. These constraints impact echocardiography the most, because of the high frame rates required to capture the motion of the heart. The intention of this section is to provide insights into the constraints and trade-offs faced by ultrasound engineers developing 3D ultrasound modes and some of the methods used to address these challenges.

2.1.1 It's all about the transmit beams

Whether 2D, 3D, color Doppler, or B-mode, the basic unit for all ultrasound datasets is the ultrasound beam. When envisioning this ultrasound beam (particularly on transmit), a good analogy would be the light beam from a flashlight (◙ Fig. 2.1).

> Scanning a room with a flashlight beam is a good analogy to 2D and 3D ultrasound.

Imagine standing in a dark room with nothing but a flashlight with a relatively narrow beam. To see what is on a shelf on the

other side of the room, one would simply point the flashlight beam on the left side of the room and scan the shelf from left to right. The light is emitted from the flashlight, transmitted across the room, reflected off the shelf, and finally received by the eye (◙ Fig. 2.2). This is a good analogy to 2D ultrasound.

However, the room is three-dimensional. Perhaps there is a table and a chair and more bookshelves in the room. For the original scan of the bookshelf, the narrow light beam had a limited diameter, say 10 cm, so all of these other structures were missed.

One approach to scanning the entire room between the flashlight and the wall is to initially place the beam in the upper left corner of the wall. Then traverse the beam from left to right (just like in a 2D scan).

When the beam reaches the upper right edge of the wall, start on the left side again, but with the beam 10 cm lower than the first pass. Repeat this sequence until the entire wall and other structures are scanned from ceiling to floor (◙ Fig. 2.3). Such a sequence is nearly identical to the scan sequence used in 3D ultrasound equipment (◙ Fig. 2.4) where each scan line corresponds to a different direction in space of the beam emitted from the flashlight.

By integrating the light over the entire scan, the entire shelf and room can be evaluated (◙ Fig. 2.5). On 3D ultrasound equipment, this integration occurs by digitizing the returning sound echoes and storing them in the system's memory. Thus, a room that is 5 m wide by 3 m tall and a light beam that is 10 cm in diameter would require 50 light beams across and 30 light beams high to scan the entire wall. Note that such numbers are not atypical of the number of transmit beams used in both 2D and 3D echocardiography. Using typical echocardiography times, it takes about 0.2 ms for the sound to emanate from the face of the probe, hit a target 15 cm deep, and return to the face of the probe. Therefore, 50 transmit beam emissions require 10 ms to scan the wall, resulting in a sustained frame rate of up to 100 Hz. This is just for the 2D B-mode.

To preserve the same image quality and line density used in 2D, 3D would require 50 horizontal/lateral beams by 30 vertical/elevation beams or 1500 transmit beams per volume, with a total scan time of 300 ms. The resulting low 3.3 Hz frame rate would be unacceptable.

Alternatively, given that adult echocardiography typically »requires« frame rates in excess of 20 Hz (50 ms), how many transmit

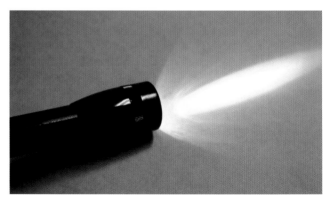

◙ **Fig. 2.1** Flashlight beam: analogy for an acoustic transmit beam

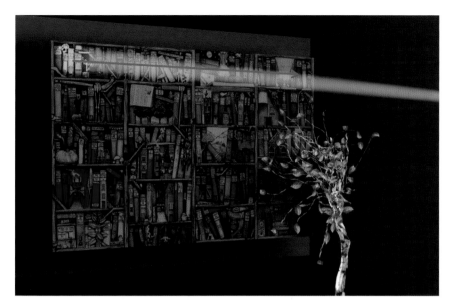

■ **Fig. 2.2** Scan of a bookshelf is analogous to a 2D B-mode scan. The illustration shows a room with bookshelf and a light beam emitted from a flashlight, transmitted through the room, and reflected off the shelf. By traversing the beam from the left to the right (*red arrow*) allows the entire upper bookshelf (just like in a 2D scan) to be scanned

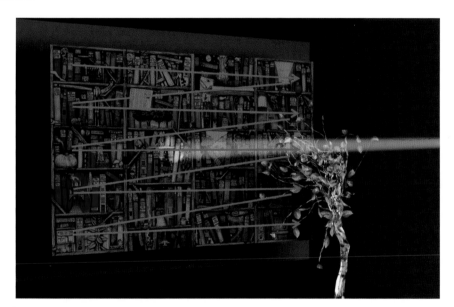

■ **Fig. 2.3** The 3D scan of bookshelf illustrating 3D ultrasound scan. The 3D scan of the room does not only illuminate the bookshelf but all objects in the three-dimensional room (like the small tree)

events (beams) could be supported in a live volume dataset? The typical transthoracic echo depth of 15 cm (with a 0.2 ms echo transit time) would limit the volume to only 250 transmit events. An example scan grid of 25 transmit beams in the lateral dimension (the 2D scan plane) by 10 transmit beams in the elevation dimension would severely sacrifice the image quality as compared to 2D with a similar lateral span. This is because the 3D line spacing would have to be significantly coarser.

This is essentially the 3D problem. One can either sacrifice frame rate for image quality (resolution) or resolution for frame rate. It is very difficult to have both. The options and trade-offs to address this problem are as follows:

- Limit the total number of beams by scanning a smaller volume (3D zoom mode).

- Tolerate the degradation in frame rate.
- Use the patient's ECG signal to acquire smaller »subvolumes« for each R-to-R interval, and then concatenate (stitch) these subvolumes to produce the larger volume (also termed full volume dataset).
- Employ spatial aliasing. This is where the ultrasound beams (on both transmit and receive) are spread far enough apart that there are gaps between the beams that are not adequately sampled. In the bookshelf/flashlight analogy, this would be illustrated by moving the 10 cm diameter beam 20 cm in each interrogation. Clearly the books located between beams would not be well illuminated. In echocardiography, this will either be observed as a scintillation of the speckle pattern (observed on older 2D B-mode scan-

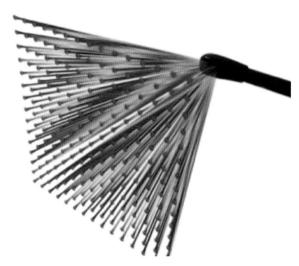

Fig. 2.4 Transmit scan lines emanating from a matrix transesophageal transducer

The 3D volumes in echocardiography are often degraded due to sparse, poorly focused, low intensity transmit beams. In the attempt to maintain acceptable frame rates, the ultrasound engineer will both spread and broaden the transmit beams. To broaden the transmit beam, there are really only two options: either reduce the active aperture (transmit on fewer elements) or defocus the beam (e.g., focus at infinity).

Perhaps worse is the impact on sensitivity and penetration. By broadening the beam (**Fig. 2.6**), the transmitted ultrasound energy is spread over a larger area. However, this is particularly constraining for tissue harmonic imaging. In order for an adequate harmonic wave to be generated, the intensity needs to be above a certain threshold. Transesophageal images, which predominantly rely on nonharmonic imaging modes, are less susceptible to the sensitivity issues caused by transmit beam broadening. Therefore, in order to maintain adequate sensitivity and image quality when scanning fast (coarse transmit beam spacing), the ultrasound engineer has to increase the acoustic energy per transmit burst.

One approach is that the engineer can »simply« increase the transmit voltage. This can have significant ramifications, since special high voltage integrated circuits will be required. This tends to increase the amount of the electronics in the probe housing, and hence the size of the probe can become quite large. In addition, the more electronics, the more heat that is generated. This then pushes the engineer towards using active cooling[1], which further enlarges the size, cost, and complexity of the matrix transducer. Such methods are often associated with the larger, transthoracic matrix transducers.

ners) or a blurring of small structures. This blurring effect can often be exacerbated by selecting the low line density option available on most 3D ultrasound machines.

— Broaden the transmit beam. In this case, the intent would be to increase the diameter of the beam from 10 cm to 20 cm. This would allow one to scan the wall twice as fast in both directions (4x faster for a volume scan). But as will be discussed later, such a technique is also not without compromise.

All of these »solutions« are employed to varying degrees by all 3D ultrasound manufacturers.

2.1.2 The need for bigger, better, faster

Anyone who has ever used 3D echocardiography clinically will inevitably request larger volumes (bigger), improved image quality (better), and faster frame rates (faster).

---

1 Active cooling refers to active methods of removing heat from the probe, often relying on pumping a fluid (such as water) down the transducer cable to a heat exchanger inside the probe housing. This is very similar to how water cooling works in a car engine. The counter approach is to use passive cooling, which relies on heat conducting materials to wick the heat into the patient, into the hand of the scanning clinician, or into the transducer cable.

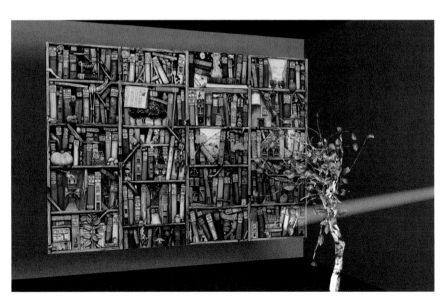

Fig. 2.5 The 3D reconstructed view of room and bookshelf

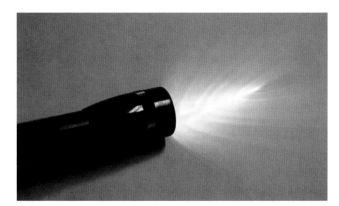

◪ Fig. 2.6 Broad beam (compare to focused beam shown in ◪ Fig. 2.1)

❯❯ The more electronics, the more heat is generated in the probe housing.

Alternatively, more acoustic energy can be transmitted by optimizing the transfer of electrical energy into acoustic energy. This could include the use of single crystalline piezoelectric materials and the use of advanced matching layer materials that facilitate the transfer of sound energy from the acoustic stack into the human body. Because of size and heat constraints, such methods of efficient design are most applicable to transesophageal matrix transducers.

2.1.3 Fully sampled matrix array transducers

Over the last 30 years, numerous ultrasound methods have been used to scan 3D volumes in the body, although with minimal clinical or market success (▶ Chapter 1). Clearly there was a need for a matrix phased array transducer, particularly given the success of phased arrays over mechanically swept transducers for routine 2D applications.

In the late 1980s, such a matrix transducer was considered unfeasible. Even a small aperture transducer would require in excess of 2500 elements (50×50). The cable connecting the transducer with the ultrasound instrument would be extremely large, bulky, and expensive. Thus, the phased array beamformer (part of the ultrasound instrument) with its 2500 processing channels would be extremely expensive to manufacture.

This impetus drove the concept of sparse arrays. In sparse matrix arrays, only a small percentage of the 2500 elements are electrically connected or acoustically active. This sparse array technology was commercialized in the mid 1990s, but has since been abandoned by most manufacturers.

There were three major problems with sparse array technology:

— Although the elements were strategically placed to mitigate obvious grating lobes, there was still degradation in side-lobe performance, which would appear as degraded contrast resolution to the clinician.
— The reduced number of elements and the reduced area of the probe face associated with transmitting and receiving ultrasound data would result in a loss of signal-to-noise ratio. This would be seen as a clinical loss in penetration.

— Emergence of tissue harmonic imaging. During the 1990s, harmonic imaging quickly became mainstream for transthoracic cardiac imaging. In order to create a harmonic echo, transmit waveforms with sufficient pressures needed to be transmitted into the body. Sparse arrays, with only a fraction of the elements transmitting, would have been incapable of creating the mechanical index (MI) necessary to create a clinically viable tissue harmonic image.

Given the practical limitations of sparse arrays, there was clearly a desire to produce a »fully sampled« matrix array, where all of the transducer elements were capable of both transmit and receive. Yet the practical limitation of supporting a transducer and system with a very large element and channel count remained.

❯❯ Given the practical limitations of sparse arrays, there was clearly a desire to produce fully sampled matrix array transducers.

This led to the development of micro-beamforming [10]. The key concept is to electrically group small arrays of elements (referred to as patches) and to coherently combine their output to a single wire going back to the »mainframe« beamformer. A typical patch for a cardiac matrix probe might contain approximately 25 elements configured in a 5×5 geometry. Assuming a 128 channel beamformer with 128 wires, connecting the transducer to the mainframe beamformer would provide a fully sampled array of 3200 elements.

In other words, micro-beamforming allows one to achieve the same uncompromised performance as a fully sampled array having 3200 wires and 3200 analog-to-digital converters, which can be achieved in a transducer with the size and cost appropriate for clinical use. A micro-beamformer acts, just as its name implies, like a very small electronic beamformer. Its sole purpose is to »point« its 25 elements (on both transmit and receive) toward the desired scan line.

In ◪ Fig. 2.7, a returning echo (wave field on the upper left) impinges on the face of the probe. For illustration purposes, there are only three elements in a patch. The sound arrives at the top element first and arrives at the bottom element last. The objective of each micro-beamformer is to time align all of the echoes from each element in its patch. Since the elements within a patch are co-located, the delay corrections can be quite small, and therefore the electronic circuitry in the matrix transducer can be small as well. Each micro-beamformer has its own output, which is wired back to the mainframe beamformer (back to the ultrasound system through the transducer cable assembly; ◪ Fig. 2.8). The roles of the mainframe beamformer are to time align the patches and to produce the parallel receive beams for each transmit beam.

There is a common misconception that a given acoustic scan beam is matched to a single element. Although a matrix array of elements might look like the CCD (digital film) of a camera, the matrix elements are better envisioned as the camera lens (which is used to focus the light).

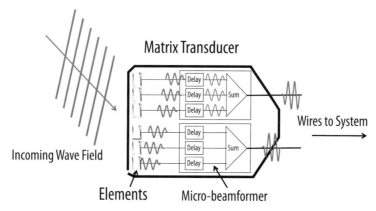

Fig. 2.7 Illustration of the principle of micro-beamforming

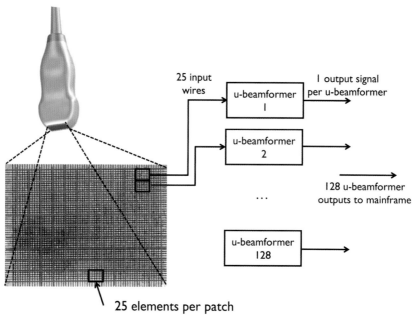

Fig. 2.8 Illustration of connection between micro-beamformers and mainframe beamformer

2.1.4 Parallel receive beam processing

One of the key ways to improve frame rate in current 3D ultrasound machines is through the use of parallel receive beam processing. Using the flashlight analogy will help illuminate how this works. In the darkened room, assume that there are four observers, but only one flashlight. The flashlight is slightly defocused to increase the spot size to 20 cm in diameter (it was 10 cm in the original scenario). Now each observer is asked to focus on a different quadrant of the light beam: observer A is asked to focus on the top left, observer B on the top right, C on bottom left, and D on the bottom right. So now, with each illuminated section of the wall, four smaller regions can be simultaneously interrogated (❑ Fig. 2.9).

❯ The use of parallel beam processing is one key way to improve frame rate in 3D ultrasound machines.

Most modern 3D phased array ultrasound machines use four or more simultaneous receive beams (the observers) for each transmitted beam (the flashlight). However, each receive beam shares the same aperture (probe face), the same elements, the same patches, and the same micro-beamformers. By using slightly different time delays in the mainframe beamformer, as applied to the micro-beamformed output, allows the »mainframe« beamformer to steer the receive beams in slightly different directions from one another.

2.1.5 Three-dimensional color flow

Unfortunately, 3D color flow inherits all of the B-mode issues (as discussed previously) and then compounds it with its own problems. Clearly the largest problem is frame rate, which can be experienced in 2D color flow. Why is color flow so much slower than B-mode?

In order to observe Doppler velocity shifts from blood, color flow imaging requires that an »ensemble« (a group) of scan lines be fired in the same direction. This is required for two reasons. The first is the need of a »wall filter«, which is used to remove the stationary tissue echoes that can be thousands of times larger than the

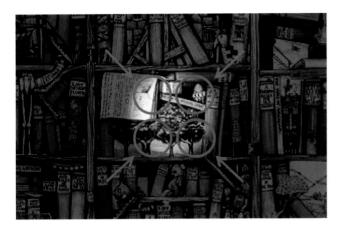

Fig. 2.9 Illustration of principle of parallel receive beam processing using the analogy of the flashlight

blood echoes. In its simplest embodiment, a wall filter can simply subtract the echoes from consecutive scan lines. Echoes that have not moved (from tissue) will be identical in both scan lines and, hence, will be eliminated. Moving echoes (from blood) will not be subtracted, since they are displaced scan line to scan line.

> Clearly the largest problem of 3D color flow is frame rate.

The second justification for having an ensemble of color flow lines is to detect the motion. By observing the time shift in the blood echoes (post wall filter) from one scan line to the next, the engineer can directly calculate the displacement distance. Dividing by the pulse repetition interval (PR=time between subsequent scan lines=~0.2 ms) will calculate the velocity, which is then encoded as a color and displayed. Note that this simple explanation can also be used to derive the Doppler equation.

Based upon the prior discussion, the smallest theoretical ensemble is three. However, for numerous practical reasons, a typical ensemble length for 2D color flow consists of 6–10 or more scan lines (for commercially available instruments). Recalling the 250 transmit events available for a real-time B-mode volume, a real-time color volume would be further limited to only 25 transmit scan directions (assuming an ensemble of ten acoustic lines per scan direction). Even at the relatively coarse transmit spacing of three degrees, the real-time 3D color would be limited to a 15×15 degree volume (lateral × elevation) using a 5×5 scan grid. This is a very small volume for routine clinical use.

There are four options available to the ultrasound engineer to make this 3D color flow volume larger:
- Coarsen the transmit line spacing. Not only will this adversely affect the color flow resolution (more lateral/elevation smearing of the color data), it will also degrade sensitivity and the ability to detect pathologic flows.
- Decrease the number of acoustic lines within an ensemble. This will also degrade color flow sensitivity.
- Sacrifice frame rate.
- Sacrifice real-time and use gating: acquire smaller subvolumes over multiple cardiac cycles.

Again, all of these techniques are used to varying degrees by the various 3D manufacturers.

2.1.6 Principle of depth volume rendering for 3D imaging

Volume rendering is a method by which a 3D matrix of numbers is composited to produce a 2D image. Although the resultant 2D image looks very similar to the 2D image produced by surface rendering (the method common to the video gaming industry), the source data and the method of compositing can be quite different.

Volume rendering is very analogous to the way in which the human eye sees the 3D world. For each rod (or cone) on the retina, a »ray cast« originates from the eye such that the light intensity on the rod will be dictated by the first opaque structure intersecting the ray cast.

In volume rendering, a »2D plane« is spatially oriented with respect to the 3D object. The 3D object (or volume) contains samples at each point in the XYZ space. Note that 3D samples are referred to as voxels, and 2D samples as pixels. For each pixel on the 2D plane, a ray cast line is created which is perpendicular to the 2D plane and which intersects the 3D object. This is shown in **Fig. 2.10. In 3D echocardiography, the voxels could either be B-mode magnitudes or color velocities as acquired from a matrix transducer.

Each sample along the ray cast, corresponding to the distance from the pixel, will be assigned the value from its intersected voxel. This is shown in **Fig. 2.11. Whereas the ray cast signal looks noisy, this is typical of ultrasound data. The high frequency variations correspond to the speckle variations seen in clinical images, which make volume rendering more difficult.

Compositing is the process that converts ray cast values into the single value assigned to a pixel. For the human eye analogy, compositing effectively assigns the light from the first opaque structure to the rod. This occurs because each voxel in 3D space has both reflective and translucent physical properties. For example, the ray cast will sample »air« voxels, but these are not visualized since they are 100% translucent.

Volume rendering of ultrasound voxels is a bit more difficult. Ultrasound voxels are not inherently translucent or opaque. Therefore, during the compositing process, the algorithm will need to calculate an opacity for each ultrasound voxel. In the case of B-mode anatomical data, it would be desirable to make the heart chambers and the blood pools translucent. Since such echoes tend to be hypo-echoic, one can use the amplitude of the B-mode data to assign the opacity. This often involves a threshold such that any ray cast value below the threshold will be considered 100% translucent. This threshold is illustrated by the red line in **Fig. 2.11.

In a very simple compositing implementation, one could simply select the first sample above the opacity threshold. In **Fig. 2.11, the first sample above the threshold has a value of 29, which would then be assigned to the 2D pixel. Repeating this operation for every pixel in the 2D plane would produce the volume rendered image similar to the one of the right in **Fig. 2.10. Actual volume rendering in commercial 3D ultrasound machines is a bit more complicated. Further insights can be gained from [11].

Recent advances in 3D visualization have involved the use of colorization, or chroma, to imbed depth information in the

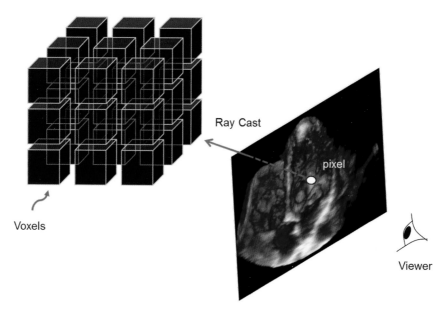

Ray Cast

pixel

Voxels

Viewer

☐ **Fig. 2.10** Volume rendering

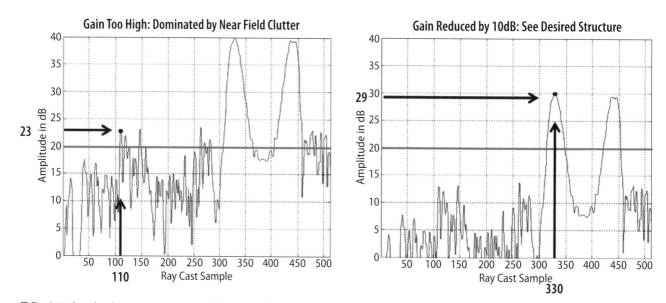

☐ **Fig. 2.11** Samples along a ray cast corresponding to a single pixel. The horizontal axis corresponds to the sample index, or to the distance from the pixel. The vertical axis corresponds to the amplitude of the B-mode echo. *Left* Illustration of a situation where the gain is too high, such that near field clutter exceeds the opacity threshold (*red line*). *Right* The gain is reduced, such that the desired anatomical structure (@ sample 330) is now visualized. Note the deeper anatomical structure located at 440. This will not be observed because it is blocked by the first structure at 330

volume rendered image [12]. This helps to increase the 3D depth perception of the image without having to resort to stereoscopic methods (e.g., 3D glasses).

Internal to the ultrasound instrument, a depth-weighted compositing algorithm will calculate two values for each ray cast line: the amplitude of the first opaque sample and its depth location. Referring to the right image in ☐ Fig. 2.11, the first opaque anatomical structure has an amplitude of 29 with a depth index of 330. From these values, two separate images are created: the first being the classic volume rendered image, which has already been described, and the second being a depth image (lower left in ☐ Fig. 2.12). The intensity of the depth image corresponds to

the depth of the sample; shallow structures (close to the viewer) are shown in black, whereas deeper structures are shown as white.

These two internal images will then be combined through a 2D look up table (LUT). It has the special properties that the intensity of the RGB (red, green, blue) colors will only be dictated by the value of the composited value, and that the hue of the RGB colors will only be dictated by the depth index. Repeating this operation for every pixel in both source images will produce the depth-rendered image as seen on the right in ☐ Fig. 2.12. This allows twice the information to be communicated in a very intuitive manner.

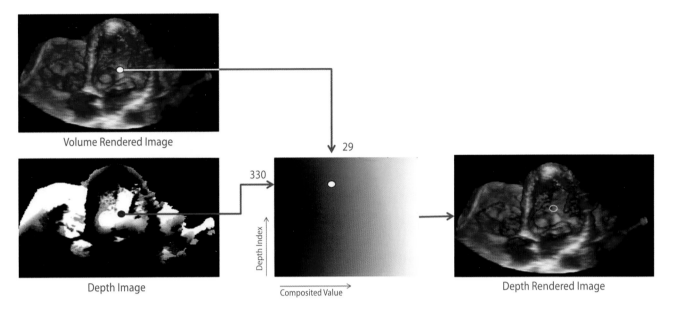

Volume Rendered Image

330

29

Depth Index

Depth Image

Composited Value

Depth Rendered Image

□ Fig. 2.12 Volume rendering using depth-weighted colorization

2.2 The probes

Today, matrix array probes exist for both transthoracic and transesophageal live 3D scanning. Compared to the first commercial matrix array probe by Volumetrics (▶ Chapter 1), the transthoracic probes have decreased significantly in size and nowadays are hard to differentiate from conventional 2D phased array probes (□ Fig. 2.13 and □ Fig. 2.14). There were several challenges to overcome in building the latest matrix array transducer generation (▶ Section 2.1). Because of the large number of ultrasound elements (2400–2500, compared to 64–128 elements in 2D phased array probes), the size of the transducer aperture became too large to scan through the narrow intercostal space. Decreasing the size of ultrasound elements and narrowing the field of ultrasound elements, however, caused increased problems with heating which have been successfully solved in present 3D transthoracic and transesophageal transducers by using more efficient piezoelectric elements and active or passive cooling techniques. Other difficulties to overcome pertained to the data transfer of the analogue high-frequency (HF) signals from the transducer via the transducer cable to the digital signal analysis unit within the ultrasound system. As mentioned in ▶ Section 2.1, computer boards for signal analysis nowadays have been miniaturized to fit into the transducer handle, which results in a relatively thin and flexible transducer cable for digital signal transfer to the ultrasound system for further analysis and display. We can expect that 3D ultrasound systems will be further miniaturized in the near future, and even cordless transducers using wireless transmission are conceivable.

❯ In the newest transesophageal and transthoracic 3D probes, all ultrasound modalities have been successfully integrated.

As a practical limitation, it should be noted that some 3D probes are still currently limited to 3D imaging only and do not provide standard 2D imaging modes and spectral Doppler acquisition. This is particularly the case in some transthoracic probes, thus, urging the examiner to change transducers during 2D and 3D scanning, whereas in 3D transesophageal probes all ultrasound modalities – 2D, 3D as well as color and spectral Doppler – have been successfully integrated as an essential requirement. The newest generation of transthoracic 3D probes combines all features of previous matrix-array 3D probes and standard 2D probes (□ Fig. 2.13). Such all-in-one-probes allow full integration of 3D imaging into a standard transthoracic echocardiographic workflow, thereby overcoming the need to change between 3D and 2D transducers. This new all-in-one matrix array transducer technology is also capable to provide full volume acquisition in one beat (one-beat full volume mode) as well as live 3D color Doppler imaging (□ Fig. 2.15).

2.3 Live 3D echocardiographic examination

In principle, there are two ways of performing a RT3D echocardiographic examination in clinical practice:
1. to perform a standard 2D echocardiographic examination and to add RT3D datasets of selected structures or regions or
2. to perform a full RT3D echocardiographic examination with standard 3D views and to add only spectral Doppler datasets with information that cannot be obtained by RT3D datasets [13](14).

Currently, the first protocol is certainly more common for several reasons. Most echocardiography laboratories are still on a learning curve and not experienced enough to fully rely on RT3D datasets yet. In a recent first recommendation paper on 3D image acquisition and display, however, prerequisites for the integration of 3D echocardiography into routine patient examinations very

Matrix-array 3D   2D

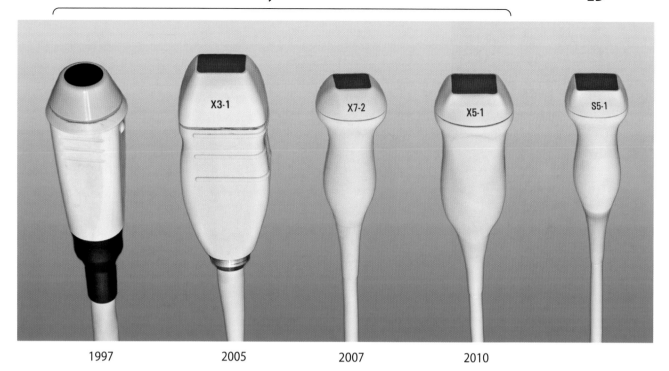

1997   2005   2007   2010

◻ **Fig. 2.13** Evolution of transthoracic real-time 3D matrix array transducers: (from *left* to *right* with year of first release). The first commercially available matrix array transducer with a sparse array of 50×60 elements and a very large transducer cable (1997, Model 314U, 3.5 MHz, Volumetrics Medical Imaging, USA) [20] [21]. The adult matrix array transducer with 2400 active elements with a relatively bulky handle due to embodied postprocessing electronics, but a relatively thin transducer cable (2005, Model X3-1, 1–3 MHz, Philips Medical Systems, USA). Further miniaturized pediatric matrix array transducer with 2500 active elements (2007, Model X7-2, 2–7 MHz, Philips Medical Systems, USA). The new all-in-one adult matrix array transducer with an ergonomic sized handle which also operates with all common 2D imaging and spectral Doppler modes (2010, Model X5-1, 1–5 MHz, Philips Medical Systems, USA). *Far right* A conventional 2D phased array transducer with 80 elements is shown (Model S5-1, 1–5 MHz, Philips Medical Systems, USA)

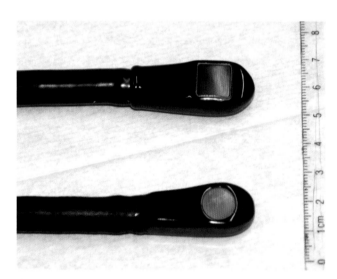

◻ **Fig. 2.14** Side-by-side illustration of a transesophageal live 3D matrix array probe with 2600 elements (*top*; Model x7-2t, 2–7 MHz, Philips Medical Systems, USA) and a standard multiplane 2D phased array probe with 64 elements (*bottom*; Model Omni 3, Philips Medical Systems, USA)

outlined as to be (1) a single transducer capable of 2D and 3D imaging, (2) accurate automated chamber quantification, and (3) automated display of standard 3D and 2D echocardiographic views [15]. With the latest all-in-one 3D matrix array probes the first requirement has been achieved. Although, analysis of 3D datasets can be time consuming, several semiautomated 3D quantification tools have been developed or will be available in the near future which addresses the second and third requirements. However, the recent recommendations on 3D image acquisition and display provide a first consensus on the use of 3D echocardiographic techniques in clinical routine practice, thus, paving the way for more standardized 3D examinations and the broader use of RT3D echocardiography. Besides the need of national and international recommendations, two other factors are important for wider clinical application of RT3D echocardiography: (1) expert-guided training courses to ease and accelerate climbing the learning curve and (2) the manufacturers to make the handling and analysis of 3D data as feasible as 2D data. In other words, the workflow of integrating 3D echocardiography into the examination needs to be made easier.

❯ There is still some uncertainty about how to integrate 3D echocardiography into the patient examination that needs to be overcome.

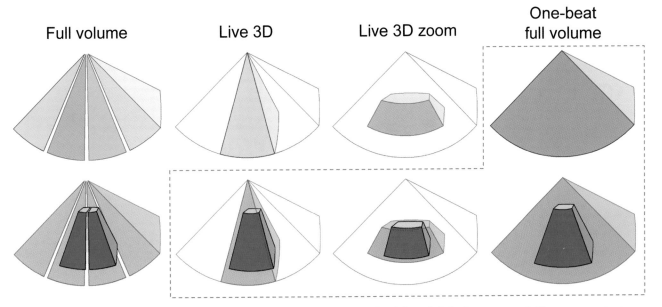

Fig. 2.15 Schematic representation of different 3D volume acquisition modes. *Top row from left to right* Full volume composed of four or seven subvolumes; live 3D mode; live 3D zoom mode; one-beat full volume. *Bottom row* The respective 3D volume acquisition modes with additional 3D color Doppler volumes are illustrated. The volume modes within the dashed line – one-beat full volume with and without color Doppler and live 3D color Doppler – are not available in all 3D systems yet. The 3D datasets included in this book were all acquired using the four 3D volume acquisition modes outside the dashed line

2.3.1 First steps and learning curve

When RT3DE with live 3D visualization became widely available for the first time in 2002 (after its introduction at the European Society of Cardiology Congress in August 2002), the majority of users discovered that the acquisition of transthoracic datasets (and later in 2008 similarly with transesophageal datasets) was feasible and relative easy to learn. However, further analysis of 3D datasets, either onboard or on an external workstation, required special knowledge and skills of 3D dataset cropping, 3D orientation, and knowledge of how to use the 3D analysis software. This was particularly important as 3D datasets often reveal their entire information only after cropping and slicing, like in a crystal geode (▶ Section 2.3.2, »Multiple-beat full volume mode«) and unlike 2D images that instantly show their information as it is acquired. Beyond this, 3D analysis is still considered to be more time consuming compared to conventional 2D image analysis. As a consequence, users acquired large numbers of 3D datasets without drawing diagnostic information from them and finally run the risk of becoming dissatisfied even before they started to move up the learning curve.

> The 3D datasets often reveal their entire information only after cropping and slicing.

Learning from this experience, 3D manufacturers and clinical experts have offered interactive 3D training courses to help novice users to overcome difficulties when learning to use 3D analysis software for cropping, orientation, and displaying of 3D images [16]. Even more, measurements in 3D datasets, including size of an atrial septal defect (ASD), left atrial (LA) volume, or quantification of global and regional left ventricular (LV) function as well as the more advanced quantification of mitral valve anatomy required initial step-by-step interactive demonstration.

2.3.2 Three-dimensional acquisition (modes and image settings)

Nowadays, 3D data acquisition, in principle, can be easily integrated into standard transthoracic and transesophageal echocardiographic examinations by using an all-in-one matrix array transducer capable of 2D, spectral Doppler and 3D imaging and switching to 3D modes by pressing a button [17]. As mentioned above, different modes of 3D volume acquisition are available. Currently, the most common modes are live 3D, live 3D zoom, full volume as well as full volume color Doppler acquisitions, which are available on both transthoracic and transesophageal matrix array probes (▢ Fig. 2.15).

However, as the diagnostic applications of live 3D in transthoracic echocardiography (TTE) and transesophageal echocardiography (TEE) are different, it is of critical importance to understand the characteristics of the different volume modes in order to choose the most appropriate one for a given setting, which is analogous to choosing the appropriate gear when driving a car instead of always driving in the same gear. Basically, we can currently state that real-time 3D TTE is more suitable for whole heart capture by gated or one-beat full volume acquisition for quantitative 3D analysis of global and regional LV function, RV volumes, and LA volumes, whereas real-time 3D TEE is especially suited for detailed 3D imaging using zoomed live 3D volume acquisitions for the analysis of valves, defects, and other structures, e.g., cardiac masses [13]. The different real-time 3D volume modes can be characterized as described below. As has been previously mentioned, there are a number of important interactions between the physical characteristics of a 3D dataset; these will now be described in more detail.

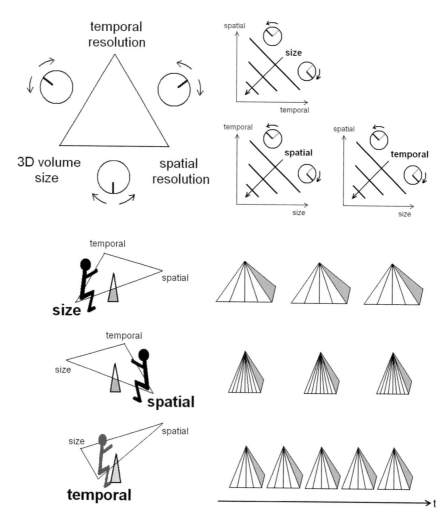

◨ Fig. 2.16 Principle of interdependency of 3D volume size, temporal and spatial resolution. *Upper left* The interdependency is expressed by a triangle where all three parameters are connected to each other. The dial knobs between each pair of parameters indicate the option for weighting more to the one or the other. *Upper right* The three diagrams illustrate the effect of the dialing for all possible settings of the three parameters. The *upper diagram* shows for a given 3D volume size the effect of dialing more towards increased spatial resolution causing lower temporal resolution and vice versa. With increasing 3D volume size (in direction of the size arrow), however, both temporal and spatial resolution have to decrease. *Lower part* Interdependency between the three parameters is illustrated by the triangle balanced on a center axis point. The preference set to a large 3D volume size (*top*) causes lower temporal resolution (as indicated by the separation between pyramids on the right) and lower spatial resolution (as indicated by the three wide-spread lines). The preference set to higher spatial resolution (*middle*) causes smaller 3D volume size at a lower temporal resolution (the higher spatial resolution indicated by a larger number of lines with higher density). The preference set to higher temporal resolution (*bottom*) causes smaller 3D volume size and lower number and density of lines

■   **The triangle of interdependency between temporal and spatial resolution and volume size**

Setting up real-time 3D volumes is fundamentally determined by a triangle of three interdependent characteristics as these are (1) the volume size, and here particularly the width in lateral and elevation dimension, (2) temporal resolution, and (3) spatial resolution (◨ Fig. 2.16). As there is only one transmit beam travelling through the scan volume of a given size and the velocity of the ultrasound beam is a constant of approximately 1540 m/s, the time required for the beam to fully travel through the entire volume is determined by two factors (1) the size of the scan volume and (2) the line density which determines the total number of scan lines in the scan volume as already emphasized in the technical part in ► Section 2.1.1. As the line density determines the spatial resolution of the 3D voxel dataset and the resulting 3D image and the total number of scan lines required to scan the volumes determines the temporal resolution the following consequences and trade-offs exist:

━   **For a larger 3D image** increasing the scan volume has the consequence of increasing the number of scan lines resulting in a longer time to scan the volume and, thus, lower temporal resolution or the consequence to accept a lower line density resulting in lower spatial resolution or a combination of both consequences (in newer systems this issue has been especially addressed by adding a dialing function that allows for weighting the trade-off to be more on temporal or more on the spatial resolution).

━   **For higher image resolution** increasing spatial resolution by increasing the line density has the consequence of decreasing the size of the scan volume or to increase the number of scan lines required to scan the volume resulting in a lower temporal resolution or a combination of both consequences.

■ **For higher temporal resolution** increasing temporal resolution by decreasing the number of scan lines required to scan the volume has the consequence of decreasing the size of the scan volume or to decrease the line density resulting in a lower spatial resolution or a combination of both consequences.

From these interdependencies and trade-offs, the following characteristics and practical recommendations for setting up 3D volume acquisition evolve.

■ One-beat 3D volume acquisition mode

In principle, in the latest generation of 3D systems one-beat 3D volume acquisition mode providing live 3D imaging can be set up to acquire volumes of almost any size from relatively narrow pryramid-shaped volumes and zoomed volumes up to large pyramid-shaped full volumes of more than 90° angle width. However, live 3D imaging with satisfactory temporal resolution requires a minimum of approximately 10–12 volumes per second. And therefore according to the interdependencies discussed above one-beat 3D volumes or live 3D volumes should be limited to a size that still provides a volume rate of at least 10–12 volumes per second and acceptable spatial resolution. For example, setting up a transthoracic one-beat full volume to a size large enough to encompass the entire left heart or even left and right heart temporal resolution in most 3D systems will drop to less than 10 beats per second or/and spatial resolution will drop such that satisfactory image quality is prevented. To address these requirements, for example, in some older 3D systems, a live 3D volume acquisition mode with a fixed narrow volume size was configured: angle width was about 30° in the elevation dimension and about 65° in longitudinal (azimuth) dimension (◘ Fig. 2.15).

Advantages of a live 3D volume of such narrow dimensions, however, are high spatial resolution (because of high line density) and high temporal resolution (because of a relative narrow scan volume). Therefore, such a narrow live 3D volume is particularly useful for visualization of structures that are small enough to fit into the narrow volume, e.g., small valves, small masses, or vegetations, which become more difficult to fit into a narrow live 3D volume the closer the structure is to the transducer. However, because in transesophageal scanning the orientation of the aortic valve plane is nearly parallel to the ultrasound beam direction, it fits very well into this narrow live 3D volume where it is located in an upright position (▸ Section 2.3.3). Compared with this, normal-sized mitral valves are oriented in a more perpendicular position and are usually too wide or too close to the transducer to fit into a narrow live 3D volume. In addition, in transthoracic live 3D scanning, the mitral valve fits better into the narrow volume because of the larger distance from the transducer (◘ Fig. 2.17). Note, however, that for a given line density visualization of a structure (i.e., valve) at a lower depth (as in transesophageal scanning) results in an effectively higher line density as the lines had a smaller distance to diverge as compared to visualization of a structure at a higher depth (as more frequent in transthoracic scanning) resulting in an effectively lower line density as the lines had a longer distance to diverge (◘ Fig. 2.18). As a practical recommendation in order to minimize this effect, the

volume depth should be set up to visualize the structure of interest rather in the center or the near field of the volume instead in the far field, in both transthoracic and transesophageal 3D scanning. The one-beat or live 3D volume mode (according to its name) provides live 3D viewing during scanning. However, because of the pyramid shape of the volume, direct viewing of valves, for example, requires extra cropping of the volume, particularly in transthoracic 3D datasets. Today, switching to 3D color Doppler in the live 3D and live 3D zoom modes is available in all 3D echocardiographic machines of the latest generation (◘ Fig. 2.15).

■ Live 3D zoom mode

Live 3D zoom or zoomed live 3D is a very practical mode particularly in transesophageal 3D scanning. It is similar to zoom modes in 2D scanning in that it allows one to manually define a volume of interest (◘ Fig. 2.15 and ◘ Fig. 2.17), which can encompass a specific region or structure. As an advantage opposed to pyramid-shaped live 3D volumes, this zoomed live 3D volume mode eliminates the need for cropping of the volume because the volume can be defined in a manner that provides direct viewing of the structures of interest, e.g., direct en face viewing of the mitral valve (◘ Fig. 2.17). However, the price to pay for the advantage of a live 3D visualization of a structure of interest (e.g., the mitral valve) in a volume wide enough to encompass the entire structure frequently is a relatively low temporal resolution with a volume rate of between 10 and 16 volumes per second depending on the width of the defined zoom volume and a lower spatial resolution due to the lower line density. The lower line density results in less detailed surface rendering of fine structures, e.g., chords or vegetations, which appear thicker compared to when a narrower live 3D volume or full volume mode are used (◘ Fig. 2.19). Despite inferior temporal and spatial resolution compared to 3D volume modes with smaller volumes or higher line density, live 3D zoom is probably the most practical and most frequently used 3D mode during transesophageal 3D scanning.

■ Multiple-beat full volume mode

The description »full volume« relates to the size of the pyramid-shaped 3D volume being large enough to encompass the full heart, reaching angles up to more than 100° in both the longitudinal (azimuth) and elevation dimensions. As described above one-beat full volumes are inherently limited by low temporal and low spatial resolution. In contrast to a one-beat full volume or other live 3D modes, a multiple-beat full volume does not consist of a single volume but of multiple 3D volumes stitched together (◘ Fig. 2.15 and ◘ Fig. 2.20). As a consequence, the multiple-beat full volume mode does not allow live 3D viewing, because the number of subvolumes is needed to be acquired over a corresponding number of heart cycles by electrocardiographic triggering, which also gives it the name »gated« 3D acquisition. As typical for large multiple-beat full volumes, pyramid-shaped datasets from a transthoracic approach look unspectacular from the outside as there is no information about the inside of the object, like in a crystal geode (◘ Fig. 2.21). By changing the settings for line density and number of subvolumes, the size of the full volume can by defined prior to acquisition. Because a multiple-beat

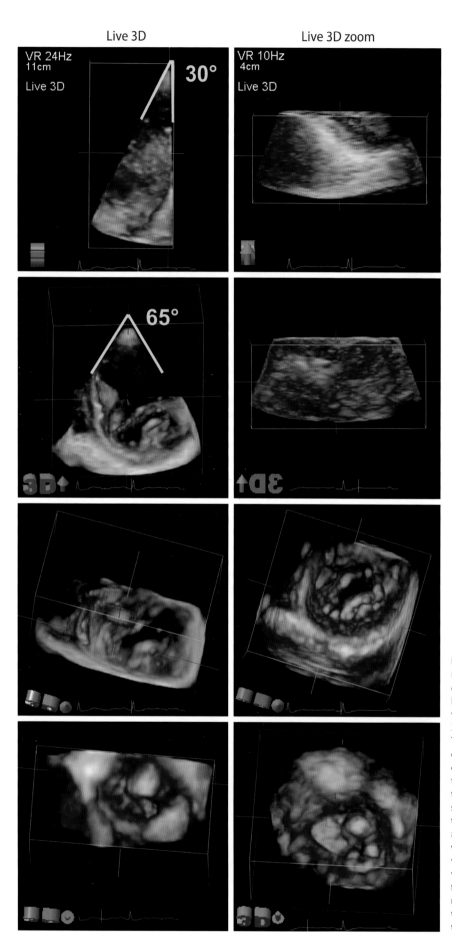

Live 3D

Live 3D zoom

■ **Fig. 2.17** Comparison of transthoracic live 3D mode (*left column*) and live 3D zoom mode (*right column*) in the same patient with mitral P2 prolapse. The two panels in the *top row* show side views of a live 3D volume with a narrow angle of 30° (*left*) and a wider live 3D zoom volume (*right*). The two panels in the *second row* show the same datasets from the other side after clockwise vertical rotation by 90°. The yellow crop box with the three axes (*red, green, blue*) helps with the orientation of the volume in space. An additional aid for spatial orientation is given by the *blue* **3D**↑ icon in the lower left corner of each figure. Panels in the *third row* show a view from the apex to the mitral valve: the live 3D volume provides a very narrow view to the mitral valve with signals of the left ventricular (*LV*) apex in between. The wider but flatter live 3D zoom volume provides a more direct view of the mitral valve. *Bottom* A view from the left atrium (*LA*) to the mitral valve with detection of P2 prolapse is shown. [→Videos 2.17A–H]

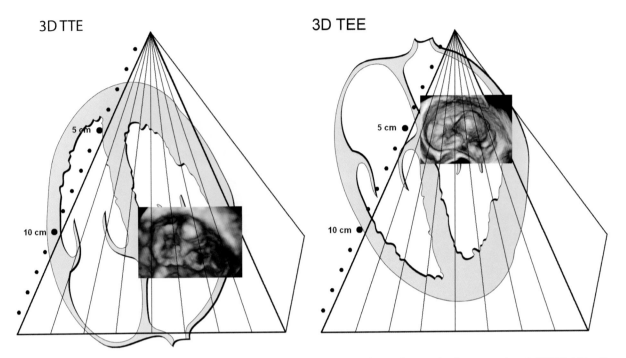

3D TTE   **3D TEE**

5 cm   5 cm

10 cm   10 cm

▣ **Fig. 2.18** Illustration of the relation between scanning depth, line density, and spatial resolution of 3D imaging from a transthoracic (3D TTE; *left*) and transesophageal approach (3D TEE; *right*). In the example of 3D scanning of the mitral valve, the schematic illustrates that due to the divergence of imaging lines with increasing depth spatial resolution and, thus, resulting 3D image quality is higher at a lower depth of 4–5 cm, which is where the mitral valve is located from a TEE approach (*right*), compared to imaging the mitral valve at a higher depth of 9–10 cm from a TTE approach (*left*)

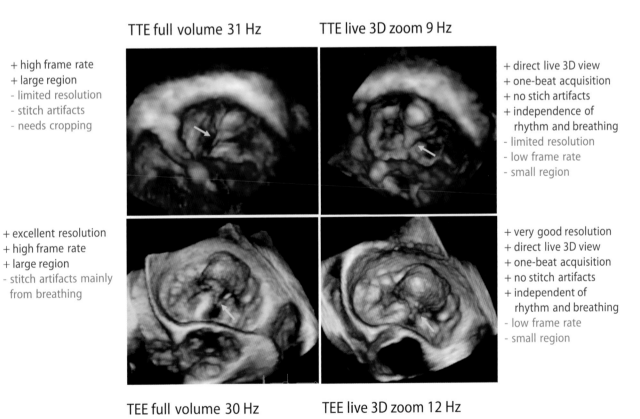

TTE full volume 31 Hz   TTE live 3D zoom 9 Hz

+ high frame rate
+ large region
- limited resolution
- stitch artifacts
- needs cropping

+ direct live 3D view
+ one-beat acquisition
+ no stich artifacts
+ independence of
   rhythm and breathing
- limited resolution
- low frame rate
- small region

+ excellent resolution
+ high frame rate
+ large region
- stitch artifacts mainly
  from breathing

+ very good resolution
+ direct live 3D view
+ one-beat acquisition
+ no stitch artifacts
+ independent of
   rhythm and breathing
- low frame rate
- small region

TEE full volume 30 Hz   TEE live 3D zoom 12 Hz

▣ **Fig. 2.19** Differences in image quality between transthoracic (*TTE, top row*) and transesophageal 3D imaging (*TEE, bottom row*) and full volume acquisition (*left column*) and live 3D zoom acquisition (*right column*) in the same patient are demonstrated. This shows an en face view from the left atrium to the mitral valve with P2 flail leaflet. For quick reference, positive (*blue*) and limiting (*red*) criteria of image quality are indicated for each 3D acquisition mode. Importantly, the different 3D acquisition modes have a significant impact on the representation of fine structures, such as a ruptured chord (*yellow arrows*) with the finest visualization of the chord in the 3D TEE full volume mode (*bottom left*) and the most blurred and thickened representation in TTE live 3D zoom mode (*top right*). [→Videos 2.19A–D]

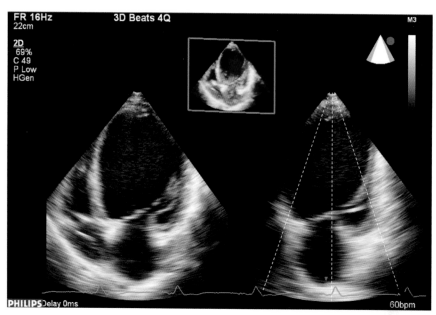

◘ Fig. 2.20 Display during transthoracic four-beat full volume acquisition using a Philips X5-1 matrix array transducer. *Bottom left* Sector view represents the standard 2D scan plan according to the transducer orientation. *Bottom right* This view is a view perpendicular to the *left,* generated simultaneously by the matrix array probe in elevation dimension. The 3D image at the *top* represents the acquired 3D volume. *Lower right* The sector view is divided by *three dashed lines* dividing the four real-time 3D volumes stitched together

full volume consists of two, four or on some 3D systems even more 3D volumes stitched together, spatial and temporal resolution of the full volume dataset is as high as for the individual 3D volumes according to the trade-offs discussed above.

However, as a practical limitation, multiple-beat full volume datasets are prone to stitching artifacts (► Section 2.6) mainly caused by translation of the heart from breathing during the volume acquisition period. Therefore, stitching artifacts can be best prevented by breath holding in both transthoracic and transesophageal examinations or pausing respiration during cardiac surgery. If the length of the heart cycles vary, e.g., in atrial fibrillation, stitching artifacts can also result. In general, multiple-beat full volume is the most appropriate mode for transthoracic acquisition of large volumes encompassing the entire heart or the entire left ventricle for heart chamber quantification. In transesophageal examinations, the multiple-beat full volume mode allows acquisition of a wide 3D image encompassing multiple valves (◘ Fig. 2.22) or large structures, e.g., large myxomas with good temporal and spatial resolution.

❯ The full volume is the most appropriate mode for transthoracic acquisition to encompass the entire heart or the left ventricle.

▪ 3D color Doppler mode

In newer 3D systems, 3D color Doppler is available in both multiple-beat full volume acquisition mode and all one-beat or live 3D volume modes. In principle, as in 2D modes, a 3D color Doppler volume is superimposed onto the 3D volume with tissue information (◘ Fig. 2.15) allowing to either turn-off color Doppler information or tissue information for visual assessment. Note that the fundamental trade-offs pertaining to volume size,

temporal, and spatial resolution as discussed above are also valid for 3D color Doppler volumes. In addition, like multiple-beat full volume acquisition, multiple-beat 3D color Doppler volumes are potentially affected by stitching artifacts.

After acquisition of a 3D color Doppler volume, various color Doppler settings can be applied to the dataset significantly affecting the image quality. Important color Doppler settings include (1) color Doppler gain, (2) smoothing, (3) color vision, (4) filter, and (5) baseline velocity. Those settings can be either changes directly on the 3D system or off-line using analysis software such as Qlab (Philips) as long as the original 3D data format with raw data information is kept. The following settings are recommended for 3D color Doppler datasets acquired on a Philips 3D system: color Doppler gain =50, smoothing =2, color vision =2, filter =4–6, and baseline velocity =6 (default).

It is important to note that in 3D color Doppler acquisition, like in 2D color Doppler, depth setting has an important impact on temporal resolution in the way that the deeper the depth of the 3D color Doppler volume is set up, the lower the temporal resolution will be, whereas the depth setting in the normal tissue mode has little effect on temporal resolution or on one of the other interdependent factors as discussed above. As in 2D color Doppler, the autocorrelation process to determine color Doppler velocities along the color Doppler scan lines in a 3D volume is a time-consuming calculation, which results in longer scan time for each 3D volume when the depth of the 3D color Doppler volume and along with this the length of the color Doppler scan line increases.

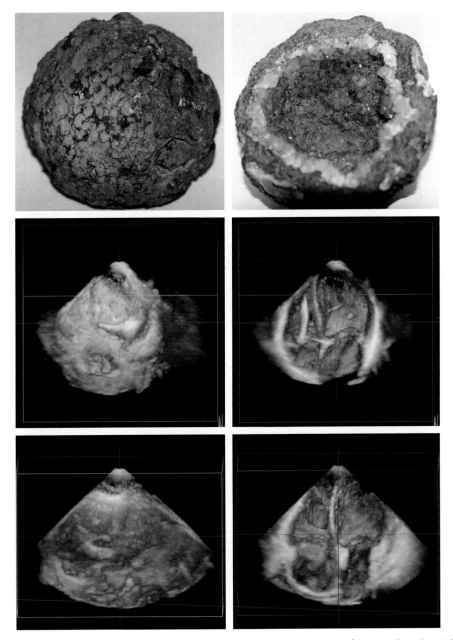

Fig. 2.21 Two examples of the full volume mode using TTE. The uncropped full volume (*left*) provides no information about the inside of the object, like a crystal geode (*top left*). Cropping the full volume towards its center provides a direct view of the important details inside. [→Videos 2.21A–D]

2.3.3 Standard 3D views and image orientation

Although live 3D echocardiography has been available since 2002, there were no unified recommendations on a standard examination protocol and standard views available until recently. This was partly because of the far more complex image information compared to 2D images. Now, a joint recommendation paper by EAE/ASE has been recently become available providing general information on how to set up 3D transthoracic and transesophageal examination protocols [15]. A first examination protocol for transthoracic RT3DE (RT3D TTE) with 3D image orientation according to anatomic cut planes of the heart in transverse, sagittal, and coronal orientation was proposed by Nanda et al. [18], where (1) a transverse cut plane orientation represents a vertical plane which is oriented almost perpendicular to the long axis of the heart and therefore provides short-axis views of the heart, for example a short axis of the LV, (2) a sagittal plane represents a vertical plane along the long axis of the heart that divides the heart into a left and right half, providing for example a long-axis view of the left ventricle, LVOT, and aortic root, and (3) a coronal plane represents a plane along the long axis of the heart but perpendicular to the sagittal plane, thus, separating the heart in an anterior and posterior half, providing for example a typical 4-chamber view (◘ Fig. 2.23). More recently, a systematic characterization of the mitral valve using RT3D TEE was proposed by Salcedo et al. [19]. In principle, definition of standard views is more difficult in 3D datasets because orientation in space is unlimited compared to transthoracic 2D echo-

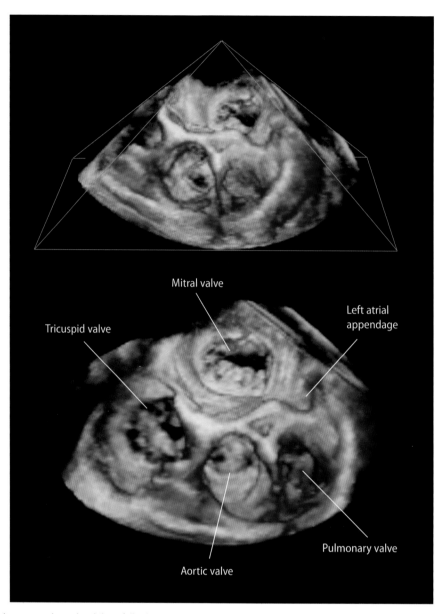

◘ Fig. 2.22 Example of a wide transesophageal multibeat full volume dataset with good spatial and temporal resolution (25 Hz). The upper image illustrates the pyramid-shaped dataset with the left atrium near the peak of the pyramid which is from where the transducer transmits the ultrasound beam through the heart. The lower image shows the dataset in an en face view to the valve plane [→Video 2.22A,B]

cardiography which is limited to parasternal and apical views, for example.

Based on the different characteristics of the 3D acquisition modes used in transthoracic echocardiography (TTE) and transesophageal echocardiographic (TEE) examinations, the following 3D views have been found to be particularly important and useful in the majority of 3D examinations. However, it is important to emphasize that »standard 3D views« are useful, on the one hand, to follow in a structured examination protocol, but, on the other hand, it is equally important to freely rotate and orient the 3D datasets to obtain the 3D view that best describes the relevant structure or region. It is important to again emphasize that a complete 3D echocardiographic examination should consist not only of 3D en face views, but should also contain cross-sectional 2D views of structures, like mitral and aortic valves, the left atrial appendage, and the interatrial septum using either standard

2D views from conventional 2D scanning or 2D planes from a multiple planar reconstruction (MPR) mode from 3D datasets as widely used in the following chapters on special pathologies. Note that 3D image acquisition and standard 3D views as proposed in the following text do for the most part, but do not fully comply with the recent recommendations on 3D image acquisition and display [15] as for the proposed standard views we did not focus on the transducer position for volume acquisition (e.g., apical, parasternal, mid-esophageal) but more on the desired 3D image and its orientation, which was acquired from any position that provided the best 3D dataset quality.

> ❯ A complete 3D echocardiographic examination should also always contain cross-sectional 2D views of structures, as 2D views add to the understanding of 3D views the same as 3D views add to the understanding of 2D views.

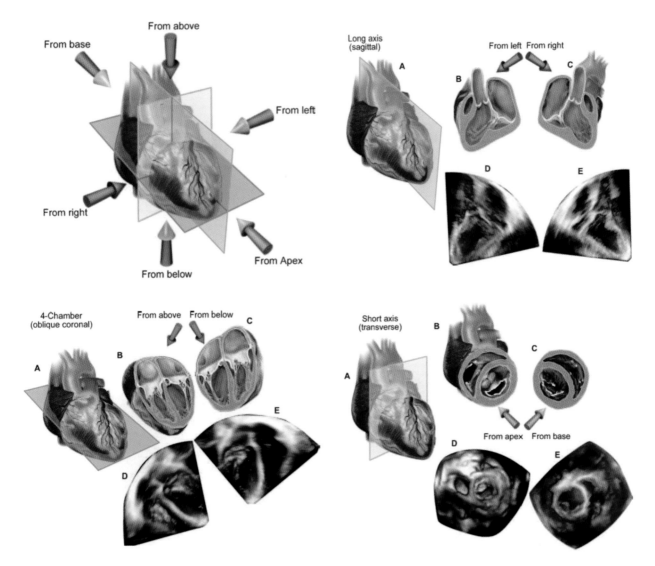

Fig. 2.23 Definition of transthoracic standard 3D views based on direct comparison of standard anatomic cut planes of the heart and corresponding 3D echocardiographic views. Reproduced from [18]; Copyright John Wiley and Sons

Standard 3D views for TTE (◘ Fig. 2.24):
— Four-chamber view using cropped full volume
(◘ Fig. 2.24.1) provides a wide view of all four chambers as well as the mitral and tricuspid valves with good image resolution and good temporal resolution (here 20 Hz).
— Two-chamber view using cropped full volume (◘ Fig. 2.24.2) provides a 2-chamber view of the LV and LA with good image resolution and good temporal resolution (here 20 Hz). Same dataset as used in ◘ Fig. 2.24.1. Provides en face view of interventricular septum for detection of VSD.
— En face mitral and tricuspid valve views from the apex using cropped full volume (◘ Fig. 2.24.3) provides en face view of mitral and tricuspid valve from the LV apex with good image resolution and good temporal resolution (here 20 Hz). Same dataset as used in ◘ Fig. 2.24.1.
— En face mitral valve view from the LV using live 3D zoom (◘ Fig. 2.24.4) provides a focused live view of the mitral valve from the LV with moderate image resolution and limited temporal resolution (here 16 Hz). Capturing part

of aortic valve helps with orientation. This view is particularly useful for assessment of incomplete mitral leaflet closure and restricted mitral leaflet motion in mitral stenosis.
— En face mitral valve view from the LA using live 3D zoom (◘ Fig. 2.24.5) provides a focused live view of the mitral valve from the LA with moderate image resolution and limited temporal resolution (here 16 Hz). Same dataset as used in ◘ Fig. 2.24.4. This view is particularly useful for assessment of organic mitral valve disease, e.g., prolapse and flail leaflet. It also provides a focused live view of the aortic valve from the aortic root. Morphologic assessment of the aortic valve, however, can be limited with current transthoracic matrix array transducer performance.
— En face aortic valve view from the LV using live 3D zoom (◘ Fig. 2.24.6) provides a focused live view of the aortic valve and the LVOT from the LV with limited image resolution and limited temporal resolution (here 16 Hz). Same dataset as used in ◘ Fig. 2.24.4.

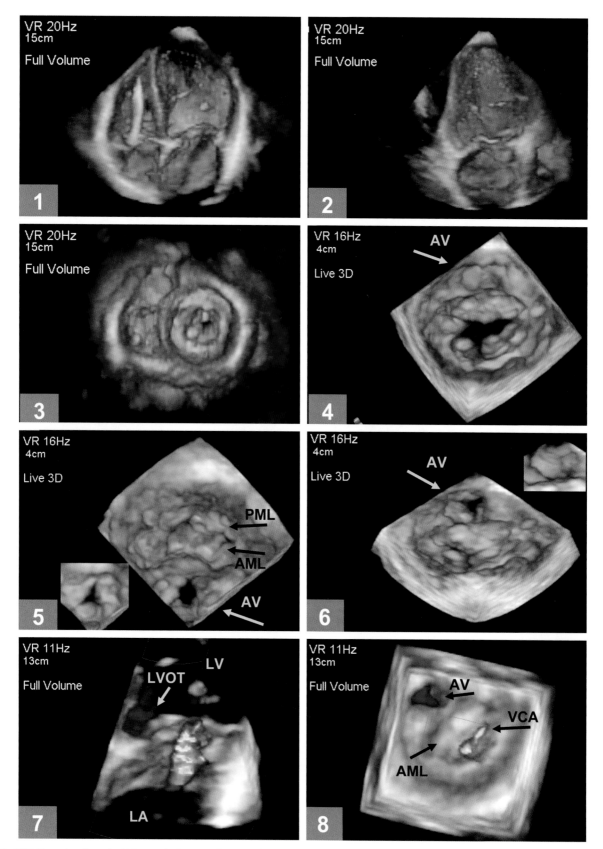

Fig. 2.24 Examples of standard 3D views for TTE according to the list given in the text. In **5** and **6**, the small pictures provide an en face view of the aortic valve in a more closed position with good depiction of the three cusps. *AV* aortic valve, *PML* posterior mitral leaflet, *AML* anterior mitral leaflet, *LVOT* left ventricular outflow tract, *LV* left ventricle, *LA* left atrium, *VCA* vena contracta area. [→Videos 2.24A–H]

- Long-axis mitral valve view using cropped full volume with color Doppler for 3D flow analysis (■ Fig. 2.24.7) provides 3D representation of mitral valve regurgitant and stenotic flow with good image resolution but limited temporal resolution (here 11 Hz).
- En face mitral valve view using cropped full volume with color Doppler for 3D flow analysis (■ Fig. 2.24.8) provides direct assessment of shape and size of vena contracta area of mitral regurgitant jet with good image resolution but limited temporal resolution (here 11 Hz). Same dataset as used in ■ Fig. 2.24.7.

Because of currently limited 3D TTE image quality, no 3D standard views can be recommended for the assessment of narrow or thin structures like the tricuspid valve, interatrial septum, and left atrial appendage. However, this will likely change as 3D TTE image quality improves.

Standard 3D views for TEE (■ Fig. 2.25):

- En face mitral valve view from the LA using live 3D zoom (■ Fig. 2.25.1) provides a focused live view of the mitral valve with good image resolution but limited temporal resolution (here 12 Hz). Optimal narrowing of the 3D volume to the mitral valve is recommended for an acceptable volume rate. Capturing part of the AV helps with orientation. This view is particularly useful to assess organic mitral valve disease, e.g., prolapse, flail leaflet, endocarditis. It is also useful for periinterventional live monitoring and guiding during paravalvular defect closure device implantation or mitral clipping.
- En face mitral valve view from the LV using live 3D zoom (■ Fig. 2.25.2) provides a focused live view of the mitral valve from the LV with good image resolution but limited temporal resolution. Same dataset as used in ■ Fig. 2.25.1. This view is particularly useful for assessment of incomplete mitral leaflet closure and restricted mitral leaflet motion in mitral stenosis.
- En face mitral valve view from the LA using full volume (■ Fig. 2.25.3) provides an increased view of the mitral valve, left atrial appendage, aortic valve, part of tricuspid valve, and interatrial septum from the LV with high image resolution and increased temporal resolution (here 27 Hz). Can be affected by stitching artifacts.
- En face mitral valve view using full volume with color Doppler for 3D flow analysis (■ Fig. 2.25.4) provides 3D representation of mitral regurgitation color Doppler jets in a relatively narrow view of the mitral valve with good image resolution but limited temporal resolution (here 14 Hz). Can be affected by stitching artifacts.
- En face aortic valve view from the aorta using a narrow live 3D mode (■ Fig. 2.25.5) provides a live view from the aortic root to the aortic valve with good temporal resolution (here 30 Hz). Because of the upright position, the aortic valve fits into the narrow live 3D volume.
- Long-axis aortic valve view using a narrow live 3D mode (■ Fig. 2.25.6) provides a long-axis live view of the aortic valve, LVOT, and aortic root with good image resolution and good temporal resolution (here 30 Hz). This live view is

particularly useful for periinterventional live monitoring during transcatheter aortic valve implantation.

- En face aortic valve view from the aorta using full volume (■ Fig. 2.25.7) provides an en face view from the aortic root to the aortic valve with high image resolution and good temporal resolution (here 27 Hz). Can be affected by stitching artifacts. Because the dataset is not live, it cannot be used for periinterventional live monitoring.
- Long-axis aortic valve view using cropped full volume (■ Fig. 2.25.8) provides a long-axis view of the aortic valve, LVOT, and aortic root with high image resolution and good temporal resolution (here 27 Hz). Same dataset as used in ■ Fig. 2.25.7 cropped to the aortic valve (can be affected by stitch artifacts and cannot be used for periinterventional live monitoring).
- Long-axis aortic valve view using cropped full volume with color Doppler for 3D flow analysis (■ Fig. 2.25.9) provides 3D representation of aortic valve regurgitant and stenotic flow with good image resolution but limited temporal resolution (here 14 Hz). Can be affected by stitch artifacts.
- Left atrial appendage view from the LA using the live 3D zoom (■ Fig. 2.25.10) provides a focused live view from the LA to left atrial appendage with good image resolution and moderate temporal resolution (here 15 Hz). Capturing part of the mitral valve (MV) helps with orientation. This view is particularly useful for periinterventional live monitoring during left atrial appendage closure device implantation.
- Atrial view to the interatrial septum using live 3D zoom (■ Fig. 2.25.11) provides a live view of the RA, LA, and interatrial septum with good image resolution but limited temporal resolution (here 11 Hz). This view is particularly useful for periinterventional live monitoring during interatrial septum closure device implantation, guiding transseptal puncture or guiding of EP catheter positioning.
- Interatrial septum view with contrast application for patent foramen ovale (PFO) testing using live 3D zoom (■ Fig. 2.25.12) provides a live view from the LA to the interatrial septum. Similar datasets, such as in ■ Fig. 2.25.11, could also be used. This view is particularly useful for detection and localization of transseptal contrast bubble passage through a PFO. This view is also useful for periinterventional live monitoring during interatrial septum closure device implantation and transseptal puncture.

The order of the views and acquisition of datasets are interchangeable according to the leading pathology.

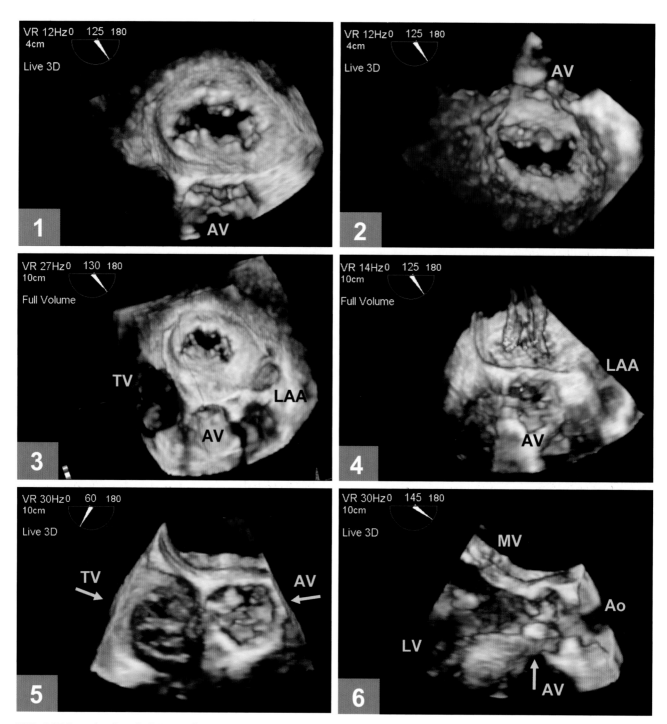

□ **Fig. 2.25** Examples of standard 3D views for TEE according to the list given in the text. *AV* aortic valve, *TV* tricuspid valve, *LAA* left atrial appendage, *MV* mitral valve, *LV* left ventricle, *Ao* aorta, *AML* anterior mitral leaflet, *LA* left atrium, *IAS* interatrial septum, *RA* right atrium, *SVC* superior vena cava. [→Videos 2.25A–L]

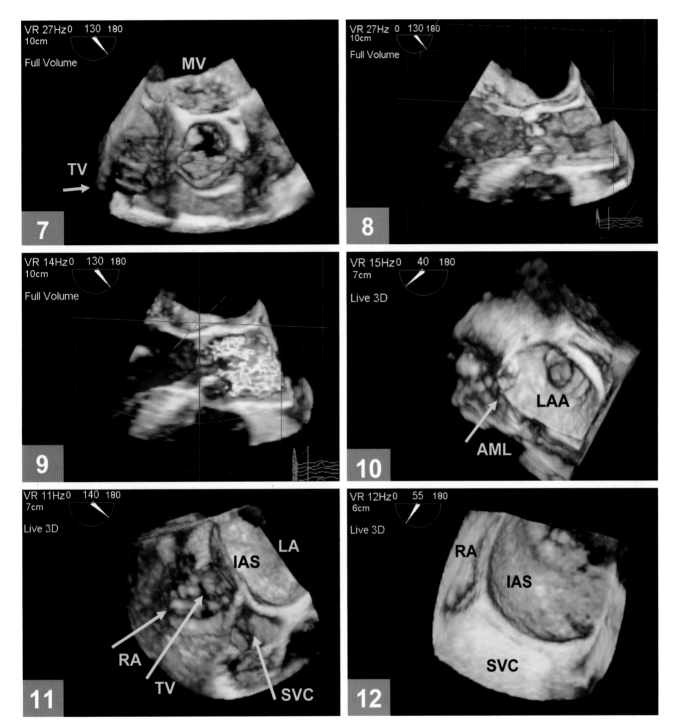

Fig. 2.25 Continuation

2.4   Basic 3D analysis: cropping and slicing

> Today, 3D analysis packages provide a rich spectrum of analysis features and are relatively easy to use.

As previously mentioned, after being acquired, 3D datasets need to be analyzed using special 3D analysis software. While in the past 3D dataset analysis was cumbersome, limited, and time consuming, today practical 3D analysis packages are integrated into standard 3D echocardiography machines. These provide a rich spectrum of analysis features and are relatively easy to use. The following basic steps of 3D dataset analysis are demonstrated using screenshots from Qlab™ version 7.0 3D analysis software (Philips Medical Systems. Note: there are no relevant differences between Qlab version 7.0 and the most recent version 10). In addition, all options of 3D analysis can be applied identically to all 3D datasets independent of the technique (TTE or TEE) or the kind of 3D dataset (live 3D, live 3D zoom, multiple-beat full volume).

2.4.1   First steps of 3D dataset cropping

The basic steps of 3D analysis include 3D orientation, cropping, and slicing. Of the three steps, 3D orientation is probably the most basic and most often used action during 3D analysis as it describes the process of manual free rotation of the dataset around a center point to provide the best perspective of the structures of the heart. Cropping describes the process of manually moving a cutting plane from outside the 3D volume towards its center, thus, providing a view from the cutting plane into the 3D volume (◘ Fig. 2.26, ◘ Fig. 2.27, ◘ Fig. 2.28, ◘ Fig. 2.29, ◘ Fig. 2.30, ◘ Fig. 2.31, ◘ Fig. 2.32, ◘ Fig. 2.33). Cropping (◘ Fig. 2.26, ◘ Fig. 2.27, ◘ Fig. 2.28, ◘ Fig. 2.29, ◘ Fig. 2.30, ◘ Fig. 2.31, ◘ Fig. 2.32) is usually possible along the three perpendicular major axes in space or using a free cropping plane (◘ Fig. 2.33). Finally, slicing describes the extraction of image planes from the 3D volume in different modes (◘ Fig. 2.34, ◘ Fig. 2.35, ◘ Fig. 2.36, ◘ Fig. 2.37).

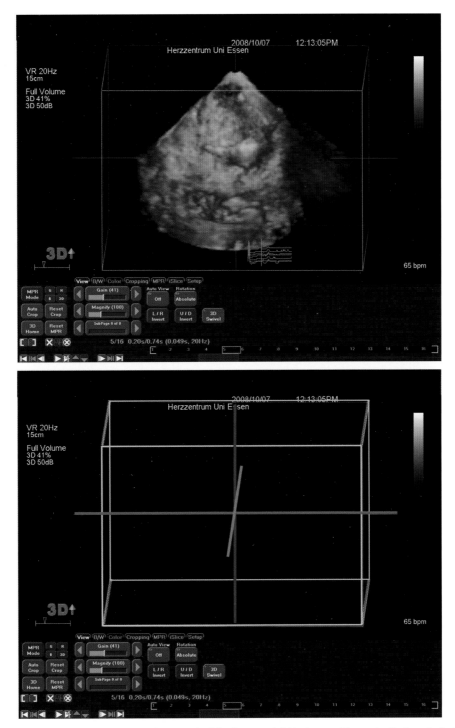

Fig. 2.26 A view from outside a pyramid-shaped 3D TTE dataset in the full volume mode [this view provides no details about the inside of the 3D dataset (◘ Fig. 2.21)] is shown. A transparent reference box (see bottom display with enhanced visualization) with *yellow lines* encompassing the 3D pyramid and three perpendicular axes in space (i.e., *red*, *green*, and *blue*) is displayed (*top*). In the lower left corner of the 3D display, the *blue* **3D**↑ icon indicates the spatial orientation of the 3D pyramid as it moves synchronously with the dataset. The *lower blue* part of the display contains the command buttons of the Qlab™ software. The most important buttons will be explained in the following figures. [→Video 2.26]

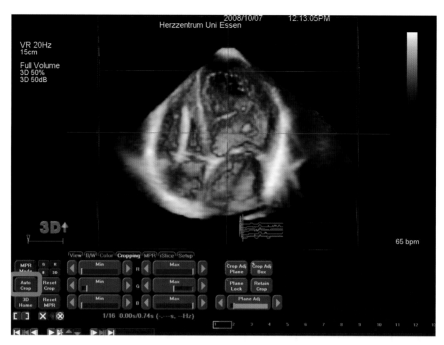

Fig. 2.27 By simply pressing the *Auto Crop* button (highlighted), the 3D dataset is vertically cut in half and shows the inner content of the dataset (■ Fig. 2.21). In this example, the cropped dataset shows a standard apical 4-chamber view (note the pacemaker lead in the right heart). [→Video 2.27]

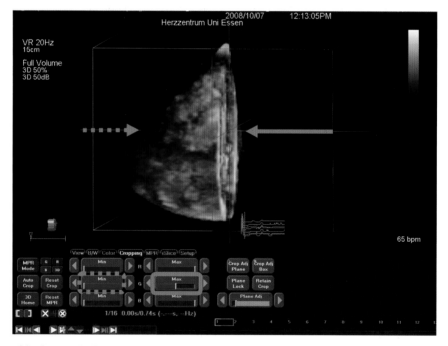

Fig. 2.28 The cropping of the dataset in half along the *green* axis as shown in ■ Fig. 2.27 is demonstrated in a view from the side of the dataset with the cropping direction indicated by the *green arrow*. Note the turned **3D**↑ icon in the lower left corner as well as the turned *green* and *red* axes indicating the different 3D orientation. Also note the highlighted *green* control bar moved to the halfway position. The dataset can of course also be cropped in the other direction, along the *green* axis (*dashed arrow*). [→Video 2.28]

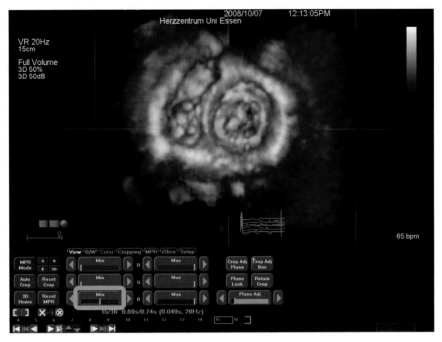

Fig. 2.29 This figure shows cropping along the vertical *blue* axis resulting in a horizontal cut through the dataset, which provides an en face view from the apex to the mitral and tricuspid valve. Note the presentation of the three cusps of the tricuspid valve. Also note the highlighted *blue* control bar moved to the halfway position. [→Video 2.29]

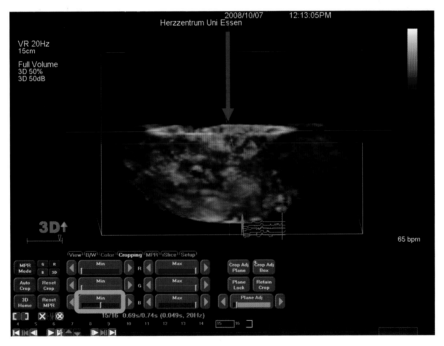

Fig. 2.30 The vertical cropping along the *blue* axis as shown in **Fig. 2.29** is demonstrated in a view from the side with the cropping direction indicated by the *blue arrow*. [→Video 2.30]

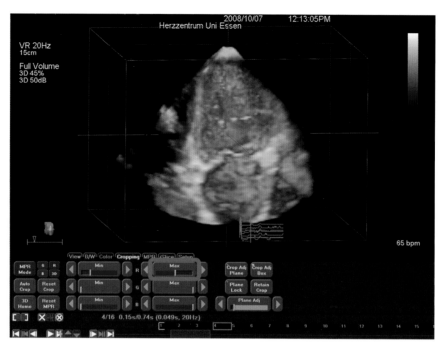

Fig. 2.31 For the third major cropping direction, the dataset is cropped along the *red* axis to create a typical 2-chamber view. Note the highlighted *red* control bar moved to the halfway position. [→Video 2.31]

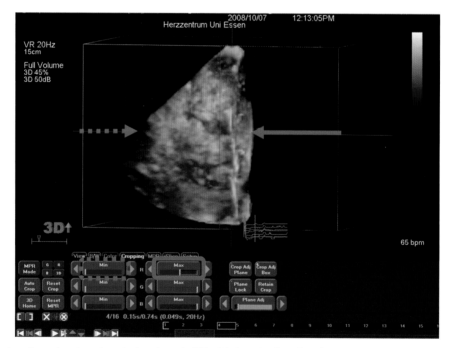

Fig. 2.32 Demonstration of cropping along the *red* axis as shown in Fig. 2.31 in a view from the side with the cropping direction indicated by the *red arrow*. [→Video 2.32]

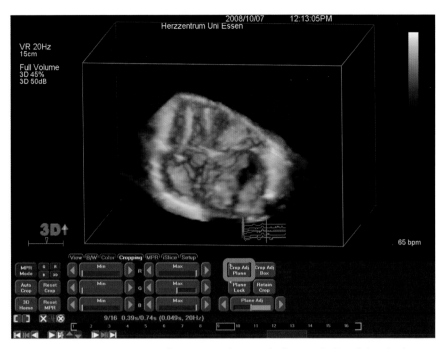

■ **Fig. 2.33** In addition to the three major cropping directions, a free cropping plane can also be moved arbitrarily into the dataset to create unique views and demonstrate anatomy which is not correctly visualized using standard cropping planes (compare the cropped dataset with the dataset shown in ■ Fig. 2.27 with the same orientation). This type of cropping is also known as anyplane mode. [→Video 2.33]

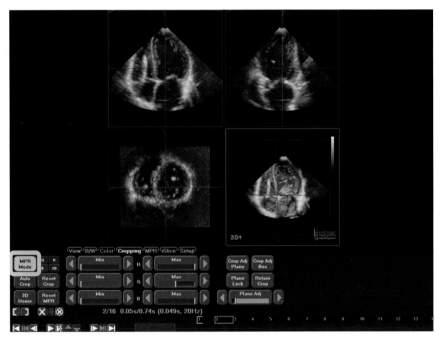

■ **Fig. 2.34** This figure demonstrates representation of multiple 2D planes (MPR mode) reconstructed from a 3D dataset. The display shows the 3D volume with three perpendicular planes in *red, blue,* and *green* (*lower right*). The *other three panels* show the 2D slice images of the three planes through the 3D volume where color of the image frame corresponds to the plane color. The planes can be manually moved and rotated. As the example shows, slicing of the 3D volume can also be used to display standard 2D views: here a standard 4-chamber view (*upper left*), a standard 2-chamber view (*upper right*), and a standard short-axis view of the left ventricle (*lower left*) have been created. [→Video 2.34]

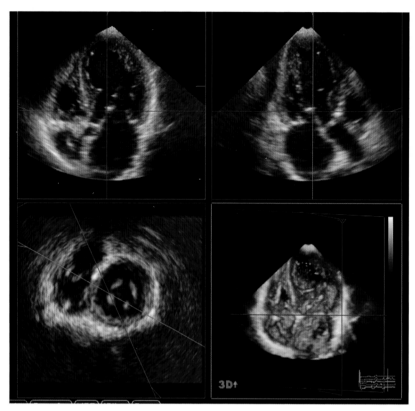

Fig. 2.35 In this example, the orientation of the *green* and *red* plane were changed by rotation (as shown in the *lower left*) to display a standard 5-chamber view (*upper left*) and a standard 3-chamber view (*upper right*). [→Video 2.35]

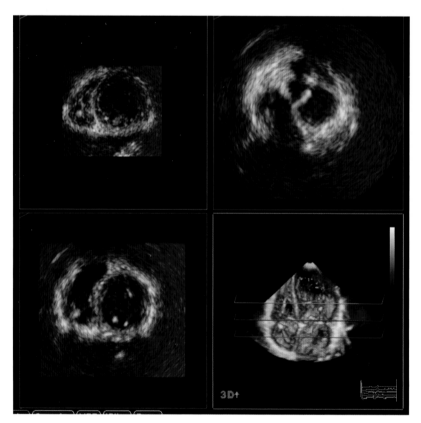

Fig. 2.36 Parallel slicing as shown here can be used to arrange the three slice planes in parallel orientation to display three short-axis views of the left ventricle at a midventricular level with papillary muscles (*upper left*), at a basal left ventricular level (*lower left*), and at a left atrial level with the aortic root (*upper right*). [→Video 2.36]

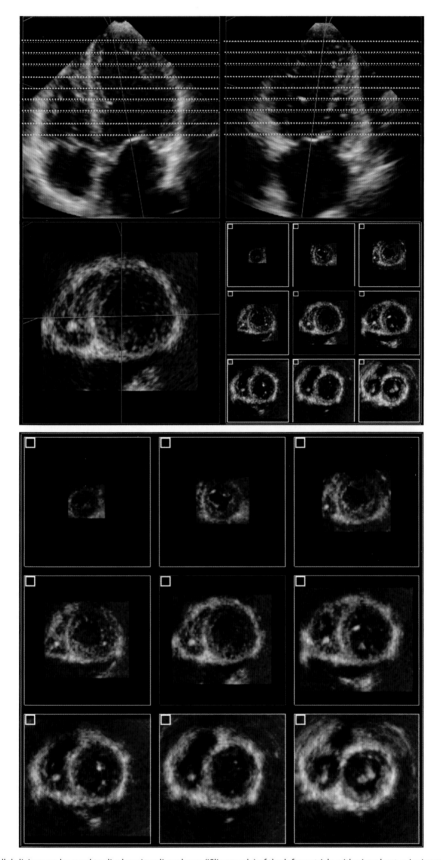

□ Fig. 2.37 Finally, parallel slicing can be used to display nine slice planes (iSlice mode) of the left ventricle with nine short-axis views from the apex to the mitral valve plane. The two *upper panels* display the nine slices in a 4-chamber (*left*) and 2-chamber view (*right*) for optimal representation of the left ventricular cavity and endocardial contours. Note that the *red axis* in the *upper left* indicates the orientation of the *red plane* (*upper right*) and the *green axis* in the *upper right* indicates the orientation of the *green plane* (*upper left*). These are aligned to the long axis of the ventricle to avoid foreshortening of the left ventricular cavity. [→Videos 2.37A,B]

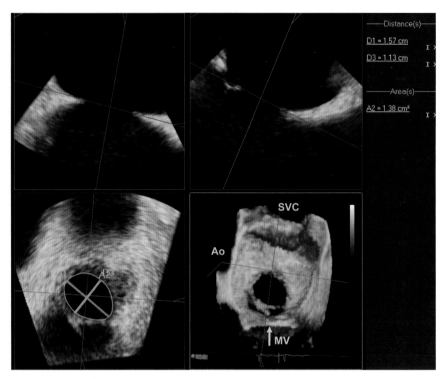

◘ Fig. 2.38 Example of basic measurements of distances (*D*) and area (*A*) in a 3D TEE dataset in a patient with a secundum type atrial septal defect (*ASD*). *Lower right* The en face view from the LA towards the interatrial septum clearly shows the ASD. The *top two panels* represent two orthogonal 2D cross-sectional views (*green* and *red* planes) perpendicular to the interatrial septum. The *blue* lines represent the orientation of the *blue* plane (*lower left*) which is exactly aligned with the interatrial septum for best possible representation and measurement of the ASD area (*yellow* circumference) and diameters (*purple* and *turquoise* diameters). *MV* mitral valve, *Ao* aorta, *SVC* superior vena cava

2.5 Basic 3D measurements

Distances and areas can be fairly easily determined within a 3D dataset and are the most basic of measurements. Until recently 3D analysis software did not allow measurements to be performed directly in a 3D image. The reason for this was that the points defining a structure the user wants to measure are not necessarily in the same plane parallel to the display surface. As a consequence, basic 3D measurements could only be performed in 2D planes in the MPR mode (see above; ◘ Fig. 2.34, ◘ Fig. 2.35, ◘ Fig. 2.36) where the plane represents the structures as best possible (◘ Fig. 2.38), but were still limited in measuring areas of structures or orifices which are not planar, like most structures and orifice borders in the heart.

The newest 3D software, however, allows direct 3D measurements of distances and areas on 3D images (◘ Fig. 2.39), which makes 3D measurements much easier and faster. However, this approach is putting the responsibility for the validity of the measurements into the hands of the user, who must assure that the display plane where the measurements are performed are parallel to the anatomic structure as a prerequisite to prevent foreshortening errors (◘ Fig. 2.39A,B). Because this measurement is performed as on a clear glass plane seeing the anatomic structure behind, the method is called »3D measurement on the glass«. However, because this measurement approach is very new and has not been validated in clinical practice yet, it will not be represented as common approach in the clinical chapters of this book. The clinical applications of basic and advanced measurements in 3D volumes will be described in the following chapters on specific heart diseases.

> ❯ To perform basic 3D measurements in a 2D plane can be challenging because areas of structures or orifices are often not planar.

2.6 Artifacts

Like in 2D echocardiography, the knowledge of artifacts is critically important to avoid misinterpretation of 3D images. The most relevant artifacts pertaining to 3D images include stitching artifacts, dropout artifacts, blurring and blooming artifacts, and artifacts related to gain settings. There are other effects such as those caused by valve prosthesis that are heavily affected by dropout artifacts in 2D. These often look better in 3D, which might be partly explained by a compensation of dropout artifacts by adjacent blurring or simply because 3D visualization of the prosthesis provides more complete visual information which compensates for focal image dropouts.

> ❯ The knowledge of artifacts is critically important to avoid misinterpretation of 3D images.

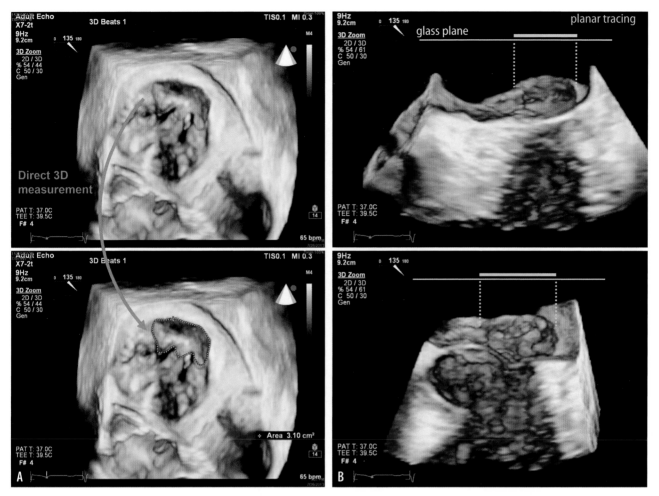

Fig. 2.39 A Illustration of direct 3D measurement in a 3D image (3D measurement on the glass). *Top* A flail leaflet of P2 segment can be clearly identified. *Bottom* The direct tracing (*dotted line*) of the area of the flail leaflet segment indicated as 3.10 cm² in the lower right. **B** Illustration of the principle of 3D measurement on the glass. The *bold yellow line* represents the planar tracing shown as the dotted line tracing in **A**, here in a view from the side (*top* long-axis view of the mitral valve with the aorta to the left; *below* 2-chamber view to the mitral valve). [→Videos 2.39A,B(a,b)]

2.6.1 Stitching artifacts

As described above, the current price to pay for full volume datasets with high spatial and high temporal resolution is to acquire a set of two, four or more narrower live 3D datasets (■ Fig. 2.15) and to stitch them together. However, the single datasets are acquired by electrocardiographic triggering at different time points in a series of consecutive heart cycles. As a consequence, the position of cardiac structures can vary between the single datasets due to translation of the heart secondary to respiration or heart motion variation because of different heart cycle lengths, e.g., atrial fibrillation. As a result, the cross-sections of two neighboring 3D datasets may not match where they are stitched together. Stitching artifacts, therefore, occur as lines of disagreement between two neighboring 3D subvolumes (■ Fig. 2.40). Depending on respiration, stitch lines can occur between only one pair of 3D subvolumes or between all pairs. Minor stitching artifacts with a small pattern of disagreement can be tolerated, whereas severe stitching artifacts cause profoundly disturbed 3D images and prevent further qualitative and quantitative analysis. Stitching artifacts can be most effectively prevented by patient breath holding or by pausing respiration during intraoperative 3D dataset acquisition.

2.6.2 Dropout artifacts

Since the beginning of 3D echocardiography, dropout artifacts have been the reason for concerns about the accuracy and reliability of 3D image information. Dropout artifacts are caused by loss of 3D surface information due to poor echo signal intensity. They typically appear as »false« holes in 3D surfaces where, in fact, no holes exist. The most common reason for dropout artifacts are structures which are too thin to reflect sufficient echo signal intensity, such as the interatrial septum, thin aortic valve cusps, or thin tricuspid valve leaflets (■ Fig. 2.41, ■ Fig. 2.42). In comparison, mitral valve leaflets are usually thicker and, therefore, are less affected by dropout artifacts. The assessment of whether a hole in a surface is a true defect or a dropout artifact can be difficult and often requires extended experience in 3D imaging interpretation. In such cases, the additional cross-sectional image information from 2D views is often helpful. In ad-

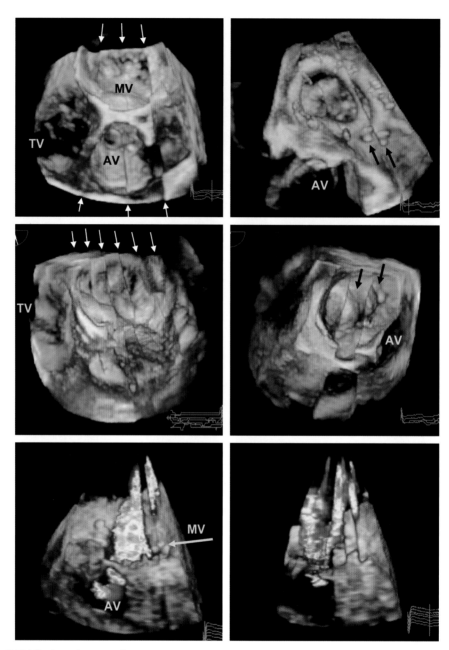

■ **Fig. 2.40** Examples of TEE full volume datasets with important stitching artifacts. *Top left* Three slices of stitching artifacts (*white arrows*) causing significant misalignment between the four subvolumes. *Top right* Severe stitching artifact causing duplication of a mitral annuloplasty ring (*black arrows* pointing to doubled knot). *Middle left* Example with six slices of stitching artifacts through a mitral and aortic valve (similar orientation as in *top left*) in a full volume of seven subvolumes. *Middle right* Severe stitching artifacts causing disruption of an en face view of the mitral valve with duplication of part of the P2 flail leaflet (*black arrows*). *Bottom* Two examples of significant stitching artifacts of full volume color Doppler datasets causing dropout artifacts within the mitral regurgitant jet. [→Videos 2.40A–F]

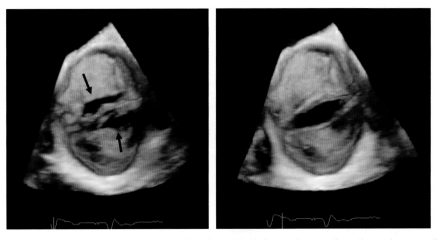

Fig. 2.41 Example of RT3DE dropout artifact. Live 3D TEE dataset with en face view of a bicuspid aortic valve with two dropout artifacts (*black arrows*) in the two cusps in an end-diastolic view (*left*) which disappeared in systole (*right*). [→Video 2.41]

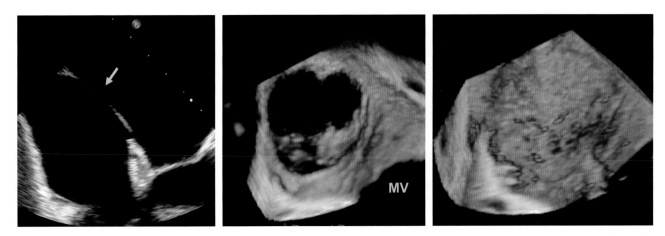

Fig. 2.42 Example of RT3DE dropout artifact at the interatrial septum (*IAS*). The 2D TEE image shows a thin interatrial septum (*arrow*) without a defect (*left*). Live 3D zoom image with a direct view from the left atrium (LA) to the IAS gives the impression almost of a defect. Filling of the RA with contrast bubbles visualized the IAS as the boundary surface between the contrast filled RA and the LA [bubbles in the LA indicate a patent foramen ovale (PFO)]. *MV* location of the mitral valve. [→Videos 2.42A–C]

dition, 2D or 3D color Doppler can help by showing the absence of flow through a »false« defect. For example, if there is no aortic regurgitation, then the defect in one or more aortic cusps must be a dropout artifact. To avoid dropout artifacts, an appropriate gain setting is critically important (i.e., mainly to avoid inappropriately low gain). Elimination of dropout artifacts by increasing the gain is difficult as this causes overgain in the rest of the 3D image (▶ Section 2.6.4). In addition to the basic image settings of gain, compress, and brightness, some 3D imaging systems also provide access to control thresholding of surface rendering; this potentially minimizes dropout artifacts. As with 2D echocardiography, attempting to orientate a structure of interest so that it is perpendicular to the transducer will also help to minimize dropout.

> The assessment of whether a hole in a surface is a true defect or a dropout artifact can be difficult.

2.6.3 Blurring and blooming artifacts

Because of voxel interpolation, 3D echocardiographic images have always been prone to blurring and blooming artifacts. These are mainly caused by inaccurate voxel interpolation between distant image lines or 2D image planes when 3D datasets were reconstructed from radial image planes. Thus, in RT3DE, blurring and blooming artifacts are strongly related to line density, with higher line density resulting in less blurring or blooming. Blurring refers to the unsharp und hazy representation of thin structures such that they appear thicker than they really are. Blurring frequently causes a thickened representation of mitral leaflets or other structures of the mitral apparatus, like the chordae tendineae and papillary muscles, but also of interventricular trabeculation (for an example of a thickened ruptured chord see ◾ Fig. 2.19). Although there is often a combination of blurring and blooming, blooming refers more to the thickened and sometimes excessive representation of structures of high echo density. This frequently occurs with artificial structures, e.g., mechanical prosthesis or pacemaker leads (◾ Fig. 2.43).

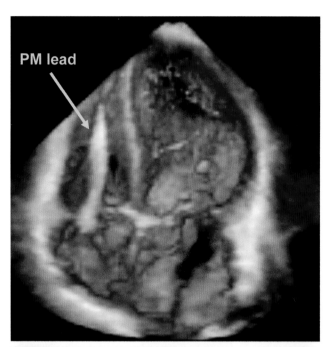

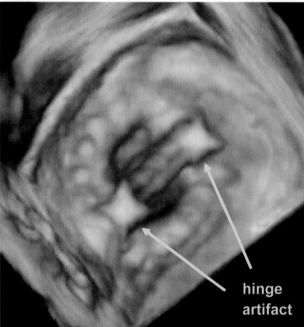

◻ Fig. 2.43 Two examples of blooming artifacts in RT3DE images. *Top* The image shows a 4-chamber view with a pacemaker (PM) lead in the right ventricle (RV), where the signal-intense lead appears much thicker than it really is. *Bottom* The image shows star-shaped blooming artifacts on the two hinge-points of a mechanical mitral valve prosthesis. [→Videos 2.43A,B]

2.6.4 Gain artifacts

For 3D imaging, an appropriate gain setting is of even greater importance compared to 2D imaging because overgain might cause an effect of dust or smoke within chamber volumes. This can obscure structures of interest. As in 2D imaging, it is important to differentiate between spontaneous echo contrast and overgain (◻ Fig. 2.44). To adjust a 3D image for appropriate gain, it is recommended to turn up the gain setting until dust appears in the cardiac chamber and then turning down the gain setting just until the dust has disappeared. Alternatively one can turn down the gain and then turn it carefully up until the first signs of dust appear. This maneuver also ensures optimal 3D surface representation. In cases with spontaneous echo contrast, this approach is more difficult as spontaneous echo contrast should not be eliminated by reducing gain. Occasionally, spontaneous echo contrast can be so severe that direct viewing of cardiac structures is impossible. An advantage of 3D datasets being stored in a raw data format is that gain settings can be adjusted and optimized even after 3D datasets have been saved.

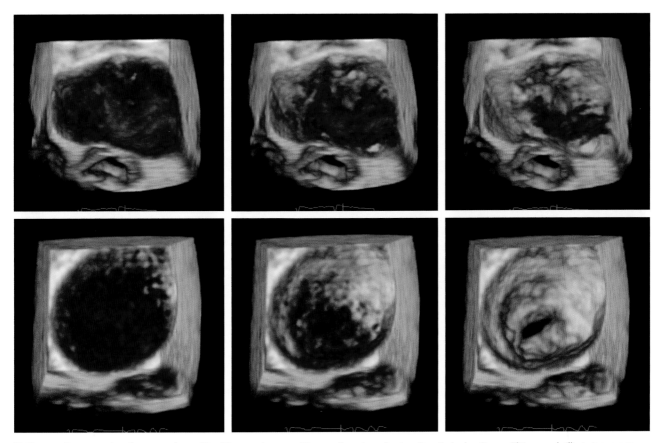

Fig. 2.44 Two examples of transesophageal live 3D zoom datasets with an en face view of a stenotic mitral valve. *Top row* This example illustrates severe spontaneous echo contrast which cannot be completely eliminated by reducing the gain setting (*left* optimal gain setting, *middle* intermediate gain setting, *right* minimal gain setting). *Bottom row* In contrast, the example shows simple overgain (*left*) which can be effectively eliminated by reducing the gain setting to obtain optimal image quality (*right*). [→Videos 2.44A–F]

References

1. Sheikh K, Smith SW, von Ramm O, Kisslo J (1991) Real-time, three-dimensional echocardiography: feasibility and initial use. Echocardiography 8:119–125

2. Stetten G, Ota T, Ohazama C et al (1998) Real-time 3D ultrasound: a new look at the heart. J Cardiovasc Diagn Procedures 15:73–84

3. Kisslo J, Firek B, Ota T et al (2000) Real-time volumetric echocardiography: the technology and the possibilities. Echocardiography 17:773–779

4. Ota T, Kisslo J, von Ramm OT, Yoshikawa J (2001) Real-time, volumetric echocardiography: usefulness of volumetric scanning for the assessment of cardiac volume and function. J Cardiol 37(Suppl 1):93–101

5. Pandian NG, Nanda NC, Schwartz SL et al (1992) Three-dimensional and four-dimensional transesophageal echocardiographic imaging of the heart and aorta in humans using a computed tomographic imaging probe. Echocardiography 9:677–687

6. Nanda NC, Pinheiro L, Sanyal R et al (1992) Multiplane transesophageal echocardiographic imaging and three-dimensional reconstruction. Echocardiography 9:667–676

7. Roelandt JRTC, Ten Cate FJ, Vletter WB, Taams MA (1994) Ultrasonic dynamic three-dimensional visualization of the heart with a multiplane transesophageal imaging transducer. J Am Soc Echocardiogr 7:217–219

8. Pandian NG, Roelandt J, Nanda NC et al (1994) Dynamic three-dimensional echocardiography: methods and clinical potential. Echocardiography 11:237–259

9. Sugeng L, Weinert L, Thiele K, Lang RM (2003) Real-time three-dimensional echocardiography using a novel matrix array transducer. Echocardiography 20:623–635

10. Savord BJ, Thiele KE (1999) Phased array acoustic systems with intra-group processors. (U.S. Patent 5997479). 7 December 1999

11. Lichtenbelt B, Crane R, Naqvi S (1998) Introduction to volume rendering. Upper Saddle River, New Jersey: Prentice-Hall, Inc.

12. Thiele K (2007) Method and apparatus for volume rendering using depth weighted colorization. USA Patent Application 20090184955, 29 May

13. Mor-Avi V, Sugeng L, Lang RM (2009) Real-time 3-dimensional echocardiography: an integral component of the routine echocardiographic examination in adult patients? Circulation 119:314–329

14. Correale M, Ieva R, Balzano M, Di Biase M (2007) Real-time three-dimensional echocardiography: a pilot feasibility study in an Italian cardiologic center. J Cardiovasc Med (Hagerstown) 8:265–273

15. Lang RM, Badano LP, Tsang W et al (2012) EAE/ASE recommendations for image acquisition and display using three-dimensional echocardiography. Eur Heart J Cardiovasc Imaging 13:1–46

16. Jenkins C, Monaghan M, Shirali G et al (2008) An intensive interactive course for 3D echocardiography: is 'crop till you drop' an effective learning strategy? Eur J Echocardiogr 9:373–380

17. Sugeng L, Shernan SK, Salgo IS et al (2008) Live 3-dimensional transesophageal echocardiography initial experience using the fully-sampled matrix array probe. J Am Coll Cardiol 52:446–449

18. Nanda NC, Kisslo J, Lang R et al (2004) Examination protocol for three-dimensional echocardiography. Echocardiography 21:763–768

19. Salcedo EE, Quaife RA, Seres T, Carroll JD (2009) A framework for systematic characterization of the mitral valve by real-time three-dimensional transesophageal echocardiography. J Am Soc Echocardiogr 22:1087–1099

20. von Ramm OT, Smith SW (1990) Real-time volumetric ultrasound imaging system. Journal of Digital Imaging 3:261–266

21. Smith SW, Pavy HG, von Ramm OT (1991) High-speed ultrasonic volumetric imaging system. Part 1. Transducer design and beam steering. IEEE Trans Ultrasonic Frequency Control 38:100–108

Left ventricular and left atrial function

Harald P. Kühl

T. Buck et al. (Hrsg.), *Three-dimensional Echocardiography*,
DOI 10.1007/978-3-642-36799-1_3, © Springer-Verlag Berlin Heidelberg 2014

3

Global left ventricular (LV) function is an important prognostic parameter and is useful for therapeutic decision-making. Since its introduction, two-dimensional (2D) echocardiography has played an important role in the quantitation of LV function. However, the limitations of 2D echocardiography for the accurate determination of cardiac volumes and function in distorted LVs soon became apparent. Therefore, since the early 1990s, considerable efforts have been undertaken to develop three-dimensional (3D) echocardiographic methods for the evaluation of LV function.

>> Use of 3D echocardiography allows the assessment of LV volumes and ejection fractions that are independent of geometric assumptions.

Three-dimensional echocardiography offers important advantages over conventional 2D echocardiography for the determination of global and regional LV function. Assessment of LV volumes and ejection fraction can be accomplished independently of geometrical assumptions which are inherently needed for 2D echocardiography [1][2][3][4]. Several studies have demonstrated that the actual geometry of severely diseased LVs only rarely coincides with the assumed geometry observed by 2D echocardiography [5][6][7]. Thus, quantitation of LV volumes by 2D echocardiography is inaccurate in severely distorted LVs [8][9]. Yet, in these hearts, accurate quantitation of LV function is of utmost importance for the cardiologist to guide treatment and make decisions. Another important drawback of 2D echocardiography is its poor reproducibility and reliability which is related to the fact that an exact positioning of the 2D imaging plane in the 3D space is not reliably possible [10][11]. Thus, the position of the 2D image plane may slightly differ during consecutive measurements of the same ventricle at different time points resulting in poor test–retest reliability of the technique [12].

A number of studies have demonstrated that 3D echocardiography is more accurate, more reproducible, and more reliable than 2D echocardiography for the quantitation of LV volumes and ejection fraction in LVs with distorted geometry [9][12][13][14][15]. The recent introduction of real-time 3D data acquisition as well as semiautomatic border detection algorithms have allowed fast, easy, and a more observer-independent quantitation of LV function, requiring only minimal interaction by the investigator [16]. However, semiautomated algorithms for 3D LV quantification requiring manual definition of anatomic landmarks of the LV are a potential source for interobserver variability as indicated in a recent study by Chang et al. [17] demanding improvements of automatic border detection algorithms to permit observer-independent LV analysis. Later in this chapter a new method called the Heart Model providing fully automated chamber detection and quantitation will be presented.

>> Accurate LV function analysis using RT3DE may strengthen the indication for cost-intensive device therapies.

Several studies have validated real-time 3D echocardiographic (RT3DE) LV quantification using cardiac magnetic resonance imaging (CMR) as the reference standard [12][18][19][20][21]. Thus, transthoracic RT3DE with semiautomatic border detection is now considered the echocardiographic method of choice

for the fast, reproducible, and reliable assessment of LV function, especially in patients with distorted LVs and in candidates for device therapy, e.g., implantable defibrillators, biventricular pacemakers. In heart failure patients with ejection fraction values close to the threshold considered appropriate for device therapy (≤35%) by 2D imaging techniques, RT3DE may be of special value to strengthen the indication for cost-intensive device therapies [22]. Moreover, the higher reproducibility and reliability promises that the technique will be the echocardiographic method of choice for the serial assessment of LV volumes and ejection fraction [23]. These findings translate into smaller numbers of patients required to observe a treatment effect in studies aimed at assessing the effects of new drugs when using 3D echocardiography compared to standard 2D echocardiography. In addition, preliminary data in patients who have survived a myocardial infarction suggest that volume estimation by RT3DE also has prognostic relevance [24].

Several case reports of patients with tako-tsubo cardiomyopathy (TTC) demonstrated feasibility of RT3DE with accurate representation of LV volumes, mass and ejection fraction compared to 2D echocardiography and left ventricular angiography [25][26][27][28]. Beside accurate visual representation and quantitation of left ventricular volumes in the presence of variations of apical, mid-ventricular or basal ballooning 3D echocardiography has been described to provide superior qualitative analysis of pathologic regional wall motion pattern [25][26][27][28] as well as advanced quantitative analysis of the course of recovery of regional wall motion abnormalities in TTC [29]. As a consequence of these advantages RT3DE quantification of LV volumes and ejection fraction has been recommended over the use of 2D echocardiography for its improved accuracy and reproducibility according to current EAE/ASE recommendations [30].

3.1   Assessment of left ventricular volumes and ejection fraction

RT3DE using the transthoracic approach is the method of choice for accurate and reliable assessment of global LV function. Until recently, the ECG-gated full volume acquisition mode has been the standard approach to capture the entire LV over several cardiac cycles. With this method, several scan sections or subvolumes are assembled automatically to form a large pyramidal volume incorporating the complete LV information (► Chapter 2). The most important disadvantage of this technique is misalignment of subvolumes due to respiratory motion or arrhythmia, creating artifacts in the composed 3D dataset [30]. Thus, the method may be inappropriate in patients unable to hold their breath or in subjects with atrial fibrillation of frequent premature beats. Recent technological developments have enabled acquisition of the entire heart in a single cardiac cycle. In a recent study, feasibility of one-beat full volume RT3DE for quantification of left ventricular volumes was 84% in 109 consecutive patients [17]. In the same study agreement for volumes and ejection fraction calculation between one-beat RT3DE and CMR was acceptable as was observer variability [17]. Thus, this novel approach will further contribute to enhance use of RT3DE for

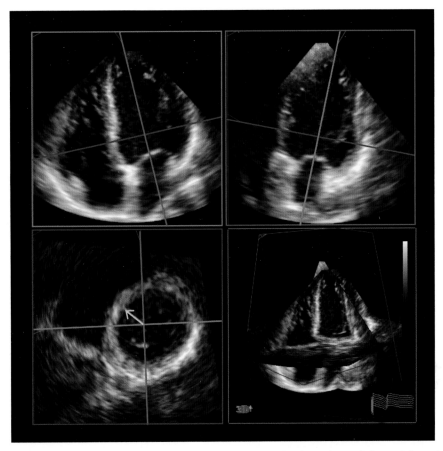

Fig. 3.1 Illustration of correct alignment of the two long-axis 2D planes indicated by the *red* and *green lines* with the true left ventricular (*LV*) long axis to represent the LV with its maximum dimension. The *yellow arrow (bottom left)* is manually directed to the mid interventricular septum for correct anatomic definition of LV segments. [→Video 3.1]

evaluation of the LV, acceleration of data acquisition, and reduction of artifacts. However, profound limitations in spatial and temporal resolution of current one-beat techniques demand future improvements to allow precise quantification of volumes and function.

> Recent technological developments have enabled full volume acquisition of the entire heart in a single heart beat.

For data acquisition using the full volume method, one has to ensure that the dataset contains the complete LV including the apex, which can be accomplished by the simultaneous visualization of the LV in two orthogonal 2D views commonly provided during 3D acquisition. Capturing the entire LV in the 3D dataset may sometimes be difficult in the severely dilated LV, e.g., in patients with dilated cardiomyopathy or apical aneurysms due to a larger anterior wall myocardial infarction. In this case, the 3D echocardiographic systems offer the possibility of acquiring multiple-beat wide-angle datasets (pyramidal volume of about 110°×110°) which allow incorporation of the entire LV, while at the same time maintaining adequate temporal and spatial resolution. However, despite these technical advancements underestimation of LV volumes by RT3DE compared with CMR has been described recently in patients with heart failure and severely dilated left ventricles [31]. After satisfactory data acquisition, the datasets need to be processed by a software program designed for

quantitative analysis of LV function. Apart from commercially available stand-alone software programs, vendor specific built-in software programs can be used allowing for analysis of datasets immediately after data acquisition.

The process of data analysis is fast, easy, and straight forward. With the analysis software already available in current 3D echocardiography systems (e.g., QLab software on Philips 3D systems), analysis of LV function takes only about 1–2 min. Initially, after definition of the end-diastolic and end-systolic stop-frame images, data are presented to define landmark points which are needed for the definition of the mitral valve plane, the apex and LV antero-posterior as well as medial–lateral orientation. At this point, it is of critical importance to align the two long-axis image planes exactly with the long axis of the LV to prevent foreshortening of the LV walls (■ Fig. 3.1). The possibility of 3D analysis to optimally adjust the LV to its maximum long axis and chamber size is an important advantage over 2D analysis prone to foreshortening error [4]. Foreshortening of the LV cross-section in 2D scanning is caused by the 2D transducer position which is most often offset to the LV apex, thus, leading to malalignment of the scan sector with respect to the LV long axis [32]. A total of ten points – five each for end-diastole and end-systole – need to be set by the investigator, defining not only the anterior and inferior as well as medial and lateral mitral annulus, but also the apex (■ Fig. 3.2).

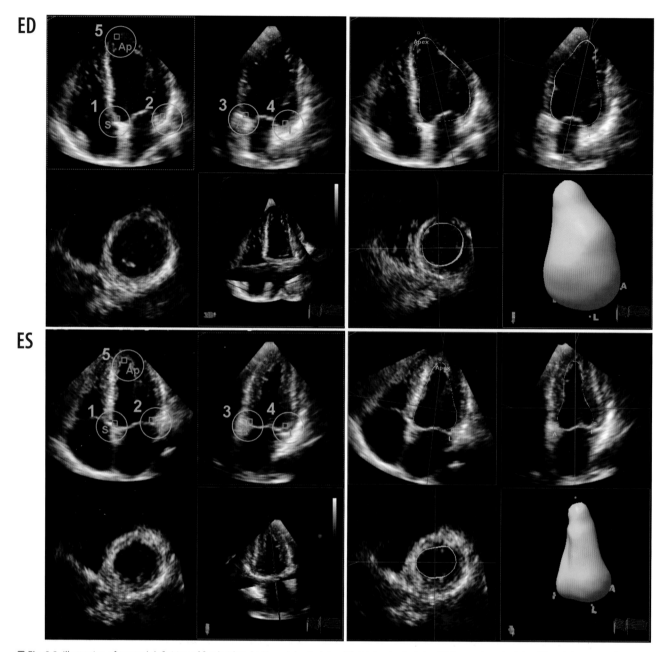

◪ **Fig. 3.2** Illustration of manual definition of five landmarks [*1:* septal mitral ring (*S*), *2:* lateral mitral ring (*L*), *3:* anterior mitral ring (*A*), *4:* inferior mitral ring (*I*), *5:* apex (*Ap*)] in each end-diastole (*ED; top row*) and end-systole (*ES; bottom row*). The two quad-panels on the right demonstrate the semiautomatically detected LV contour and the 3D surface reconstruction of LV contour

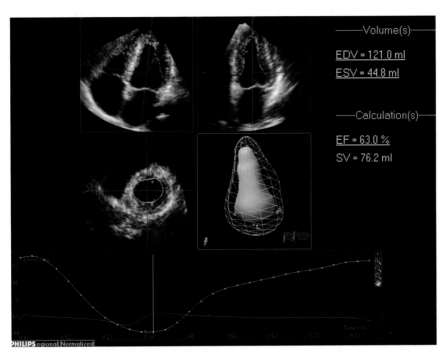

◘ **Fig. 3.3** Illustration of global volume–time curve (*bottom*) as well as results of global 3D volume analysis with ejection fraction in the same patient as shown in ◘ Fig. 3.1 and ◘ Fig. 3.2. *Bottom right* The end-systolic LV contour (*yellow*) in relation to the end-diastolic contour represented by a transparent wire mesh is shown. [→Video 3.3]

❯ **Compared to 2D analysis, optimal adjustment of the LV to its maximum long axis in a 3D volume eliminates fore-shortening.**

With this information, the system automatically tracks the complete LV endocardial borders in the 3D dataset for each acquired time frame. Thus, after processing of the data, a global volume–time curve is obtained, which displays the dynamic course of the global volume change during the cardiac cycle with an end-diastolic maximum and an end-systolic minimum (◘ Fig. 3.3).

From these data, the global ejection fraction is automatically calculated and displayed (◘ Fig. 3.3). The accuracy of the technique has been largely validated against cardiac MRI [12][18][20][33]. Although underestimation of volumes has been reported in comparison to cardiac MRI results [18][20], the difference is likely the consequence of different tracing algorithms between the two imaging methods, including LV trabeculae in the LV volume using MRI versus excluding them using echocardiography [33]. However, for ejection fraction calculation no significant under- or overestimation has been reported in different studies [12][18][19].

❯ **Good image quality is a prerequisite for accurate quantification of LV volumes using semiautomated border detection in 3D datasets.**

As a rule, good image quality is a prerequisite for accurate quantitation of global LV function using the semiautomatic border detection approach. Before acquiring the 3D dataset, meticulous care has to be taken to visualize the endocardial borders of most of the myocardial segments in the preparatory apical biplane view [30]. This may be challenging for the basal lateral as well as basal and mid-ventricular anterior myocardial segments in the

simultaneous 4- and 2-chamber views, respectively. When more than two myocardial segments cannot be visualized in the apical biplane view, correction of the image plane position as well as correction of the breath-hold position should be sought until this goal is met. To ensure good visibility of the endocardial borders, it may be very helpful to ask the patient to breathe in slowly during imaging to find a breath-hold position that allows for optimal delineation of all LV segments in the apical biplane view. Since acquisition of the 3D data only takes about four to seven heartbeats, data acquisition can be started immediately after finding the optimal breath-hold position. This procedure is subject to a steep learning curve and should be learned at the beginning of 3D echocardiography training.

In patients with suboptimal image quality, manual editing of the semiautomatically derived endocardial contours may be required to ensure adequate tracing of the endocardial boundaries. Changing of contours made in 2D sections out of the 3D dataset is subsequently propagated throughout the 3D dataset in such a way that correction of endocardial borders is translated to the complete LV. Although slightly more time-consuming compared to biplane Simpson's method, this approach is more accurate and reproducible because it takes advantage of all 3D information generated by RT3DE [19]. Left heart contrast administration has been used to enhance border detection in patients with poor endocardial visibility (◘ Fig. 3.4). Contrast-enhanced RT3DE has proven superior to contrast-enhanced and noncontrast-enhanced 2D echocardiography as well as to noncontrast-enhanced 3D echocardiography compared with MRI for assessing volumes in patients with previous myocardial infarction [34].

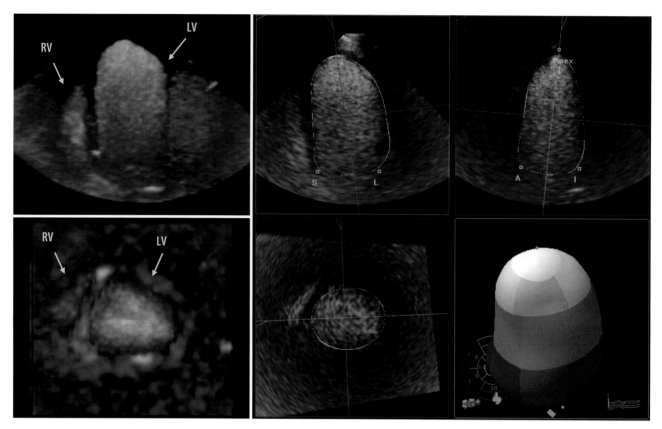

Fig. 3.4 Example of RT3DE LV contrast application. *Left* The dark space between the contrast-filled LV (*right*) and the contrast-filled RV (*left*) represents the interventricular septum. *Right* Multiplanar representation of LV contour. *LV* left ventricle, *RV* right ventricle. [→Videos 3.4A,B]

■ **Heart Model volume segmentation**

Very recently, a new method for fully automating the segmentation of all four heart chambers has been introduced. The Heart Model method is capable of detecting all four heart chambers – the two atria and the two ventricles – in an apical transthoracic 3D dataset without any interaction by the user.

The method uses a parameterized model of the heart, which was customized for echocardiography using knowledge gained from a large, expert-annotated ultrasound training database of normal and abnormal hearts.

Post-acquisition of a full volume apical data set, which at a minimum includes both the LV and LA, the Heart Model performs the following automated steps:

— identify the ES (end-systolic) and ED (end-diastolic) volumes,
— orient and align the internal representation of the heart model with the 3D ultrasound data,
— adjust the global Heart Model parameters so that the boundaries provide a best fit with the endo- and epicardial borders based on the detection of the observed blood–tissue borders, and
— locally deform the heart model borders to minimize any residual border location errors specific to the current heart.

Once the search process for the four heart chambers was successful and the displayed automated border definition was confirmed by the operator ◘ Fig. 3.5, the Heart Model tool visualizes all four chambers with a graphical surface reconstruction and instantly reports quantitative volumetric data of end-systolic and end-diastolic LV volumes, ejection fraction (EF), and LV stroke volume as well as LA end-systolic volume (◘ Fig. 3.6 and ◘ Fig. 3.7). Potentially the Heart Model tool can automatically report all volumetric data for all four chambers including those of the difficult to measure right ventricle and also LV mass, in addition to accepted clinical measures of distance and area.

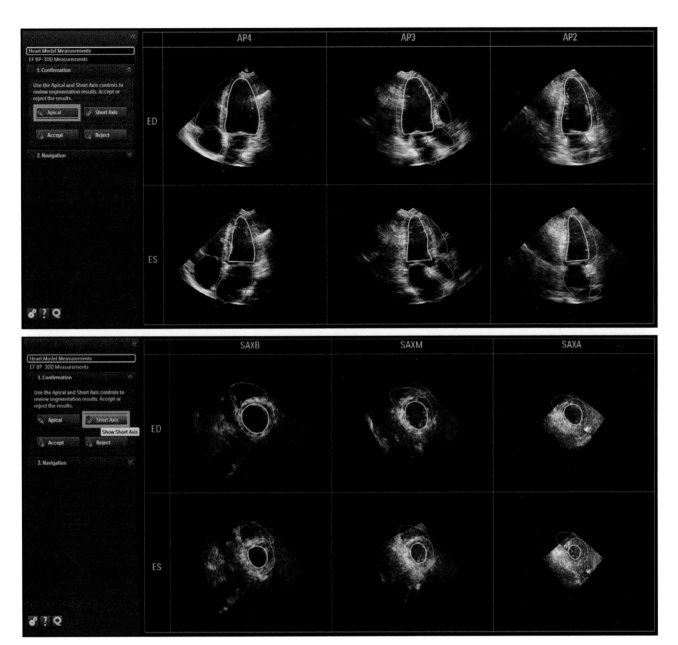

■ **Fig. 3.5** Illustration of the Heart Model tool for automated segmentation and quantification of heart chambers. The *upper image* shows the step of confirmation of the endocardial and epicardial border definition in the apical views in end-diastole (*upper half*) and end-systole (*lower half*) and the *lower image* in the short-axis views. Note that all four chambers – including the asymmetric right ventricle – are segmented accurately

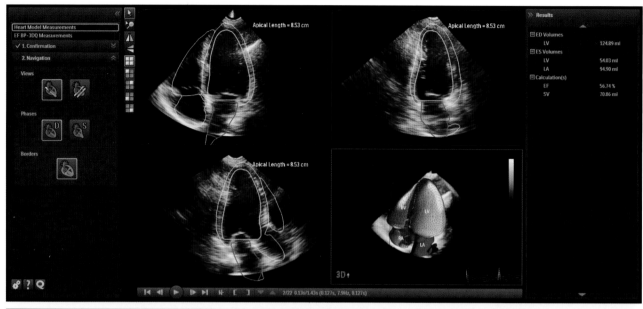

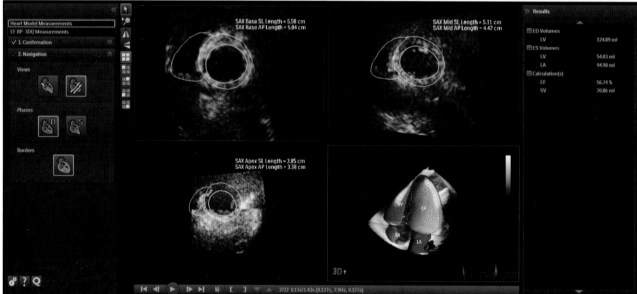

◘ Fig. 3.6 Illustration of the second phase of the automated Heart Model analysis presenting the graphical surface reconstruction of all four chambers shown in different colors and quantification of end-diastolic and end-systolic volume of the left ventricle (*LV*) and the end-systolic volume of the left atrium (*LA*) as well as LV ejection fraction and stroke volume

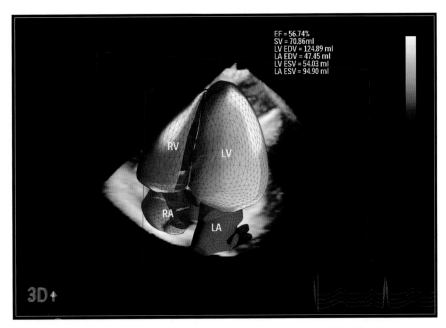

EF = 56.74%
SV = 70.86ml
LV EDV = 124.89 ml
LA EDV = 47.45 ml
LV ESV = 54.03 ml
LA ESV = 94.90 ml

RV   LV

RA   LA

3D↑

☐ **Fig. 3.7** Presentation of the Heart Model's detailed surface reconstruction of all four chambers embedded in the 3DE image dataset. *LV* left ventricle, *LA* left atrium, *RV* right ventricle, *RA* right atrium

3.2 Evaluation of left ventricular mass

In addition to accurately quantifying LV volumes and ejection fraction, RT3DE allows precise calculation of LV mass [4][35][36]. Determination of LV mass requires tracing of both endocardial and epicardial boundaries preferably in end-diastolic images which is more challenging compared to volume measurements, owing to the difficult definition of the epicardial boundary in echocardiographic images (☐ Fig. 3.8, ☐ Fig. 3.9, ☐ Fig. 3.10). Similar to 3D analysis of LV volumes, LV mass analysis using 3D datasets provides the advantage of accurate definition of the LV long axis, which has been demonstrated to yield significantly larger LV long-axis dimensions and measurements of LV mass compared to the 2D method (☐ Fig. 3.8) [36].

Nevertheless, in comparative studies, RT3DE has proven to be more accurate compared with 1D or 2D echocardiographic methods to calculate LV mass when compared with MRI as the standard of reference (☐ Tab. 3.1) [35][36][37][38][39][40][41].

Moreover, in patients with pure severe aortic stenosis undergoing valve replacement therapy, differences in the extent of LV mass regression in relation to the implanted valve size has been reported using 3D echocardiography [42], demonstrating the high precision of 3D echocardiography to assess LV mass.

3.3 Assessment of regional left ventricular function

For the visual interpretation of regional myocardial function in long-axis views, the full volume dataset can be cropped in any plane to depict the different myocardial segments of the LV wall; thus, it is possible to comprehensively study regional myocardial function of the American Society of Echocardiography (ASE)-de-

fined LV segments. Errors in image plane positioning related to angulation or foreshortening, which is frequently encountered with 2D echocardiography, are avoided using 3D echocardiography since the complete 3D information can be used. The echocardiographic system allows long-axis slices of variable thickness (so-called thick slice) to be created, which may aid in the interpretation of regional myocardial function, since it contains more tissue information, when compared with the thin-sliced standard 2D echocardiographic images.

> ❯ Echocardiography developed into a tomographic imaging technique once 3D volumes became available.

Another practical approach to evaluate regional myocardial function is the multiple slice technique, which allows myocardial function to be assessed in short-axis cross-sections. Since the full volume dataset contains the complete dynamic information of the LV during one cardiac cycle, it can be manipulated in such a way that a stack of evenly distributed short-axis slices of variable thickness are created (☐ Fig. 3.11). This tomographic view onto the LV resembles the stack of short-axis cut planes well known from cardiac MRI. The short-axis technique bears the advantage that regional myocardial function can be studied in more detail in the circumference of short-axis slices compared with long-axis cut planes. For example, evaluation of slightly rotated long-axis cut planes may miss minor regional contraction abnormalities apparent in short-axis slices only, thus, giving the false impression of preserved regional myocardial function. This may also be of special importance when interpreting the results of stress echocardiograms using 3D echocardiography (▶ Chapter 4).

In addition to visually analyzing regional myocardial function in long- and short-axis cut planes, a more objective evaluation of regional function can be accomplished. For this tech-

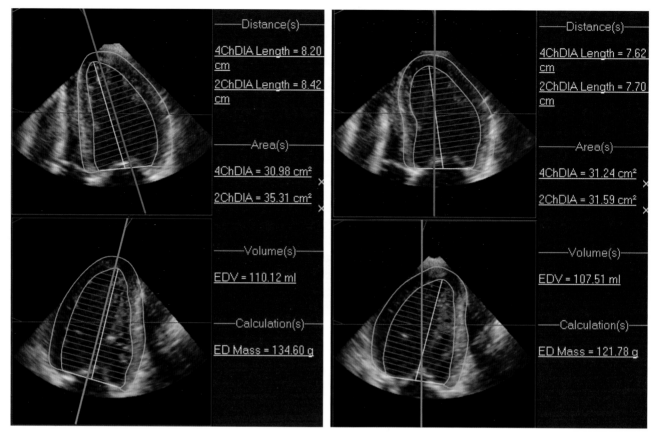

Fig. 3.8 Demonstration of the effect of optimal long-axis alignment (*left*) on the determination of left ventricular (*LV*) dimensions with larger LV length, LV volume, and LV mass compared to results without alignment (*right*). The fast biplane disk method in a RT3DE dataset provides 'pseudo' 3D LV mass analysis

Epicardial 3D surface   Endocardial 3D surface

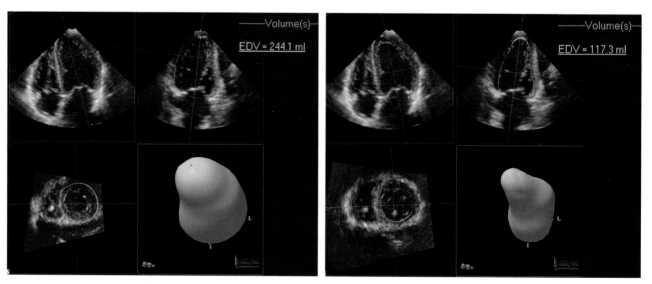

3D LVM = Vol-Epi – Vol-Endo x Density (Myoc) = 244 ml -117 ml x 1.04 g/ml = 132 g

Fig. 3.9 Example of full 3D analysis of end-diastolic epicardial left ventricular (*LV*) volume (*left*) and end-diastolic endocardial LV volume (*right*) for calculation of LV mass (*bottom line*) using the standard 3D LV volume analysis tool. This method, however, is fundamentally limited because epicardial and endocardial contours cannot be shown simultaneously for representation of myocardial thickness. Note that LV mass measurements in ■ Fig. 3.8, ■ Fig. 3.9, and ■ Fig. 3.10 were made in the same RT 3DE dataset of the same patient

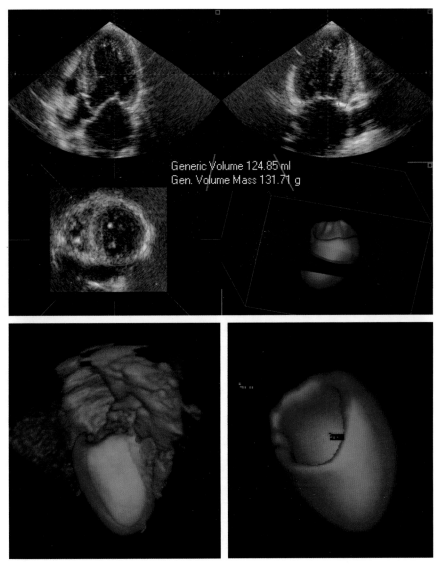

Generic Volume 124.85 ml
Gen. Volume Mass 131.71 g

Fig. 3.10 Example of full 3D analysis of left ventricular (*LV*) mass with the advantage of simultaneous definition of epicardial and endocardial borders (4D LV-Analysis©, TomTec, Germany). This analysis allows intuitive illustration of 3D contours of the LV and spatial pattern of LV hypertrophy. [→Videos 3.10A,B]

Tab. 3.1 Comparison of 3D left ventricular (LV) mass analysis compared to MRI in the recent literature. Indicated values of LV mass were determined by 3D echocardiography

First author [ref]	n	LV mass (g)	Method	r
Kühl [38]	20	202±66	3° rot	0.99
Chuang [41]	25	177±56	Freehand	0.99
Mor-Avi [36]	21	126±39	RT3DE	0.90
Oe [40]	21	288±90	RT3DE	0.95
Bosch [35]	20	145±55	RT3DE	0.94
Pouleur [39]	83	149±42	RT3DE	0.94
Takeuchi [37]	55	153±65	RT3DE	0.94

n number, *r* correlation coefficient, *3° rot* rotation of image planes in steps of 3°, *RT3DE* real-time 3D echocardiography, *Freehand* freehand 3D echocardiography, *LV* left ventricle.

nique, the semiautomatic border-tracking procedure of the complete LV endocardium during the cardiac cycle is needed. The procedure of semiautomatic border tracking has been described above. Based on the landmark information set for the quantitation of global function, the LV is automatically subdivided into 16 segments according to ASE guidelines [4]. For each of these volume segments, a volume–time curve is displayed, demonstrating maximum and minimum volumes of that specific segment during the cardiac cycle. Hypo- or noncontractile segments can easily be identified based on the pattern of the curve, while diseased segments have a flattened curve (**Fig. 3.12**). This approach has been validated using MRI as the standard of reference [43].

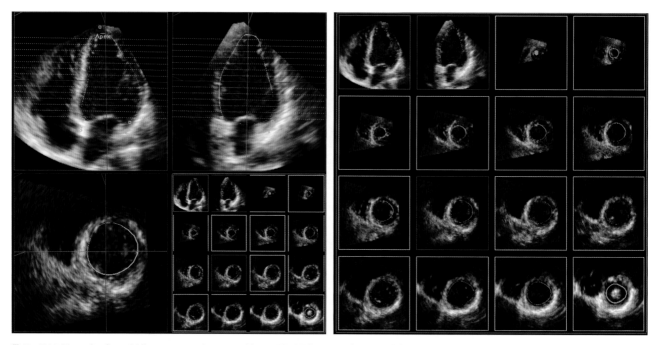

◻ Fig. 3.11 Example of a multislice representation created from a RT3DE dataset. *Left* Manual definition of orientation and distribution of multiple slices represented as a stack of parallel lines oriented perpendicular to the LV long axis. *Right* A 4×4 panel multislice representation with two long-axis views and fourteen short-axis views. [→Video 3.11]

3.4 Determination of left ventricular dyssynchrony

An important aspect of assessing regional myocardial function by echocardiography is the evaluation of LV dyssynchrony. Patients with left bundle branch block (LBBB) may demonstrate marked dyssynchrony with early contraction of the septum and delayed contraction of postero-lateral myocardial segments. Clinical studies have demonstrated a mortality benefit of cardiac resynchronization therapy (i.e., implantation of a biventricular pacemaker) in patients with LBBB and poor LV function (ejection fraction: ≤30 to 35%) on optimal medical treatment [44] [45]. Yet, a nonresponder rate of approximately 30% in patients has been reported. Conventional and novel echocardiographic imaging parameters, such as tissue Doppler indices, have failed to reliably identify candidates who may benefit from resynchronization therapy [46]. In principle, 3D echocardiography may play an important role in assessing regional LV dyssynchrony, since it allows evaluation of the complete LV in near real time. Several studies have demonstrated the potential of 3D echocardiography to assess LV dyssynchrony by calculating a systolic dyssynchrony index (SDI) based on regional volume–time curves [47][48] where the SDI is defined by the standard deviation of time to maximal velocity of all 16 LV segments (Tmsv 16-SD; ◻ Fig. 3.12). A more detailed approach to the use of RT3DE in the assessment of mechanical dyssynchrony is provided in ► Chapter 4.

> **❯** The 3D analysis of regional LV function may play an important role in assessing regional dyssynchrony.

3.5 Parametric imaging

Assessing regional myocardial function in 16 or 17 segments is a rather coarse and imprecise way of describing segmental myocardial contraction of the LV. This is especially true since the full volume 3D dataset contains much more spatial information. For this purpose, a more finely resolved approach has been developed. More than 800 endocardial data points are used to develop a polar map of the endocardial surface of the LV. Based on an end-diastolic and end-systolic map of LV endocardial surface, a parametric image of regional LV endocardial motion can be obtained (◻ Fig. 3.13).

Endocardial motion is displayed as shades of blue (for positive excursion values representing inward motion), red (for negative excursion values representing outward motion), and black (representing no motion). Thus, an akinetic or dyskinetic myocardial region would be displayed as black or red color, while a normal or hypokinetic contracting segment would be displayed in shades of light to dark blue. This fine-tuned regional myocardial motion information is mapped on a polar plot with the superimposed American Heart Association (AHA)-defined 17-segment model (◻ Fig. 3.13). Examples of a patient with normal endocardial excursion demonstrating almost homogenous distribution of endocardial motion through the LV and of a patient with an anterior wall myocardial infarction showing akinesia to dyskinesia of the apex, apical septum, and apical anterior wall are shown in ◻ Fig. 3.13.

Apart from displaying absolute endocardial excursion, timing of regional endocardial motion can also be displayed in a parametric image. For this purpose, the time to maximal endsystolic excursion is assessed for each endocardial data point. From these data, a polar map is created displaying the average

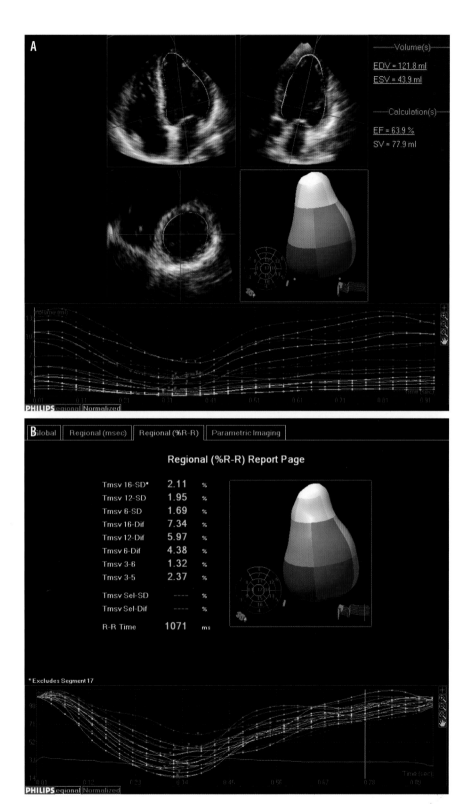

◧ **Fig. 3.12** **A** Three-dimensional regional LV analysis with illustration of segmental volume–time curves (*bottom*) and dynamic 3D visualization of LV segments during contraction (*lower right*) with a bull's eye representation of LV segments. The example shows a healthy subject (same subject as in ◧ Fig. 3.1, ◧ Fig. 3.2, and ◧ Fig. 3.3) with normal segmental contraction and synchronous timing as indicated by the small deviation of *red points* of maximal systolic contraction. **B** Visualization of percentage segmental volume change (*bottom*) in the same normal subject as shown in **A**. The numbers (*top*) represent results of standard deviation of time to maximal velocity (*Tmsv*) for different selections of segments for assessment of segmental timing and dyssynchrony (▶ Chapter 5) with a Tmsv 16-SD of 2.11 indicating normal synchrony.

3

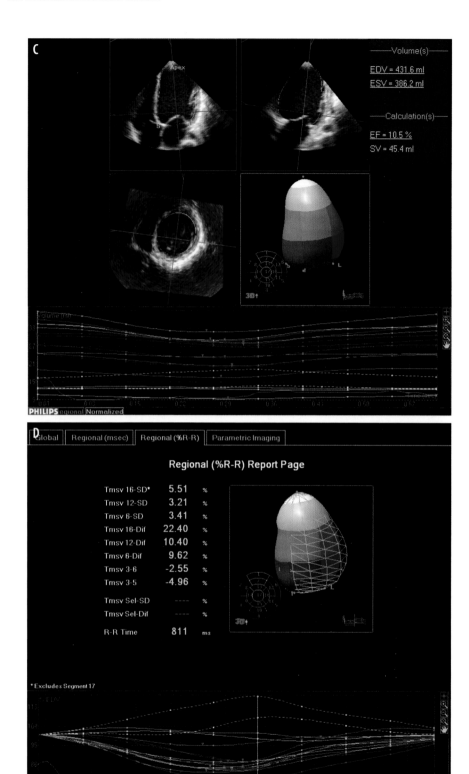

□ **Fig. 3.12 Continued. C** Compared to **A** and **B**, this example shows the 3D regional LV analysis in a patient with dilated cardiomyopathy with an ejection fraction (*EF*) of 10% and left bundle branch block. *Bottom* Due to poor regional contraction segmental volume–time curves are markedly flattened and the *red points* that indicate segmental maximum contraction are significantly dispersed, thus, indicating dyssynchrony. **D** Visualization of percentage segmental volume change (*bottom*) in the same subject with severe dilated cardiomyopathy as shown in **C**. Volume–time curves above the 100% threshold indicate dyskinesia. *Top* The Tmsv 16-SD of 5.51 indicates significant dyssynchrony. [→Videos 3.12A,C]

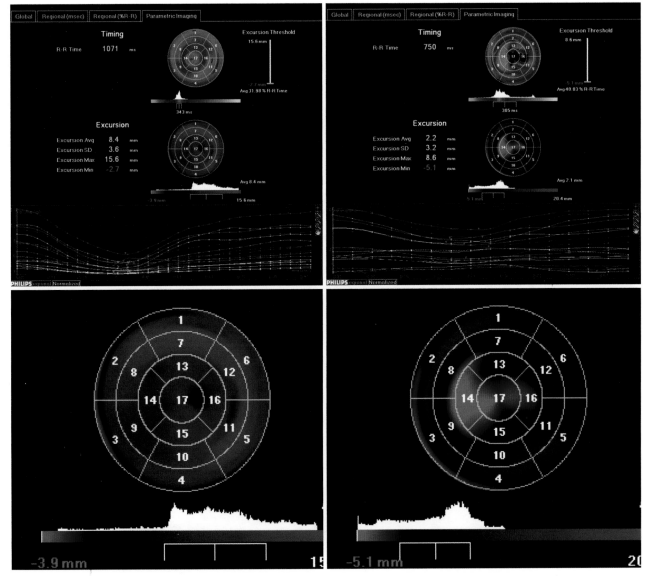

Fig. 3.13 Two examples of parametric imaging representing segmental endocardial excursion in a normal subject (*left*) and a patient after myocardial infarction (*right*) with apical, apical septal, and apical anterior akinesia (*black*) and dyskinesia (*red*). The parametric imaging report pages with segmental volume–time curves are shown (*top*)

timing of endocardial motion in green. Events happening before average motion are displayed in shades of blue, while events happening after average motion are displayed in shades of red to yellow. ▪ Fig. 3.14 shows an example of a patient with synchronous timing of endocardial excursion demonstrating almost homogeneous distribution of green color throughout the polar plot and for a patient with LBBB showing asynchronous early contraction of the septum (blue color) and delayed contraction of the antero-lateral wall (red color). Software from different vendors may display alternative color schemes and also display endocardial excursion in a moving image termed contraction front mapping. However, limited data on the clinical value of this approach are available; hence, it is not discussed here.

3.6 Transesophageal real-time 3D echocardiography

All of the above presented methods and techniques do, in principle, also apply to transesophageal RT3DE (RT3D TEE). This is of special importance for the assessment of global LV function and hemodynamics in intubated and ventilated patients with cardiogenic shock or decompensated heart failure in the intensive care unit. Image quality is generally good in these patients due to the unrestricted transesophageal window of the LV and the stable probe position in the esophagus during data acquisition; however, sometimes obtaining a full volume dataset of the entire LV from the midesophageal position can be challenging (▪ Fig. 3.15). A short maneuver of respiratory hold of the ventilator should be sought during data acquisition to avoid respiratory motion artifacts. Apart from global volumes and ejection fraction, cardiac

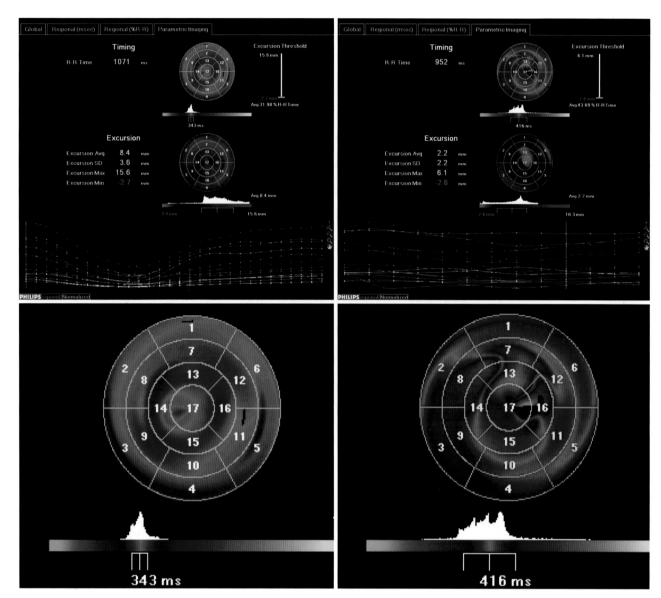

Fig. 3.14 Two examples of parametric imaging representing segmental contraction timing in a normal subject (*left*) and a patient with poor LV function and LBBB (*right*) with early contraction of the septum (*blue*) and delayed contraction of the anterolateral wall (*red*). The parametric imaging report pages with segmental volume–time curves are shown (*top*)

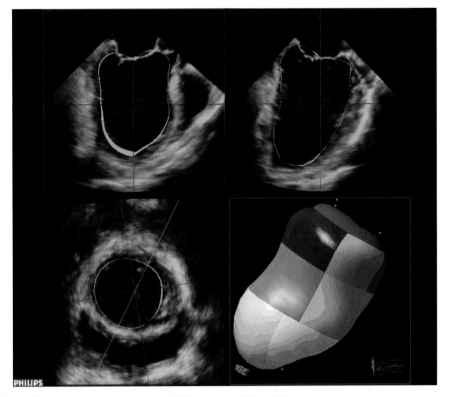

☑ **Fig. 3.15** Example of RT3D TEE analysis of global and segmental LV function. [→Video 3.15]

output measurements can be readily obtained with this technique, which may obviate the need for placement of invasive catheters (e.g., a Swan–Ganz catheter), thus, avoiding complications of the invasive approach. Moreover, the method allows for serial assessment of cardiac function very accurately guiding therapy in these difficult patients. More data are still needed to prove the benefit and advantages of this approach compared to a more invasive strategy [49].

❯ Accurate assessment of LV function using transesophageal RT3DE plays an important role in intensive care patients.

3.7 Three-dimensional assessment of left atrial volume and function

Recently, growing interest in left atrial (LA) volume measurement has evolved because an association with adverse cardiovascular outcomes has been shown [50][51]. Current guidelines for chamber quantification recommend use of either a biplane area–length method or a biplane disk method [4]. However, 3D evaluation of LA volume has been considered to be most accurate [4]. Early studies validated the accuracy of LA volume measurement by reconstructive 3D echocardiography compared to 2D echocardiography and MRI [52][53][54]. With the use of RT3DE, however, 3D analysis of LA volumes became more accurate in clinical practice by applying the same semiautomated algorithm previously described for 3D LV volume analysis (☑ Fig. 3.16) [55] [56][57].

In a recent study, Miyasa et al. [58] found improved correlation (r=0.95) of LA volume measurements by RT3DE and 64-slice multidetector computed tomography with an underestimation of 8% by RT3DE compared to 2D measurements of LA volumes (r=0.86) with a more pronounced underestimation of 19%. In a large meta-analysis of 14 studies Shimada et al. [59] found nearly similar underestimation of LA volumes of 9.4 ml by 3D echocardiography compared to MRI, where they identified existence of cardiac disease and lower number of 2D planes as significant sources of underestimation. Importantly, in a very recent multicenter study by Mor-Avi et al. [60], LA volume quantification from multibeat real-time full volume 3D datasets using a semiautomated 3D quantification algorithm revealed excellent agreement with MRI with an underestimation of only 1±14 ml for maximal end-systolic volume and 0±21 ml for minimal end-diastolic volume [60].

Moreover, recent studies demonstrated the prognostic value of RT3DE-based estimates of LA volume in patients at risk for cardiovascular events compared to conventional parameters [61, 62] as well as in patients undergoing ablation of atrial fibrillation [63, 64]. Beyond the estimation of systolic LA volume, 3D echocardiography has been demonstrated to provide advanced analysis of LA function by temporal analysis of the phasic changes of LA volumes throughout the cardiac cycle [53][65][66][67]. The assessment of phasic changes of LA volumes in a normal subject and a patient with restrictive cardiomyopathy is shown in ☑ Fig. 3.16. In the normal subject, the end-systolic LA volume of 47.0 ml (indexed to body surface=27.6 ml/m^2) is in the range of normal values, whereas the end-systolic LA volume of 86.7 ml (62.0 ml/m^2) in the patient with restrictive cardiomyopathy

3

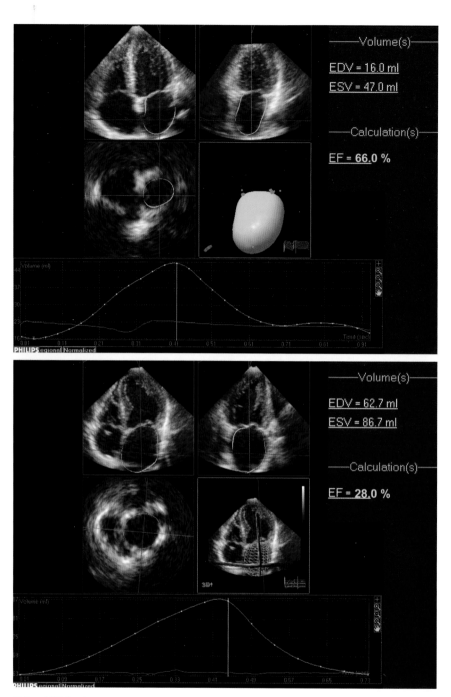

□ **Fig. 3.16** Assessment of left atrial (*LA*) volumes using RT3D TTE in a normal subject (*top*) and a patient with restrictive cardiomyopathy (*bottom*). The end-systolic LA volume is visualized by a 3D surface reconstruction (*top*), or it can be represented by a 3D wire mesh within the 3D dataset (*bottom*). Using the same semiautomated algorithm used for LV analysis, LA volume changes are detected throughout the cardiac cycle and represented by a volume–time curve (see text for further interpretation). [→Videos 3.16A,B]

(CMP) indicates severe LA enlargement [4]. Values for the ejection fraction (EF) also differed significantly with an EF of 66.0% in the normal subject compared to an EF of 28.0% in the patient with restrictive CMP, indicating severe LA dysfunction or impaired LV diastolic function. Recently, normal reference ranges for left (and right) atrial ejection fractions obtained with RT3DE have been proposed by Aune et al. [68].

❯ The 3D analysis of LA volume and function should be performed using transthoracic RT3DE, because transesophageal 3D datasets do not encompass the entire LA.

For practical application, 3D LA volume analysis should be performed using RT3D TTE full volume datasets because datasets from a transesophageal approach do not encompass the entire left atrium [30]. According to the recommendation for the application of LA area–length method, the basis of the LA volume is defined at the level of the mitral annulus. As a consequence, the five landmark points required for semiautomated endocardial border detection will be set at the septal, lateral, anterior, and inferior mitral annulus and finally at the roof of the LA (instead of the LV apex in ventricular volume determination). LA volumes by RT3DE should be indexed to body surface area as is the case for 2D LA volumes [4].

References

1. Lang RM, Mor-Avi V, Sugeng L et al (2006) Three-dimensional echocardiography: the benefits of the additional dimension. J Am Coll Cardiol 48: 2053–2069

2. Gopal AS, Keller AM, Rigling R et al (1993) Left ventricular volume and endocardial surface area by three-dimensional echocardiography: comparison with two-dimensional echocardiography and nuclear magnetic resonance imaging in normal subjects. J Am Coll Cardiol 22:258–270

3. Siu SC, Rivera JM, Guerrero JL et al (1993) Three-dimensional echocardiography. In vivo validation for left ventricular volume and function. Circulation 88:1715–1723

4. Lang RM, Bierig M, Devereux RB et al (2005) Recommendations for chamber quantification: a report from the American Society of Echocardiography's Guidelines and Standards Committee and the Chamber Quantification Writing Group, developed in conjunction with the European Association of Echocardiography, a branch of the European Society of Cardiology. J Am Soc Echocardiogr 18:1440–1463

5. Buck T, Schon F, Baumgart D et al (1996) Tomographic left ventricular volume determination in the presence of aneurysm by three-dimensional echocardiographic imaging. I: Asymmetric model hearts. J Am Soc Echocardiogr 9:488–500

6. Sapin PM, Schroder KM, Gopal AS et al (1994) Comparison of two- and three-dimensional echocardiography with cineventriculography for measurement of left ventricular volume in patients. J Am Coll Cardiol 24:1054–1063

7. King DL, Gopal AS, Keller AM et al (1994) Three-dimensional echocardiography. Advances for measurement of ventricular volume and mass. Hypertension 23:I172–I179

8. Jiang L, Vazquez de Prada JA, Handschumacher MD et al (1995) Quantitative three-dimensional reconstruction of aneurysmal left ventricles. In vitro and in vivo validation. Circulation 91:222–230

9. Buck T, Hunold P, Wentz KU et al (1997) Tomographic three-dimensional echocardiographic determination of chamber size and systolic function in patients with left ventricular aneurysm: comparison to magnetic resonance imaging, cineventriculography, and two-dimensional echocardiography. Circulation 96:4286–4297

10. King DL, Harrison MR, King DL Jr et al (1992) Improved reproducibility of left atrial and left ventricular measurements by guided three-dimensional echocardiography. J Am Coll Cardiol 20:1238–1245

11. King DL, Harrison MR, King DL Jr et al (1992) Ultrasound beam orientation during standard two-dimensional imaging: assessment by three-dimensional echocardiography. J Am Soc Echocardiogr 5:569–576

12. Jenkins C, Bricknell K, Hanekom L, Marwick TH (2004) Reproducibility and accuracy of echocardiographic measurements of left ventricular parameters using real-time three-dimensional echocardiography. J Am Coll Cardiol 44:878–886

13. Gopal AS, Shen Z, Sapin PM et al (1995) Assessment of cardiac function by three-dimensional echocardiography compared with conventional noninvasive methods. Circulation 92:842–853

14. Qin JX, Shiota T, McCarthy PM et al (2000) Real-time three-dimensional echocardiographic study of left ventricular function after infarct exclusion surgery for ischemic cardiomyopathy. Circulation 102:III101–III106

15. Qin JX, Jones M, Shiota T et al (2000) Validation of real-time three-dimensional echocardiography for quantifying left ventricular volumes in the presence of a left ventricular aneurysm: in vitro and in vivo studies. J Am Coll Cardiol 36:900–907

16. Monaghan MJ (2006) Role of real time 3D echocardiography in evaluating the left ventricle. Heart 92:131–136

17. Chang SA, Lee SC, Kim EY et al (2011) Feasibility of single-beat full-volume capture real-time three-dimensional echocardiography and auto-contouring algorithm for quantification of left ventricular volume: validation with cardiac magnetic resonance imaging. J Am Soc Echocardiogr 24:853–859

18. Kuhl HP, Schreckenberg M, Rulands D et al (2004) High-resolution transthoracic real-time three-dimensional echocardiography: quantitation of cardiac volumes and function using semi-automatic border detection and comparison with cardiac magnetic resonance imaging. J Am Coll Cardiol 43:2083–2090

19. Gopal AS, Chukwu EO, Mihalatos DG et al (2007) Left ventricular structure and function for postmyocardial infarction and heart failure risk stratification by three-dimensional echocardiography. J Am Soc Echocardiogr 20: 949–958

20. Jacobs LD, Salgo IS, Goonewardena S et al (2006) Rapid online quantification of left ventricular volume from real-time three-dimensional echocardiographic data. Eur Heart J 27:460–468

21. Sugeng L, Mor-Avi V, Weinert L et al (2006) Quantitative assessment of left ventricular size and function: side-by-side comparison of real-time three-dimensional echocardiography and computed tomography with magnetic resonance reference. Circulation 114:654–661

22. Hare JL, Jenkins C, Nakatani S et al (2008) Feasibility and clinical decision-making with 3D echocardiography in routine practice. Heart 94:440–445

23. Jenkins C, Bricknell K, Chan J et al (2007) Comparison of two- and three-dimensional echocardiography with sequential magnetic resonance imaging for evaluating left ventricular volume and ejection fraction over time in patients with healed myocardial infarction. Am J Cardiol 99:300–306

24. Mannaerts HF, van der Heide JA, Kamp O et al (2004) Early identification of left ventricular remodelling after myocardial infarction, assessed by transthoracic 3D echocardiography. Eur Heart J 25:680–687

25. Grabowski M, Piatkowski R, Scislo P et al (2008) Real-time three-dimensional echocardi-ography in transient left apical ballooning syndrome. Int J Cardiol 129:e69–e70

26. Fujikawa M, Iwasaka J, Oishi C et al (2008) Three-dimensional echocardio-graphic assessment of left ventricular function in takotsubo cardiomyopathy. Heart Vessels 23:214–216

27. Schoof S, Bertram H, Hohmann D et al (2010) Takotsubo cardiomyopathy in a 2-year-old girl: 3-dimensional visualization of reversible left ventricular dysfunction. J Am Coll Cardiol 55:e5

28. Shimada Y, Maeda K, Ogawa K et al (2010) Three dimensional echocardiography of tako-tsubo cardiomyopathy with atrial myxoma. BMJ Case Rep 2010

29. Breithardt OA, Becker M, Kalsch T, Haghi D (2008) Follow-up in Tako-tsubo cardiomyopathy by real-time three-dimensional echocardiography. Heart 94:210

30. Lang RM, Badano LP, Tsang W, Adams DH et al (2012) EAE/ASE recommendations for image acquisition and display using three-dimensional echocardiography. Eur Heart J Car-diovasc Imaging 13:1–46

31. Moceri P, Doyen D, Bertora D et al (2012) Real time three-dimensional echocardiographic assessment of left ventricular function in heart failure patients: underestimation of left ventricular volume increases with the degree of dilatation. Echocardiography 29:970–977

32. Muller S, Bartel T, Katz MA et al (2003) Partial cut-off of the left ventricle: determinants and effects on volume parameters assessed by real-time 3-D echocardiography. Ultrasound Med Biol 29:25–30

33. Mor-Avi V, Jenkins C, Kuhl HP et al (2008) Real-time 3-dimensional echocardiographic quantification of left ventricular volumes: multicenter study for validation with magnetic resonance imaging and investigation of sources of error. JACC Cardiovasc Imaging 1:413–423

34. Jenkins C, Moir S, Chan J et al (2009) Left ventricular volume measurement with echocardiography: a comparison of left ventricular opacification, three-dimensional echocardiography, or both with magnetic resonance imaging. Eur Heart J 30:98–106

35. van den Bosch AE, Robbers-Visser D, Krenning BJ et al (2006) Comparison of real-time three-dimensional echocardiography to magnetic resonance imaging for assessment of left ventricular mass. Am J Cardiol 97:113–117

36. Mor-Avi V, Sugeng L, Weinert L et al (2004) Fast measurement of left ventricular mass with real-time three-dimensional echocardiography: comparison with magnetic resonance imaging. Circulation 110:1814–1818

37. Takeuchi M, Nishikage T, Mor-Avi V et al (2008) Measurement of left ventricular mass by real-time three-dimensional echocardiography: validation against magnetic resonance and comparison with two-dimensional and m-mode measurements. J Am Soc Echocardiogr 21:1001–1005

38. Kuhl HP, Bucker A, Franke A et al (2000) Transesophageal 3-dimensional echocardiography: in vivo determination of left ventricular mass in comparison with magnetic resonance imaging. J Am Soc Echocardiogr 13:205–215

39. Pouleur AC, le Polain de Waroux JB, Pasquet A et al (2008) Assessment of left ventricular mass and volumes by three-dimensional echocardiography in patients with or without wall motion abnormalities: comparison against cine magnetic resonance imaging. Heart 94:1050–1057

40. Oe H, Hozumi T, Arai K et al (2005) Comparison of accurate measurement of left ventricular mass in patients with hypertrophied hearts by real-time three-dimensional echocardiography versus magnetic resonance imaging. Am J Cardiol 95:1263–1267

41. Chuang ML, Beaudin RA, Riley MF et al (2000) Three-dimensional echocardiographic measurement of left ventricular mass: comparison with magnetic resonance imaging and two-dimensional echocardiographic determinations in man. Int J Card Imaging 16:347–357

42. Kuhl HP, Franke A, Puschmann D et al (2002) Regression of left ventricular mass one year after aortic valve replacement for pure severe aortic stenosis. Am J Cardiol 89:408–413

43. Corsi C, Lang RM, Veronesi F et al (2005) Volumetric quantification of global and regional left ventricular function from real-time three-dimensional echocardiographic images. Circulation 112:1161–1170

44. Cleland JG, Daubert JC, Erdmann E et al (2005) The effect of cardiac resynchronization on morbidity and mortality in heart failure. N Engl J Med 352:1539–1549

45. Moss AJ, Hall WJ, Cannom DS et al (2009) Cardiac-resynchronization therapy for the prevention of heart-failure events. N Engl J Med 361:1329–1338

46. Chung ES, Leon AR, Tavazzi L et al (2008) Results of the predictors of response to CRT (PROSPECT) trial. Circulation 17:2608–2616

47. Kapetanakis S, Kearney MT, Siva A et al (2005) Real-time three-dimensional echocardiography: a novel technique to quantify global left ventricular mechanical dyssynchrony. Circulation 112:992–1000

48. Takeuchi M, Jacobs A, Sugeng L et al (2007) Assessment of left ventricular dyssynchrony with real-time 3-dimensional echocardiography: comparison with Doppler tissue imaging. J Am Soc Echocardiogr 20:1321–1329

49. Kuhl HP, Franke A, Janssens U et al (1998) Three-dimensional echocardiographic determination of left ventricular volumes and function by multiplane transesophageal transducer: dynamic in vitro validation and in vivo comparison with angiography and thermodilution. J Am Soc Echocardiogr 11:1113–1124

50. Tsang TS, Barnes ME, Gersh BJ et al (2002) Left atrial volume as a morphophysiologic expression of left ventricular diastolic dysfunction and relation to cardiovascular risk burden. Am J Cardiol 90:1284–1289

51. Tsang TS, Abhayaratna WP, Barnes ME et al (2006) Prediction of cardiovascular outcomes with left atrial size: is volume superior to area or diameter? J Am Coll Cardiol 47:1018–1023

52. Rodevan O, Bjornerheim R, Ljosland M et al (1999) Left atrial volumes assessed by three- and two-dimensional echocardiography compared to MRI estimates. Int J Card Imaging 15:397–410

53. Poutanen T, Ikonen A, Vainio P et al (2000) Left atrial volume assessed by transthoracic three dimensional echocardiography and magnetic resonance imaging: dynamic changes during the heart cycle in children. Heart 83:537–542

54. Keller AM, Gopal AS, King DL (2000) Left and right atrial volume by freehand three-dimensional echocardiography: in vivo validation using magnetic resonance imaging. Eur J Echocardiogr 1:55–65

55. Artang R, Migrino RQ, Harmann L et al (2009) Left atrial volume measurement with automated border detection by 3-dimensional echocardiography: comparison with Magnetic Resonance Imaging. Cardiovasc Ultrasound 7:16

56. Jenkins C, Bricknell K, Marwick TH (2005) Use of real-time three-dimensional echocardiography to measure left atrial volume: comparison with other echocardiographic techniques. J Am Soc Echocardiogr 18:991–997

57. Buechel RR, Stephan FP, Sommer G et al (2013) Head-to-Head Comparison of Two-Dimensional and Three-Dimensional Echocardiographic Methods for Left Atrial Chamber Quantification with Magnetic Resonance Imaging. J Am Soc Echocardiogr 2013; 26:428–435

58. Miyasaka Y, Tsujimoto S, Maeba H et al (2011) Left atrial volume by real-time three-dimensional echocardiography: validation by 64-slice multidetector computed tomography. J Am Soc Echocardiogr 24:680–686

59. Shimada YJ, Shiota T (2012) Underestimation of left atrial volume by three-dimensional echocardiography validated by magnetic resonance imaging: a meta-analysis and investigation of the source of bias. Echocardiography 29:385–390

60. Mor-Avi V, Yodwut C, Jenkins C et al (2012) Real-time 3D echocardiographic quantification of left atrial volume: multicenter study for validation with CMR. JACC Cardiovasc Imaging 5:769–777

61. De Castro S, Caselli S, Di Angelantonio E et al (2008) Relation of left atrial maximal volume measured by real-time 3D echocardiography to demographic, clinical, and Doppler variables. Am J Cardiol 101:1347–1352

62. Suh IW, Song JM, Lee EY et al (2008) Left atrial volume measured by real-time 3-dimensional echocardiography predicts clinical outcomes in patients with severe left ventricular dysfunction and in sinus rhythm. J Am Soc Echocardiogr 21:439–445

63. Marsan NA, Tops LF, Holman ER et al (2008) Comparison of left atrial volumes and function by real-time three-dimensional echocardiography in patients having catheter ablation for atrial fibrillation with persistence of sinus rhythm versus recurrent atrial fibrillation three months later. Am J Cardiol 102:847–853

64. Delgado V, Vidal B, Sitges M et al (2008) Fate of left atrial function as determined by real-time three-dimensional echocardiography study after radiofrequency catheter ablation for the treatment of atrial fibrillation. Am J Cardiol 101:1285–1290

65. Shin MS, Fukuda S, Song JM et al (2006) Relationship between left atrial and left ventricular function in hypertrophic cardiomyopathy: a real-time 3-dimensional echocardiographic study. J Am Soc Echocardiogr 19:796–801

66. Saraiva RM, Yamano T, Matsumura Y et al (2009) Left atrial function assessed by real-time 3-dimensional echocardiography is related to right ventricular systolic pressure in chronic mitral regurgitation. Am Heart J 158:309–316

67. Buechel RR, Sommer G, Leibundgut G et al (2013) Assessment of left atrial functional parameters using a novel dedicated analysis tool for real-time three-dimensional echocardiography: validation in comparison to magnetic resonance imaging. Int J Cardiovasc Imaging 2013; 29:601–608

68. Aune E, Baekkevar M, Roislien J et al (2009) Normal reference ranges for left and right atrial volume indexes and ejection fractions obtained with real-time three-dimensional echocardiography. Eur J Echocardiogr 10:738–744

Three-dimensional stress echocardiography

Andreas Franke

T. Buck et al. (Hrsg.), *Three-dimensional Echocardiography*,
DOI 10.1007/978-3-642-36799-1_4, © Springer-Verlag Berlin Heidelberg 2014

Over the last 25 years, stress echocardiography has become a widely used technique for diagnosis and risk stratification of patients with suspected or known coronary artery disease. However, relevant methodological limitations of conventional two-dimensional (2D) stress echocardiography still exist. It remains difficult to acquire high-quality data and to analyze the images with reproducible results which may lead to reduced test accuracy and a lack of ability to detect regional myocardial ischemia.

Image acquisition in 2D echocardiography may be impaired by (1) probe positioning errors resulting in inadequate image planes, e.g., LV foreshortening, (2) reduced image quality with poor visualization of especially anterior and lateral left ventricular (LV) walls, and (3) the time-consuming serial acquisition of different image planes (parasternal short and long axis, apical 4- and 2-chamber views as well as the apical long axis) in a narrow time window, during peak stress, while wall motion abnormalities are present. Even after successful image acquisition, subjectivity of image interpretation remains a major problem, causing limited interobserver agreement and relevant examiner-dependency [1].

Knowing all these limitations, several attempts have been undertaken to make stress echocardiography easier and more accurate. The use of pharmacological protocols (dobutamine plus atropine) instead of physical exercise protocols improves image quality and increases the time available for image acquisition at peak level. Harmonic imaging without use of contrast (tissue harmonics) has been demonstrated to improve endocardial visibility and test accuracy, which can be further increased by the additional application of left heart contrast for LV opacification.

Other advanced echocardiographic modalities such as tissue Doppler imaging or strain analysis may help obtain independence from subjective image interpretation, because they provide more objective and quantifiable information on wall motion abnormalities. Although promising, most of these techniques have not made their way into clinical routine mainly due to complexity. Not only technical factors may improve the accuracy of stress echocardiography, but training and increased experience of the individual examiner lowers interobserver variability and increases test sensitivity [2].

With the availability of matrix array transducers, the simultaneous acquisition of two or three image planes (bi- or triplanar imaging) or even the acquisition of a complete pyramidal volume dataset became possible (► Chapter 2). This new modality dramatically decreases the necessary number of serially acquired heart beats. Several of the above mentioned limitations of conventional 2D stress echocardiography can be potentially solved using this technique.

> ❯ Matrix array transducer technology dramatically decreases the necessary number of serially acquired heart beats.

4.1   Method

Matrix array transducers allow different approaches to perform stress echocardiography: Rotating »monoplanar«, biplanar, triplanar or full volume mode.

Most vendors developed stress echo acquisition software that takes advantage of matrix array's potential to electronically rotate an image plane. As a consequence, the image plane can be changed – as a rotation around a stable central axis – without moving the transducer (iRotate mode). Once the echo window is found, the ultrasound probe can be held still which makes acquisition easier and more robust for beginners but also for experienced examiners. Nevertheless, serial acquisition of all image planes still remains time consuming. However, in newer three-dimensional (3D) echocardiography systems, stress echocardiography software has been included, allowing to program the iRotate angles for each 2-, 3-, and 4-chamber view. During the stress protocol, then, the software automatically rotates the scan plane with each push-button for acquisition to the next view in each stress level. This stress protocol can even programmed to include 3D full volume datasets at each stress level, however, without the ability to dem-

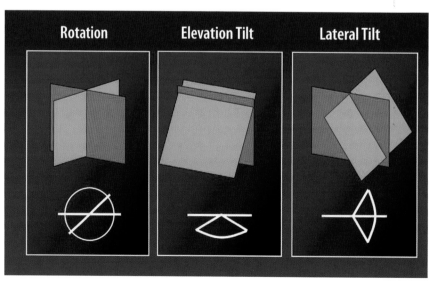

◻ **Fig. 4.1** Schematic drawing of the different spatial orientations of biplanar imaging

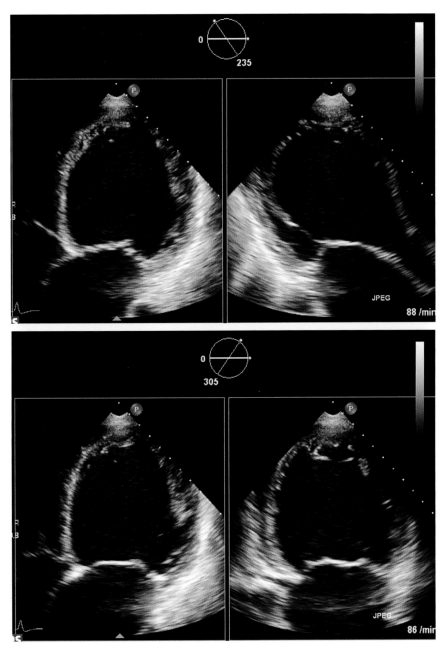

Fig. 4.2 Electronic rotation of 2D image planes during the stress echocardiographic protocol using the xPlane mode. *Top* The image shows simultaneously a 4-chamber view (*top left*) and at 235° rotation a long-axis view (*top right*). The electronic rotation of the right image relative to the left is indicated by the rotation symbol on top. *Bottom* Without rotating the matrix array transducer, the image plane on the right can be electronically rotated. Here a standard 2-chamber view is shown at 305° rotation. During a stress echocardiographic protocol, identical image plane rotations can be easily reproduced at any protocol step. [→Videos 4.2A,B]

onstrate 3D data of different stress level in a quad screen for side-by-side comparison (▶ Section 4.3).

Biplanar imaging (xPlane mode) allows the simultaneous visualization and acquisition of two image planes: the first oriented in a conventional way, the second in any desired angle of rotation or tilt (lateral and elevation tilt) which can be electronically steered by command panel buttons without changing the position of the transducer during the stress protocol (◘ Fig. 4.1 and ◘ Fig. 4.2). Typically, the biplanar mode from the parasternal echo window allows the simultaneous acquisition of a long axis and of an adapted short axis, and from the apical echo window a

simultaneous apical 4-chamber and 2-chamber view [3][4]. Finally – using the rotation of one of the image planes – in a third heartbeat the apical long axis can be acquired (◘ Fig. 4.2). Image plane orientation can be stored in the echocardiographic system as an individual setting so that after acquisition of all planes, side-by-side visualization and synchronization is possible.

Other vendors allow the simultaneous scanning of three image planes (»triplanar«; mostly in 60° increments). Acquisition of triplanar data is typically only performed from a single apical echo window. Furthermore – when omitting parasternal recording – triplanar scanning facilitates a single transducer position

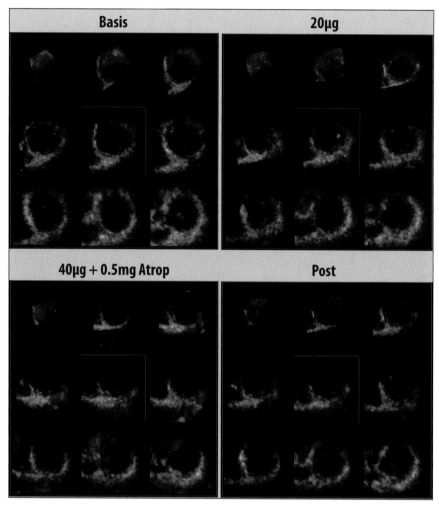

◘ Fig. 4.3 Side-by-side analysis of a nine-slice view from baseline conditions (*upper left* set of short-axis slices), low dose dobutamine (*20 µg, upper right*), peak dose dobutamine (*40 µg +0.5 mg Atropine; lower left*), and during recovery (*5 min Post; lower right*). [→Videos 4.3A–D; see also →Videos 4.3E,F demonstrating a second dobutamine 3D stress study]

for acquisition of only one heartbeat at each stress stage [5]. Loops from all three image planes are stored separately and can be presented and analyzed side-by-side comparable to conventional 2D stress echocardiography. Bi- and triplanar techniques may serve as a first step toward »complete« 3D stress echocardiography.

The acquisition of wide-angle 3D datasets (so-called »full volume mode«) is based on the serial recording of four to seven narrow subvolumes in consecutive heartbeats (▶ Chapter 2, ▶ Fig. 2.15, and ▶ Fig. 2.20). Immediately after acquisition the subsegments are combined to a pyramidal 3D dataset with an overall angle of maximally 104°×104°, which can comprise a complete cavity even in patients with dilated left ventricles. There are also new approaches to acquire wide-angle 3D datasets with only a single heartbeat (one-beat acquisition; see ▶ Chapter 2). Of course, this accepts a trade-off in spatial and temporal resolution because line density is decreased, which results in poorer lateral image resolution, and time for sweeping the complete sector is increased, which also results in a somewhat decreased time resolution. Therefore, one-beat acquisition of full volume data still remains unsatisfactory and its image quality may not yet be optimal for 3D stress echocardiography.

As in conventional 2D stress echocardiography, the acquisition of 3D datasets in the stress echocardiographic workflow is performed at rest, at low and peak stress, and during recovery. Both physical stress (either bicycle or treadmill exercise) and pharmacological stress (mainly dobutamine plus atropine, rarely dipyridamole) have been used in combination with 3D techniques. Several studies described the additional use of left heart contrast agents for better endocardial delineation [6][7].

❯ Besides the extraction of long-axis views from stress 3D datasets, multiple parallel short-axis slices allow systematic regional wall motion analysis.

Once the 3D dataset is acquired, image planes can be created in every desired orientation independent of the transducer position and beam direction during dataset acquisition. Besides the extraction of conventional 2-, 3-, and 4-chamber views (▶ Fig. 2.35 in Chapter 2), multiple parallel short-axis slices can be used for systematic regional wall motion analysis. These slices can be extracted semiautomatically as a set of three to nine parallel apical to basal slices of the LV (▶ Fig. 2.37 in Chapter 2 and ▶ Fig. 3.11 in Chapter 3). However, analysis of stress echocardiographic data – also in 3D – still remains a subjective interpretation of wall

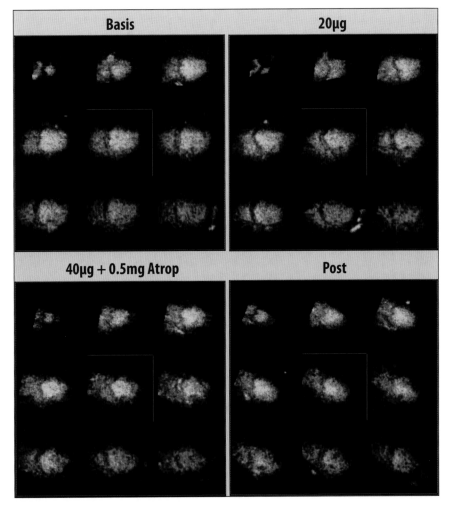

Fig. 4.4 Side-by-side analysis of a contrast-enhanced nine-slice view. Same orientation as in ▢ Fig. 4.3. [→Videos 4.4A–D]

motion analysis, optimally using a side-by-side display of the extracted image planes at different exercise levels (▢ Fig. 4.3 and ▢ Fig. 4.4). For better visualization, the endocardial border can be highlighted by a yellow contour line which represents the 3D LV chamber surface after semiautomated 3D volume analysis (▶ Fig. 3.11 in Chapter 3).

New quantitative tools, e.g., parametric imaging of endocardial displacement, regional timing of endocardial motion, or parameters of left ventricular dyssynchrony such as the systolic dyssynchrony index (SDI), may serve as objective measures of regional ischemia (▢ Fig. 4.5 and ▢ Fig. 4.6).

4.2   Clinical studies on 3D stress echocardiography

In the late 1990s, early studies using first-generation 3D equipment demonstrated that 3D volumetric imaging can be used to analyze regional left ventricular wall motion [8]. Other studies even claimed a high sensitivity and superiority over conventional 2D stress echocardiography [9][10]. However, the overall poor image quality of the purely 3D-dedicated echocardiographic sys-

tem at that time prevented this first approach from widespread clinical use.

❯ A major advantage of 3D stress echocardiography is that it requires significantly shorter scan times.

Since the advent of today's matrix array transducers, several studies have used bi- and triplanar techniques as a first step towards »complete« full volumetric 3D stress echocardiography. Most of them performed comparative studies versus conventional 2D echocardiographic or nuclear imaging [3][5] and found similar accuracy of 3D stress echocardiography compared with 2D and nuclear imaging. The major difference between 3D and 2D stress echocardiography was a significantly shorter scanning time to acquire a triplanar dataset covering the complete LV (=one loop in 4-chamber view, 2-chamber view and apical long-axis from a single apical window) compared to the serial scanning of three different 2D image planes. Importantly, a shorter scanning time did not reduce test accuracy.

Several studies on the use of full volume 3D echocardiography [4][11][12][13][14][15][16] described good correlation between conventional 2D and 3D stress echocardiography with nearly identical sensitivity, specificity, and accuracy. Again, the

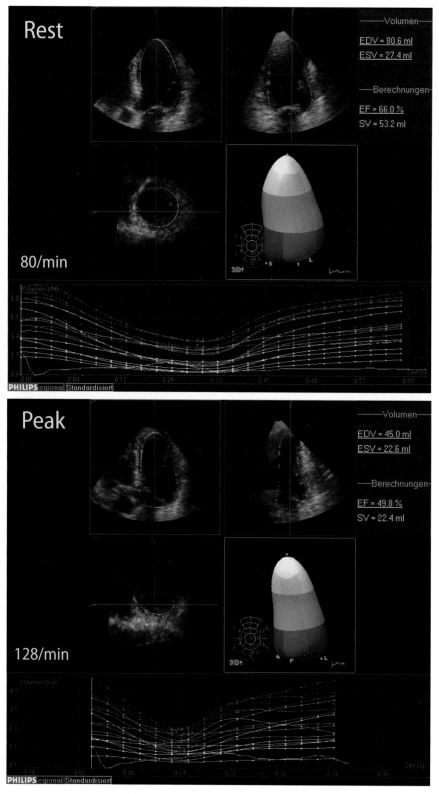

■ **Fig. 4.5** Regional volume–time curves at rest (*top*) and during peak dobutamine stress (*bottom*). Precise analysis of wall motion excursion and temporal contraction patterns become possible

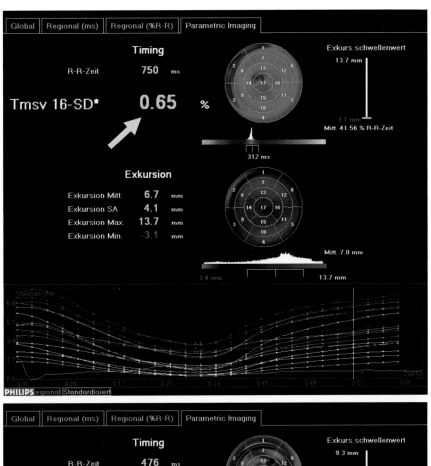

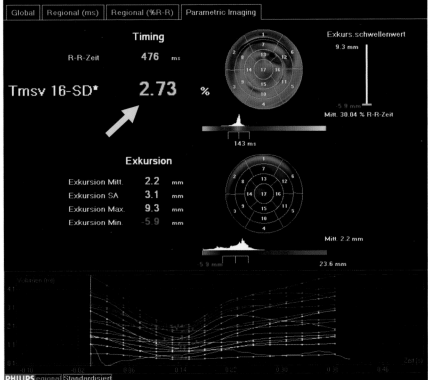

Fig. 4.6 Dyssynchrony and parametric imaging of regional contraction timing and excursion (same patient as in ■ Fig. 4.5). Volume–time curves at rest (*top*) and during peak stress (*bottom*). During peak stress the systolic dyssynchrony index (*SDI*) increases from 0.65 to 2.73%, while a new anterior/anteroseptal wall motion abnormality occurs. The parametric color-coded image of contraction timing demonstrates regions of delayed contraction as *red* areas (both upper bull's eye views), whereas analysis of wall motion excursion (second row of bull's eyes in *blue*) shows no significant change

major difference between the 2D and 3D techniques was a dramatically shorter scanning time to cover the complete LV compared to the serial scanning of three or more 2D image planes.

Analysis of 3D data in the majority of the published studies was performed using manually extracted cut planes from the LV (i.e., normally three long-axis planes and at least three short-axis planes). The examiner then looked for regional wall motion abnormalities in all stress levels separately. Some authors of recent studies used the multislice view integrated into most 3D machines today and performed a side-by-side comparison of loops at rest and at different stress levels (◘ Fig. 4.3 and ◘ Fig. 4.4). Independent of how the analysis was performed, duration tended to be longer than just looking at the conventional 2D stress echocardiography quad screen. This is, however, not due to difficulties of the image quality, the 3D data, or the observer but is caused by the lack of software solutions to automatically extract comparable image cut planes, to arrange them in a side-by-side manner, and to synchronize them.

> Dedicated 3D stress analysis software is urgently required to automatically extract image planes at different stress levels and to arrange them synchronized side-by-side.

As a consequence of these early studies, a skeptical question may evolve: is the benefit of 3D stress echocardiography worth all the trouble? Although sensitivity and specificity are similar to conventional 2D echocardiography, there are specific advantages of a 3D stress echocardiographic workflow:

- There is no need to change the transducer position during apical scanning once the echo window is found. This leads to easier acquisition for both beginners and expert echocardiographers. Moreover, image plane positioning errors including LV foreshortening, which might lead to false positive or negative 2D stress echocardiographic results, can be avoided.
- The narrow time window at peak stress can be used much more effectively when acquiring a complete 3D dataset. An earlier publication on biplanar stress echocardiography [3] demonstrated that this results in a higher heart rate during exercise stress acquisition, which is a prerequisite for the detection of ischemia.
- Three-dimensional stress echocardiography will result in a shorter scanning time at peak stress and perhaps also in a more sensitive monitoring, because more segments can be observed online using the multiple image plane (multislice mode) approach. This may reduce the potential risk of prolonged myocardial ischemia for the individual patient. Beyond this, reduction of stress echocardiography examination time may reduce costs and increase throughput in the stress echocardiography lab.
- Finally, there seem to be advantages not only during acquisition but also in the analysis of regional LV wall motion abnormalities. As in other imaging techniques (e.g., magnetic resonance imaging), interpretation of wall motion abnormalities is easier in short-axis slices instead of long-axis planes. In addition, quantitative parameters such as systolic dyssynchrony index (SDI) or parametric images of LV contraction patterns may reduce inter- and intraobserver variability compared to conventional 2D stress echocardiography.

4.3   Limitations

Despite all potential advantages of 3D echocardiography in combination with stress testing, there are also relevant limitations. Some recently developed matrix array transducers already provide a 2D image quality comparable to high-end 2D transducers. Nevertheless, overall image quality in full volume data sets is still inferior compared to 2D equipment. This is especially true for short-axis slices extracted from apically acquired 3D data caused by a limited line density and lateral resolution. The matrix array probes of several other vendors even today are relatively large and interfere with narrow intercostal spaces – thus, resulting in artifacts or dropouts.

Some authors, therefore, claim that 3D stress echocardiography cannot be performed without using left heart contrast for adequate endocardial delineation [7][16]. However, most recently published studies have used no contrast.

Time resolution of 3D full volume acquisition at present is limited to about 40–50 s (20–25 volumes/s) which is unsatisfactory especially during peak stress with high heart rates and will influence test sensitivity. Increasing time resolution without losing angle width of the acquired pyramidal 3D data set always means accepting a certain trade-off in line density (► Chapter 2). This is equivalent to reduced image quality. In a standard setting most 3D devices today allow the above mentioned temporal resolution – even in single beat acquisition. Using triggered mode (4–7 beats) or reduced acquisition angle (e.g., 80° instead of 108°) and reduced depth will allow significantly higher time resolution up to 100 volumes/s (=10 ms). However, the quality of triggered data always depends on the stability of heart rate, patients' breath hold, and probe position. Thus, the potential advantage of short acquisition time in 3D stress echocardiography may be reduced by the difficulties in obtaining an artifact-free data set.

The limited sector width in earlier versions of 3D echocardiographic equipment was sometimes not wide enough to encompass the complete LV in the ultrasound sector. This was especially true in patients where follow-up of LV function is crucial – those with an apical aneurysm or dilated ventricles. Nowadays, large sector angles up to 104° allow this problem to be circumvented in most cases.

Although acquisition of 3D data is faster than that of 2D images, the analysis requires more time [14]. This is due to the need for manual selection of the analyzed image planes, the larger number of myocardial regions analyzed, and the lack of a commercially available solution for synchronous display of rest, low, and peak dose as well as recovery loops. To date, nearly all vendors of the present 3D echocardiographic systems have not yet achieved internal software solutions that allow an easy-to-use method for the alignment of data at rest and during stress levels. In conventional 2D stress echocardiography, it is a standard technique to have side-by-side visualization of the corresponding image planes at rest and stress levels. With the completeness of 3D data, it becomes a new task to find the same image plane during different stress levels. An improper selection of image planes may add a new and unexpected source of error in the interpretation of 3D stress echocardiography.

Finally, the interpretation of image planes generated from the complete 3D data set remains subjective. The addition of more reliable quantitative tools such as speckle tracking or »3D strain« – at least at the present – is still scientific and challenging, and is still not clinical routine [17].

4.4 New approaches and future perspectives

In principle, a combination of 3D echocardiography with other new modalities such as contrast for myocardial perfusion imaging or strain imaging will open a variety of interesting and promising approaches. The combination of three modalities – 3D, contrast, and stress echocardiography – is challenging and remains difficult. Inherent problems like shadowing due to contrast application itself, rib and lung artifacts causing reduced image quality may interfere significantly with the ability to perform 3D myocardial contrast echocardiography. Nevertheless, there are early studies on the feasibility of such a combined approach which demonstrated not only the feasibility in principle [18] but also that pathological findings can be identified with good agreement to 2D echocardiography.

Tools for automated and quantifiable analysis of wall motion patterns will be helpful to overcome the inherent subjectivity of stress echocardiographic interpretation. This holds true not only for 2D but also for 3D echocardiography. Several approaches for quantitative global and regional wall motion analysis already exist in 3D echocardiography (segmental volume–time curves, systolic dyssynchrony index, parametric imaging; ▶ Chapter 3 and ▶ Chapter 5).

Several studies evaluating the diagnostic value of stress echocardiography demonstrated that not only the severity of stress-induced regional wall motion abnormalities is predictive of outcome, but changes in ejection fraction and ventricular volume are at least equally important [19][20]. As many other studies have shown over the last two decades, 3D echocardiography permits a much more accurate assessment of left ventricular volume and ejection fraction especially in patients with resting wall motion abnormalities. Thus, 3D echocardiography has another potential to further improve the accuracy of 2D stress echocardiography, particularly if LV volume quantification becomes automated as presented for the Heart Model analysis (▶ Chapter 3).

Intraventricular dyssynchrony may also be a marker for stress-induced ischemia. Three-dimensional echocardiography is one of several techniques that have been demonstrated to be capable of detecting dyssynchrony and 3D stress studies are currently underway to evaluate the potential of this technique. Moreover, studies using dynamic maps of contraction, which are derived from full volume datasets, during stress appear promising to more accurately localize and estimate severity of stress-induced ischemia by identifying areas of delayed contraction (▶ Chapter 5) [21].

Another perspective for future use of 3D echocardiography in stress testing is the combination with perfusion imaging which has already been described in a few preliminary studies [22] but still remains difficult. Furthermore, several approaches have been used to quantify dysfunctional myocardial segments [23] to visualize dysfunctional myocardium based on parametric imaging [22], to improve temporal resolution using high volume–rate techniques [25] to analyze regional diastolic properties as an early marker of ischemia [26], or to use speckle tracking for 3D deformation imaging [17].

References

1. Hoffmann R, Lethen H, Marwick T et al (1996) Analysis of interinstitutional observer agreement in interpretation of dobutamine stress echocardiograms. J Am Coll Cardiol 27:330–336
2. Picano E, Lattanzi F, Orlandini A et al (1991) Stress echocardiography and the human factor: the importance of being expert. J Am Coll Cardiol 17:666–669
3. Sugeng L, Kirkpatrick J, Lang RM et al (2003) Biplane stress echocardiography using a prototype matrix-array transducer. J Am Soc Echocardiogr 16:937–941
4. Yang HS, Pellikka PA, McCully RB et al (2006) Role of biplane and biplane echocardiographically guided 3-dimensional echocardiography during dobutamine stress echocardiography. J Am Soc Echocardiogr 19:1136–1143
5. Eroglu E, D'hooge J, Herbots L et al (2006) Comparison of real-time tri-plane and conventional 2D dobutamine stress echocardiography for the assessment of coronary artery disease. Eur Heart J 27:1719–1724
6. Pulerwitz T, Hirata K, Abe Y et al (2006) Feasibility of using a real-time 3-dimensional technique for contrast dobutamine stress echocardiography. J Am Soc Echocardiogr 19:540–545
7. Takeuchi M, Otani S, Weinert L et al (2006) Comparison of contrast-enhanced real-time live 3-dimensional dobutamine stress echocardiography with contrast 2-dimensional echocardiography for detecting stress-induced wall-motion abnormalities. J Am Soc Echocardiogr 19:294–299
8. Collins M, Hsieh A, Ohazama CJ et al (1999) Assessment of regional wall motion abnormalities with real-time 3-dimensional echocardiography. J Am Soc Echocardiogr 12:7–14
9. Ahmad M, Xie T, McCulloch M et al (2001) Real-time three-dimensional dobutamine stress echocardiography in assessment of ischemia: comparison with two-dimensional dobutamine stress echocardiography. J Am Coll Cardiol 37:1303–1309
10. Zwas DR, Takuma S, Mullis-Jansson S et al (1999) Feasibility of real-time-3-dimensional treadmill stress echocardiography. J Am Soc Echocardiogr 12:285–289
11. Matsumura Y, Hozumi T, Arai K et al (2005) Non-invasive assessment of myocardial ischaemia using new real-time three-dimensional dobutamine stress echocardiography: comparison with conventional two-dimensional methods. Eur Heart J 26:1625–1632
12. Yang HS, Bansal RC, Mookadam F et al (2008) Practical guide for three-dimensional transthoracic echocardiography using a fully sampled matrix array transducer. J Am Soc Echocardiogr 21:979–989
13. Aggeli C, Giannopoulos G, Misovoulos P et al (2007) Real-time three-dimensional dobutamine stress echocardiography for coronary artery disease diagnosis: validation with coronary angiography. Heart 93: 672–675
14. Varnero S, Santagata P, Pratali L et al (2008) Head to head comparison of 2D vs. 3D dipyridamole stress echocardiography. Cardiovasc Ultrasound 6:31
15. Nemes A, Geleijnse ML, Krenning BJ et al (2007) Usefulness of ultrasound contrast agent to improve image quality during real-time three-dimensional stress echocardiography. Am J Cardiol 99:275–278
16. Krenning BJ, Nemes A, Soliman OI et al (2008) Contrast-enhanced three-dimensional dobutamine stress echocardiography: between Scylla and Charybdis? Eur J Echocardiogr 9:757–760

17. Seo Y, Ishizu T, Enomoto Y (2011) Endocardial surface area tracking for assessment of regional LV wall deformation with 3D speckle tracking imaging. JACC Cardiovasc Imaging 4:358–365

18. Bhan A, Kapetanakis S, Rana BS et al (2008) Real-time three-dimensional myocardial contrast echocardiography: is it clinically feasible? Eur J Echocardiogr 9:761–765

19. Kort S, Mamidipally S, Madahar P et al (2010). Segmental contribution to left ventricular systolic function at rest and stress: a quantitative real time three-dimensional echocardiographic study. Echocardiography 27:167–173

20. Walimbe V, Garcia M, LaLude O et al (2007) Quantitative real-time 3-dimensional stress echocardiography: a preliminary investigation of feasibility and effectiveness. J Am Soc Echocardiogr 20:13–22

21. Jenkins C, Haluska B, Marwick TH (2009) Assessment of temporal heterogeneity and regional motion to identify wall motion abnormalities using treadmill exercise stress three-dimensional echocardiography. J Am Soc Echocardiogr 22:268–275

22. Abdelmoneim SS, Bernier M, Dhoble A et al (2010) Assessment of myocardial perfusion during adenosine stress using real time three-dimensional and two-dimensional myocardial contrast echocardiography: comparison with single-photon emission computed tomography. Echocardiography 27:421–429

23. Leung KY, van Stralen M, Danilouchkine MG et al (2011) Automated analysis of three-dimensional stress echocardiography. Neth Heart J 19:307–310

24. Ahmad M, Dimmano M, Xie C (2008) Advances in parametric 3D echocardiography in quantitative estimation of dobutamine stress induced ischemia. Circulation 118:S850–851

25. Badano LP, Muraru D, Rigo F et al (2010) High volume-rate three-dimensional stress echocardiography to assess inducible myocardial ischemia: a feasibility study. J Am Soc Echocardiogr 23:628–635

26. Kort S, Mamidipally S, Madahar P et al (2011) Real time three-dimensional stress echocardiography: a new approach for assessing diastolic function. Echocardiography 28:676–683

Cardiac dyssynchrony

Mark J. Monaghan, Shaumik Adhya

T. Buck et al. (Hrsg.), *Three-dimensional Echocardiography*,
DOI 10.1007/978-3-642-36799-1_5, © Springer-Verlag Berlin Heidelberg 2014

Cardiac dyssynchrony refers to an uncoordinated pattern of electrical activation, mechanical contraction, and relaxation of the heart. The substrate for dyssynchrony lies in dysfunction of the specialized electrical conduction tissue of the heart, or impaired conduction of electrical signals through working myocardium, or in delayed mechanical contraction or relaxation of the myocardium. Real-time 3-dimensional echocardiography (RT3DE) has enabled the whole of the left ventricle to be imaged simultaneously and allowed the development of a method to quantify intraventricular mechanical dyssynchrony.

5.1   Technique

5.1.1   Acquisition of 3D volumes

The acquisition of three-dimensional (3D) volumes that incorporate the whole left ventricle can be challenging on most commercially available 3D systems, because the whole heart cannot yet be acquired in a single heartbeat with adequate temporal and spatial resolution. In order to improve temporal resolution, small subvolumes are acquired in succession, which are stitched together by software. A minimum of four subvolumes is generally required to encompass the entire left ventricle. It is possible to increase the number of subvolumes to create a larger full volume dataset for use in patients with large ventricles. The size of the subvolumes can also be decreased, and therefore the number of segments required increased in order to increase the frame rate of acquisition. To minimize respiratory translation artifact, breath-holding is required during the acquisition sequence [1]. Patients in whom the length of the cardiac cycle varies, such as in atrial fibrillation are more likely to have significant stitching artifacts. Frequent ventricular ectopy also causes stitching artifacts, as well as not representing cardiac contraction during a sinus beat. The very latest generation of 3D ultrasound systems have the ability to acquire a full volume dataset in one cardiac cycle (one-beat full volume; ► Chapter 2.3.2), which helps to overcome these issues. However, experience with these new systems is currently limited.

In centers that have published their work with 3D echocardiography, the proportion of subjects who have inadequate quality datasets is low with a rate between 0% [2] and 8.3% [3]. In patients with heart disease, the proportion increases to between 7% [4] and 19.5% [5]. Even in patients who are deemed to have adequate scans, not every segment may be visible. The most difficult area to image is the anterior wall. Most of the published work has not described the approach to poorly visible single segments, but it is our practice to allow the software to interpolate the image, but to disregard this if it seems discordant with the 2D imaging of the same segment. Contrast may also be used in difficult to image patients since some software versions are able to accurately track the endocardium in contrast enhanced datasets.

The published experience is summarized in ◼Tab. 5.1.

5.1.2   Measures of intraventricular dyssynchrony

Kapetanakis et al. [5] developed a method using 3D echocardiography to quantify intraventricular dyssynchrony. Full volume datasets including the whole left ventricle (LV) are analyzed using semiautomated software. This requires the user to define three cut planes through the 3D dataset, and define a few points of the endocardial border in each plane, at both end systole and end diastole. Use of an edge-detection algorithm allows the extrapolation of these points to define the endocardial border accurately in each frame. This produces a mathematical cast of the left ventricle and the center of contraction of this cast can be calculated. The cast can be segmented into 16 volumes that correspond to the American Society for Echocardiography classification [6], and a curve produced for each segment of volume over time as a percentage of the cardiac cycle. The standard deviation of the time to minimum volumes, expressed as a percentage of the R-R interval, has been termed the systolic dyssynchrony index (SDI-16).

❯ The standard deviation of the time to minimum volumes of the LV segments has been termed the systolic dyssynchrony index.

Other investigators have used variations on this technique, using the same index but generated by alternative software [4][7][8]. This particular software requires the user to determine five points of the endocardial border, edit the endocardial border in systole and diastole if necessary, and then this automatically tracks the border throughout the cardiac cycle. The software also divides the left ventricular cast into 17 segments and excludes the apical segment to give a value that is confusingly also termed SDI-16. Since there are important differences in how the SDI is derived between different 3D analysis software, we will append Q to make it apparent where the latter software has been used, i.e., SDI-16Q. Although both types of software aim to generate the same index, there are differences in the amount of user involvement, segmentation, definition of the center of gravity and edge-detection algorithms, which means that the values generated are not necessarily directly comparable.

Even when using the same software packages, different measures may be used. Calculation of the SDI-16 as a percentage of the cardiac cycle allows comparison of this value between patients with differing heart rates [5]. However, some investigators have used absolute times to calculate the SDI-16, giving a result that is denominated in milliseconds [8]. Comparison with tissue Doppler imaging assessments of dyssynchrony has led some investigators to ignore the apical region and calculate the SDI of the 12 basal and mid ventricular segments [9]. Yet others have divided the LV cast into 17 segments to give the SDI-17 [10]. So there have been a number of variations on the same theme in terms of performing 3D echocardiographic assessment of dyssynchrony.

The use of 3D echocardiography to assess dyssynchrony has been validated against other imaging modalities including cardiac MRI [11] and gated myocardial perfusion single photon emission computed tomography [12]. These studies demonstrated a close correlation between the methods in the assessment of

LV function and regional wall motion. Also when the same semi-automated software used for 3D echocardiographic analysis is used to analyze cardiac MRI, the results are comparable to that of an expert interpreter of cardiac MRI [11].

Speckle tracking has recently been extended into three dimensions. This methodology uses the inherent echo-texture of the myocardium to identify speckles and track these points throughout the cardiac cycle. Perez de Isla et al. [13] have published their experience of 30 consecutive patients with good echocardiographic windows and this technique. The user defines the apex and two mitral valve hinge points in two orthogonal planes. The thickness of the myocardium is then defined and the software identifies tissue speckles and tracks them throughout the cardiac cycle. The percentage of segments with this 3D method was greater than that with 2D speckle tracking (72.4% vs. 52.0%; p<0.001). The total study time was significantly shorter with 3D than with 2D echocardiography (5.1±1.1 vs. 14.0 ± 1.9 min; p<0.001), and this was the case for both acquisition time and analysis time. There were also no differences between 2D and 3D wall motion tracking for radial strain (20.32±8.22% vs. 19.49±7.86%; p=0.66) and longitudinal strain (2.47±0.95% vs. 2.14±0.15%; p=0.10). This suggests that 3D strain assessment is feasible and quicker than 2D assessment.

The dyssynchrony indices derived from 3D speckle tracking include those evaluated in 2D speckle or tissue Doppler imaging, namely the dispersion of time to peak strain in any direction across a number of myocardial segments. Area strain has been developed as a novel 3D speckle tracking-derived index for the quantitative assessment of global and regional function [14, 15]. This divides the endocardial surface into multiple segments and measures the percentage change in area throughout the cardiac cycle compared to the reference area of the segment at end-diastole. This is therefore not a directional change unlike conventional radial, circumferential, and longitudinal strains. Again, similar to SDI, the standard deviation of the time to minimum segmental area can be used as a measure of dyssynchrony. This measure has been termed area strain–systolic dyssynchrony index (ASDI).

5.1.3 Performing 3D analysis

Here, we will work through the steps required for 3D analysis. Although the software packages vary slightly, the principle remains the same. Our practice is to acquire at least three 3D volumes and to briefly examine them offline to choose the best image quality volume for analysis. For robust analysis, several volumes may be analyzed and the results averaged. The first step of the analysis is to align the left ventricle so that the central axis runs through the apex and the middle of the mitral valve, as in ◘ Fig. 5.1 and ▶ Video 5.1A. This is performed in all cut planes to ensure that the axis is defined correctly in three dimensions. Then the user marks a number of points of the endocardial border at both end-systole and end-diastole. This is illustrated in a healthy patient in the 4-chamber view in ◘ Fig. 5.1 and ▶ Video 5.1B. This figure contains four panels: the top left shows the short-axis cut plane, the top right the 4-chamber view at end-systole, the bottom left the moving image of the 4-chamber cut plane, and the bottom right the 4-chamber view at end-diastole. We mark the border at end-systole, and assess its accuracy on the

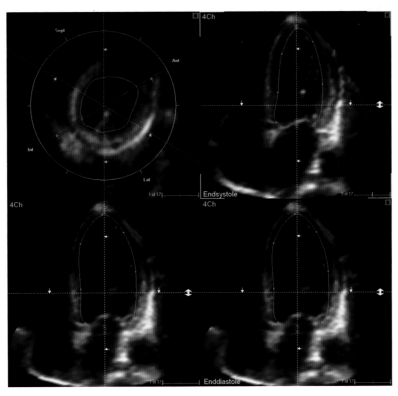

◘ **Fig. 5.1** Marking the endocardial border in the 4-chamber cut plane in a healthy patient. See text for details. *Sept* septal, *Ant* anterior, *Inf* inferior, *Lat* lateral. [→Video 5.1 A, B]

Tab. 5.1 Summary of published data on populations, echocardiographic equipment, and measurement variability

Author	Subjects	Echo hardware	Software	Dyssynchrony index	Normal exclusion rate	Patient exclusion rate	Intrapatient variability of SDI (n)	Intraobserver variability of SDI (n)	Interobserver variability of SDI (n)
Kapetanakis et al. [5]	89 normal 174 patients	Philips Sonos 7500	Tomtec	SDI-16	10.30%	19.50%	4.6% (15)	8.1% (20)	6.4% (20)
Burgess et al. [9]	100 patients with ischemic cardiomyopathy	Philips Sonos 7500	Tomtec	SDI-12	n/a	23%	n/a	14% (10)	18% (10)
Takeuchi et al. [8]	21 normal, 100 patients	Philips iE33	Qlab 4.2	SDI-16, SDI-12, SDI-6, all in ms	n/a	n/a	n/a	32% (8)	56% (8)
Marsan et al. [4]	60 patients with heart failure referred for CRT	Philips iE33	Qlab 5.0	SDI-16	n/a	7%	n/a	0.03±0.5% (mean difference ± SD)	0.1±1% (mean difference ± SD)
Delgado et al. [7]	10 normal, 50 patients	Philips Sonos 7500	Qlab 4.0	SDI-16	0%	12%	n/a	2.5% (18)	3.8% (18)
Van Dijk et al. [2]	17 normal 45 with LBBB	Philips Sonos 7500	Tomtec	SDI-16	0%	18%	n/a	1.5% (15)	6.7% (18)
Gimenes et al. [3]	131 normal	Philips iE33	Qlab	SDI-16	8.30%	n/a	n/a	ICC 0.8659 (30)	ICC 0.8218 (30)
Baker et al. [37]	9 normal children, 9 with LV dysfunction	Philips iE33 & Sonos 7500	Qlab 4.2	SDI-16	18%	0%	n/a	n/a	n/a
Conca et al. [18]	120 normal	GE Vivid 7	Tomtec	SDI-16	15%	n/a	n/a	negligible	negligible
Soliman et al. [17]	60 normal, 84 patients with HF	Philips iE33	Qlab 6.0	SDI-16	0%	16%	n/a	10.2% (50)	12% (50)
Ten Harkel et al. [21]	73 normal adolescents	Philips iE33	Qlab	SDI-16	8%	n/a	n/a	0.3±0.2% (mean difference ±SD)	0±0.27% (mean difference ±SD)
Cui et al. [22]	125 normal children	Philips iE33	Qlab	SDI-16	18%	n/a	n/a	5.10%	7.60%
Yang et al. [42]	25 patients with AMI	Philips Sonos 7500	Tomtec	SDI-16	n/a	24%	n/a	5.2% (10) for EF	6.6% (10) for EF
Porciani et al. [45]	20 patients with CRT	Philips iE33	Qlab 5.0	SDI-16, SDI-12, Sdi-6	n/a	n/a	n/a	n/a	n/a
Becker et al. [47]	58 patients with CRT	Philips iE33 & Sonos 7500	Tomtec	SDI-16	n/a	n/a	n/a	n/a	n/a
Marsan et al. [12]	40 patients with HF	Philips iE33	Qlab 5.0	SDI-16	n/a	n/a	n/a	0.03±0.4% (mean difference ±SD), (20)	0.1±1% (mean difference ±SD), (20)
Van Dijk et al. [10]	17 referred for CRT	Philips iE33 & Sonos 7500	Tomtec	SDI-17	n/a	n/a	n/a	n/a	n/a

◻ Tab. 5.1 (continued)

Author	Subjects	Echo hardware	Software	Dyssynchrony index	Normal exclusion rate	Patient exclusion rate	Intrapatient variability of SDI (n)	Intraobserver variability of SDI (n)	Interobserver variability of SDI (n)
Nesser et al. [11]	31 patients	Philips Sonos 7500	Tomtec	SDI-16	n/a	6.10%	n/a	n/a	n/a
Soliman et al. [27]	90 patients with CRT	Philips iE33	Qlab 6.0	SDI-16	n/a	6%	n/a	n/a	11%
De Castro et al. [23]	116 healthy, 22 athletes, 35 with LV dysfunction & 84 with LV dysfunction & LBBB	Philips iE33	Tomtec 2.0	SDI-16	n/a	4.50%	n/a	0.02±0.44% (mean difference ±SD), (50)	−0.04±0.52% (mean difference ±SD), (50)
Zeng et al. [24]	24 healthy, 24 DCM	Philips iE33	Qlab 4.2	SDI-16	n/a	n/a	n/a	n/a	n/a
Liu et al. [32]	35 patients with SSS	Philips Sonos 7500	Tomtec 2.0	SDI-16	n/a	n/a	n/a	ICC 0.905 (9)	ICC 0.892 (9)
Raedle-Hurst et al. [39]	30 adults with CHD, 30 controls	GE Vivid 7	Tomtec	SDI-16 & 17	n/a	n/a	n/a	n/a	n/a
Miyazaki et al. [28]	131 patients EF<35%	Philips iE33 & Sonos 7500	Not Specified	SDI-16 (TmsV)	n/a	20.60%	n/a	23.7% (18)	23.1% (18)
Kapetanakis et al. [29]	187 patients undergoing CRT	Philips iE33 & Sonos 7500	Tomtec 2.0	SDI-16	n/a	7%	n/a	n/a	7.6% (62)
Fang et al. [34]	93 patients with SSS, 93 healthy controls	Philips iE33	Qlab 6.0	SDI-16 (TmsV)	n/a	n/a	n/a	4.4% (15)	6.5% (15)
Tanaka et al. [36]	57 patients undergoing CRT, 10 healthy controls	Toshiba Artida	Toshiba	SD-16 time to peak strain, maximal opposing wall delay	n/a	overall 6% of LV segments excluded	n/a	9% (n/a)	9% (n/a)
Thebault et al. [20]	60 patients undergoing CRT	Toshiba Artida	Toshiba UltraExtend	SD-16 time to peak strain	n/a	15.00%	n/a	6% (20)	10% (20)

CRT cardiac resynchronization therapy, *n/a* not available, *SSS* sick sinus syndrome, *EF* ejection fraction, *CHD* congenital heart disease, *DCM* dilated cardiomyopathy, *SD* standard deviation, *LV* left ventricle, *HF* heart failure, *AMI* acute myocardial infarction, *LBBB* left bundle branch block.

moving image, before marking the border at end-diastole. This software package requires this process to be repeated in other cut planes. The software uses these points, together with edge-detection algorithms to define the endocardial border, and track this border through the cardiac cycle. This generates the mathematical cast, which should be inspected for accuracy and adjusted if necessary as seen in ◘ Fig. 5.2 and ► Video 5.2. The volume of each segment is plotted against time, and the time to minimum volume identified as shown in ◘ Fig. 5.3 and ► Video 5.3. The standard deviation of these times, corrected for the duration of the cardiac cycle, is termed the systolic dyssynchrony index. The numerical results of the analysis in a healthy patient are illustrated in ◘ Fig. 5.4. The software also allows the analysis of many more points than the standard 16- or 17-segment models and can generate a plot demonstrating contraction spreading through the ventricle. As the contraction front spreads through the ventricle, the color changes from blue through white to red. This allows areas of late contraction to be easily identified. This is illustrated in the lower left panel of ◘ Fig. 5.3 and ► Video 5.3. This intuitive method of visualization has been termed contraction front mapping, although its clinical utility is as yet uncertain.

In large, dilated, dyssynchronous ventricles, analysis can be more challenging. As the LV becomes more spherical, the apical segment enlarges, and it can be difficult to define the central axis of the ventricle. It is also necessary to check that the software has correctly identified the end-systolic and end-diastolic frames. Care needs to be taken with border marking,

as there is less difference between the borders at end-systole and end-diastole than in a normal ventricle, which may be confusing. This is illustrated in ◘ Fig. 5.5, and ► Video 5.5. Inspection of the cast is shown in ◘ Fig. 5.6 and ► Video 5.6, and contraction front mapping and volume time curves are illustrated in ◘ Fig. 5.7 and ► Video 5.7. The final results are illustrated in ◘ Fig. 5.8.

Development of software packages has led to increasing automation of the above process. This has the advantage of speed and intuitively should lead to less intra- and interobserver variability. However, it is important to visually confirm the automatic border detection is correct and, if necessary, manually adjust it. Similarly, it is important to visually assess tracking throughout the cardiac cycle. Any advantage in terms of variability using automatic over manual techniques will be lost if manual adjustment is necessary.

5.1.4 Measurement variability

Any method that purports to measure dyssynchrony must be reliable and reproducible. This is particularly important for those techniques that have a significant learning curve. Three-dimensional echocardiography requires expertise not only in the acquisition of datasets, but also in their analysis. In the era after the PROSPECT trial [16], where even core laboratories had poor agreement between measures, this is highly pertinent.

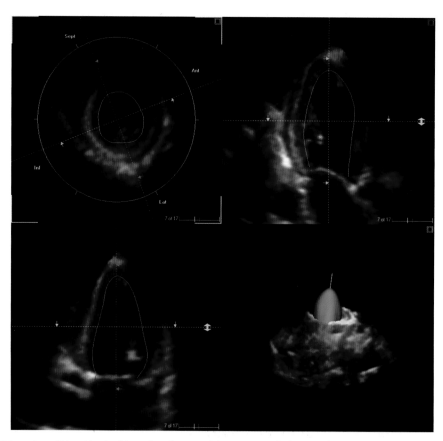

◘ **Fig. 5.2** Inspection of the endocardial cast in a healthy patient. *Sept* septal, *Ant* anterior, *Inf* inferior, *Lat* lateral. [→Video 5.2]

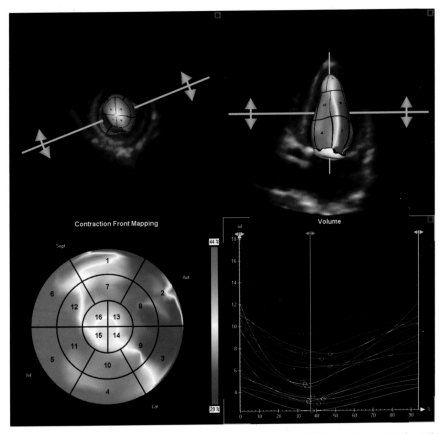

Fig. 5.3 Volume–time curve for the 16 segments in a healthy patient. *Sept* septal, *Ant* anterior, *Inf* inferior, *Lat* lateral. [→Video 5.3]

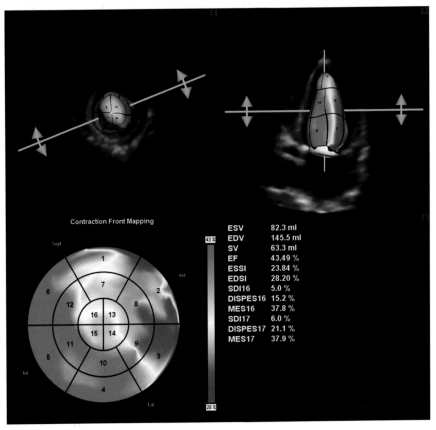

Fig. 5.4 Final results in a healthy patient. *Sept* septal, *Ant* anterior, *Inf* inferior, *Lat* lateral

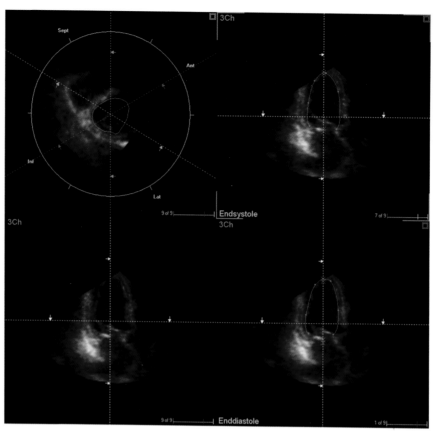

◘ **Fig. 5.5** Marking the LV endocardial border in 3-chamber cut plane in a dyssynchronous ventricle. *Sept* septal, *Ant* anterior, *Inf* inferior, *Lat* lateral. [→Video 5.5]

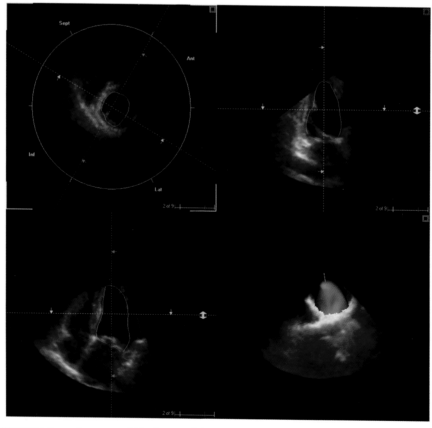

◘ **Fig. 5.6** Inspection of LV cast in a dyssynchronous ventricle. *Sept* septal, *Ant* anterior, *Inf* inferior, *Lat* lateral. [→Video 5.6]

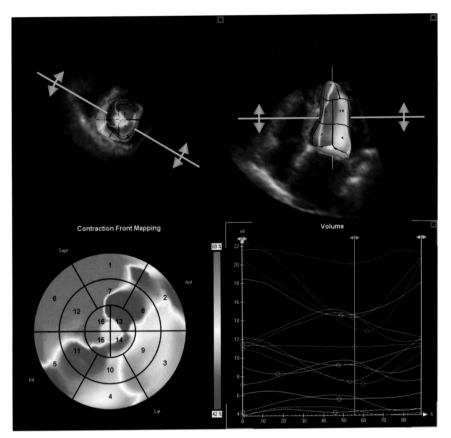

◘ **Fig. 5.7** Contraction front mapping and volume–time curves in a dyssynchronous ventricle. *Sept* septal, *Ant* anterior, *Inf* inferior, *Lat* lateral.
[→Video 5.7 A, B]

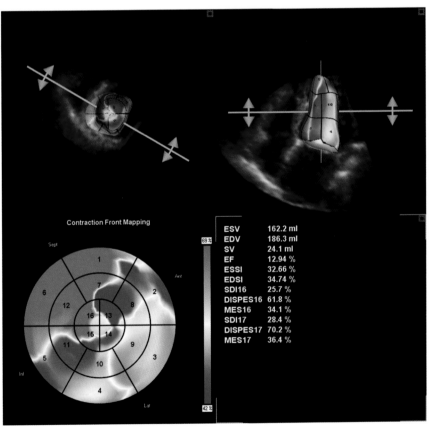

◘ **Fig. 5.8** Final results in a dyssynchronous ventricle. *Sept* septal, *Ant* anterior, *Inf* inferior, *Lat* lateral

Few studies have looked for intrapatient reproducibility but one observer studied 15 patients within 24 h and showed good intraclass correlation coefficients (ICC) and variability for end-diastolic volume (EDV), left ventricular ejection fraction (LVEF), and SDI-16 with 0.99 and 1%, 0.98 and 3.7%, and 0.88 and 4.6%, respectively [5]. Soliman et al. [17] also performed test–retest reproducibility on 10 subjects and showed an ICC of 0.951, and a variability of 10%.

Intraobserver and interobserver reproducibility has been reported by most groups, with a range of intraobserver correlation coefficients for SDI-16Q between 0.8659 [3] and 0.996 [17], and interobserver correlation of between 0.818 [3] and 0.993 [17]. Reproducibility is also better in patients with good quality datasets when compared to moderate quality datasets [17].

> Reproducibility of SDI measurements has been shown to be better in patients with good quality 3D datasets.

Interinstitutional variability for SDI-16Q has also been reported [18]. This group recruited 120 normal subjects in Switzerland, and their datasets were analyzed in both Switzerland and in Minnesota, USA. Although the mean values and 95% confidence intervals of SDI-16Q did not overlap, the concordance correlation coefficient and the limits of agreement suggested that there was no significant difference in the measurements between the two institutions.

Data for 3D speckle tracking-derived dyssynchrony indices are lacking. Tanaka et al. [19] reported on the intra- and interobserver variability for 3D derived radial strain dyssynchrony, which were 9±7% and 9±8% respectively. Thebault et al. [20] also reported variability data but for global area strain, rather than for any 3D strain-derived dyssynchrony indices.

5.2   Normal values

Normal values for dyssynchrony and ejection fraction by 3D echocardiography have been generated by a number of groups who have studied varying numbers and ages of patients. The studies have varied as to those using normal volunteers or patients referred for routine echocardiography who were deemed to be normal. Four studies have attempted to define normal ranges in adults by taking large samples of normal subjects, but most studies have used a small sample as a control group against whom to compare the results from their patients. Published values are summarized in ▢ Tab. 5.2.

Two major studies have been performed in children. Ten Harkel et al. [21] reported on 73 adolescents aged 12–18 years and found a mean SDI-16Q of 1.26%. Cui et al. [22] reported on 125 normal children aged from 1–19 years with a mean SDI-16Q of 1.16%. Both Ten Harkel et al. and Cui et al. found no significant effect of age or patient size on these results and Cui et al. also reported that dyssynchrony was independent of heart rate and left ventricular end-diastolic volume.

Kapetanakis et al. [5] studied 89 healthy adults and suggested that the upper limit of normal SDI-16 was 8.3% because this value was three standard deviations above the mean value of 3.5%. Gimenes et al. [3] investigated 131 subjects, 73 were male and the average age was 46±14 years. These subjects did not have any structural cardiac abnormalities or history of cardiac disease, but had been referred for routine echocardiography. The mean SDI-16Q was 1.59±0.99%. The frequency distribution of SDI-16Q values are appreciably skewed to the left (▢ Fig. 5.9).

Conca et al. [18] published results of their investigation of 120 normal subjects in an attempt to define normal ranges for 3D

▢ Tab. 5.2 Summary of published normal values for left ventricular ejection fraction and SDI

First author	Normal volunteers, n	Software	Mean ejection fraction (%)	SDI-16
Baker [37]	9 children	Qlab 4.2	60.8 (range 44.3–72.1)	2.1 (range 0.71–2.78)
Brunekreeft [48]	23	Tomtec	62.7±6.7	2.5±1.3
Conca [18]	120	Tomtec	67	2.7±1.1
Cui [22]	125 children	Qlab	68.3±7.1	1.16±0.58
De Castro [23]	116 20 athletes	Tomtec	59.2±4.5 59.4±4.3	2.37±0.81 2.89±0.59
Delgado [7]	10	Qlab 4.0	62±4	1.5±0.7
Gimenes [3]	120	Qlab	66.1±7.1	1.59±0.99
Kapetanakis [5]	78	Tomtec	61±6.4	3.5±1.8
Liu [32]	9	Tomtec	58.9±5.5	SDI 17 5.28±1.64
Soliman [17]	60	Qlab 6.0	60±8	4.1±2.2
Takeuchi [8]	21	Qlab 4.2	>60 by definition	17ms±10ms
Ten Harkel [21]	73 adolescents	Qlab	60±8	1.26±0.53
Van Dijk [2]	16	Tomtec	54±5	5.6±3.6
Zeng [24]	25	Qlab 4.2	66.2±6.0	1.1±0.6

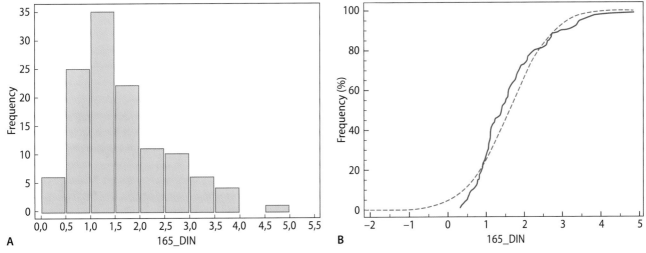

Fig. 5.9 Histogram (**A**) and cumulative frequency distribution (**B**) of SDI-16 in 120 healthy individuals. Modified from [3]; Copyright J Am Soc Echocardiogr

SDI-16Q, as well as tissue Doppler and radial strain imaging. This study was powered to be able to define 90% confidence intervals around the mean value. Although they investigated 120 normal subjects, they were only able to perform 3D assessment in 102 patients. They proposed a normal range for SDI-16Q of 1–4.8%, based on the 97.5% confidence intervals for their population. Interestingly, they found that there was little concordance between the two centers for tissue Doppler and radial strain imaging, but significant concordance in SDI-16Q.

De Castro et al. [23] studied 116 healthy volunteers and 20 elite athletes. They validated their results by performing cardiac MRI on 20 of these subjects. In healthy volunteers the mean SDI-16 was 2.37±0.8%. They also describe the pattern of contraction seen in these subjects. The apex appears the most synchronous and contracts earliest, whilst the basal segments are slightly less synchronous and contract later. Thus, they describe a contraction time gradient from apex to base.

> Most studies agree that the normal value of SDI-16 is approximately 3% and that most healthy individuals have values below 6%.

While the normal ranges for any test should be determined locally, most studies agree that the normal value of SDI-16 in adults is approximately 3% and that most healthy individuals have values below 6%. Normal values in children appear to be lower at less than 2%. There do not appear to be significant differences in the normal range dependent upon the software used to generate SDI-16. There is an overlap between this normal range and the values seen in mild left ventricular dysfunction. However, values in the context of cardiac disease are discussed below.

5.3 Dyssynchrony in heart failure and left bundle branch block

5.3.1 Relationship between left ventricular function and dyssynchrony

Studies in this area have focused on several heterogeneous groups of patients. These include patients with any form of cardiovascular disease, patients with heart failure (HF) and impaired ejection fraction (EF), patients with left bundle branch block (LBBB) with and without symptoms, and patients who are candidates for cardiac resynchronization therapy (CRT). The goal has been to describe the distribution of dyssynchrony in disease, as well as to see if 3D measures of dyssynchrony can help to better select patients who might benefit from CRT than the QRS duration alone.

Most groups that have looked at patients with cardiovascular disease and a range of cardiac function have demonstrated a strong negative correlation between EF and SDI-16 [5][8][9][24][25]. This is illustrated in ▪ Fig. 5.10.

> A strong negative correlation between EF and SDI-16 has been demonstrated in several studies.

However, this correlation may be weaker in patients with drug-refractory symptomatic HF. In 40 patients referred to a heart failure clinic there was no significant difference in SDI-16Q between patients with an EF<30% (6.9±3%) as compared to patients with an EF>30% (8.8±6.3%) [12]. The QRS width may be a confounding factor in this study as this cohort contained patients with both narrow and broad QRS and the distribution of broad QRS is unclear between the two groups with EF>30% and EF<30%.

It is difficult to separate dyssynchrony induced by LBBB alone with that seen in impaired left ventricular function, especially as LBBB is rare in healthy individuals. One group addressed this question by analyzing the difference in dyssynchrony indices between normal subjects, asymptomatic subjects with LBBB, and patients with HF and LBBB [2]. In the normal subjects, mean

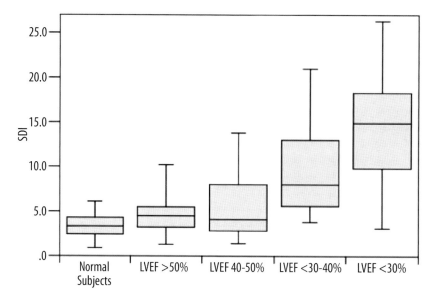

■ **Fig. 5.10** Box plot displaying 10th, 25th, 50th, 75th and 90th percentiles of systolic dyssynchrony index (*SDI*) in normal subjects, patients with normal left ventricular ejection fraction (*LVEF*), and patients with mild, moderate, or severe left ventricular function (p<0.001 for trend). Modified from [5]; Copyright American Heart Association

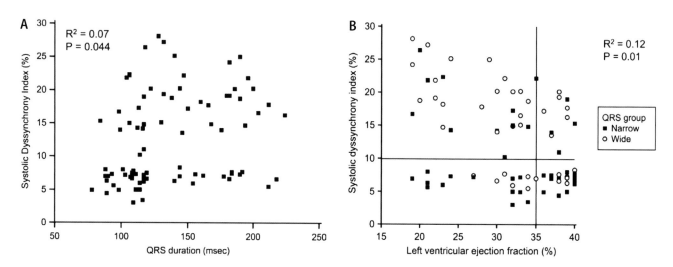

■ **Fig. 5.11** Linear regression plot displaying the relationship between the left ventricular SDI (systolic dyssynchrony index) and (**A**) QRS duration and (**B**) left ventricle ejection fraction in 84 patients with heart failure. Modified from [27]; Copyright Elsevier

LVEF was 54±5% and SDI-16 was 5.6±3.6%, in patients with asymptomatic LBBB the LVEF was 50±9%, and SDI-16 7.3±3.2%, and in heart failure patients with LBBB the LVEF was 29±9% and SDI-16 12.8±4.8%. SDI-16 was significantly higher in HF patients than both other groups, but although the mean SDI-16 in subjects with asymptomatic LBBB was higher than normal subjects, this difference did not reach statistical significance (p=0.08). In addition, the mean QRS duration in the asymptomatic LBBB group was less than that of patients with HF and LBBB, which also did not quite reach statistical significance (p=0.052). This suggests there may be a correlation between QRS width and SDI-16.

However, another study found this correlation between QRS width and SDI-16 in patients with HF to be weak. Soliman et al.

[17] studied 84 patients with HF and either a narrow (mean QRS 98±12 ms, 30 patients) or wide QRS (mean QRS 157±26 ms, 54 patients). The SDI-16Q was significantly larger in the wide QRS group (15.0±7.9%) than in the narrow QRS group (10.5±7.7%, p<0.01). The correlation between the QRS duration and the SDI-16Q was weak (r^2=0.07, p<0.05), as was the correlation between the SDI-16Q and the LVEF (r^2=0.12, p<0.01). Of this cohort, 20% of the patients with HF with LVEF less than 35% had a narrow QRS and high SDI-16Q, and 14% of the patients with HF with LVEF greater than 35% had narrow QRS and high SDI-16Q. This is illustrated in ■ Fig. 5.11.

5.3.2 Patterns of dyssynchrony

Three-dimensional echocardiography has revealed some insights into the pattern of dyssynchrony in patients with left ventricular dysfunction. A comparative study of tissue Doppler and 3D dyssynchrony found that 3D echocardiography was less sensitive than tissue Doppler at detecting significant dyssynchrony and that the areas of maximum delay varied by tissue Doppler and 3D echocardiography [9]. The anteroseptal and septal walls were more frequently the most delayed in 3D echocardiography, while by tissue Doppler it was the lateral and posterior walls. This is illustrated in ◘ Fig. 5.7, in which the lower left panel shows contraction front mapping and the septal wall to be red indicating delayed contraction. This variation occurred even in patients deemed to have good images. When 3D echocardiography and TDI assessment of maximal delay was compared to delay by anatomical M-mode, the correlation was higher with 3D than TDI. In this population of patients, the average ejection fraction was 37% by 2D echocardiography and average SDI-12 was 8.3%.

Furthermore, De Castro et al. [23] studied 39 patients with left ventricular dysfunction and narrow QRS (24 ischemic heart disease, 15 DCM), and 90 patients with left ventricular dysfunction and LBBB. They found that patients with left ventricular dysfunction had more dyssynchrony than normal and that patients with LBBB were more dyssynchronous than those with narrow QRS. The pattern of contraction also differed between the groups, with a time gradient from apical to basal contraction in patients with narrow QRS, but not in patients with LBBB in whom the mid segment often contracted before the apical segments. This emphasizes the importance of assessing apical contraction and dyssynchrony, as many methods such as tissue Doppler imaging do not interrogate the apex. It is also important to realize that some 3D analysis software excludes the apical cap in their 16-segment model, though it still appears to have useful predictive value.

5.3.3 SDI as a predictor of outcome of cardiac resynchronization therapy

Cardiac resynchronization therapy (CRT) is a useful therapy in some patients with heart failure but it is acknowledged that up to a third of patients who meet current criteria for CRT implantation do not improve symptomatically [26]. A variety of techniques have been assessed to evaluate whether they can better predict outcome than current conventional criteria [16]. Several small studies with 3D echocardiography have shown that patients with high SDI-16 values do better with CRT than their counterparts with lower SDI-16. These studies have mainly used echocardiographic improvements in LV function as their endpoints.

> Several studies with 3D echocardiography have shown that patients with high SDI values do respond clinically better with CRT than those with lower SDI values.

Kapetanakis et al. [5] studied 26 patients who fulfilled standard criteria for CRT. These patients had 3D echocardiography performed before and 10 months after CRT implantation. Clinical responders differed significantly in SDI-16 but not LVEF before implantation, with higher SDI-16 ($16.6\pm1.1\%$ vs. $7.1\pm2\%$; p=0.0005) but similar LVEF ($18.6\pm2.8\%$ vs. $23.9\pm2.4\%$; p=0.4) and NYHA class (3.4 ± 1.8 vs. 3.0 ± 1.7; p=0.09).

Delgado et al. [7] studied 27 patients with DCM scheduled for CRT and performed echocardiography before, 24–48 h after, and at 6 months. Twenty-two patients had datasets that were adequate for analysis, and 11 patients were followed up at 6 months. The most delayed segment was the basal and mid infero-posterior segments. Prior to CRT, the EF was $26\pm8\%$, SDI-16Q was $14.3\pm7.5\%$; immediately after CRT, the EF was $32\pm7\%$, SDI-16Q was $9.7\pm6.8\%$; at 6 months the EF was $39\pm14\%$, SDI-16Q was $4.9\pm3.1\%$. These improvements were statistically significant. They found that responders to CRT (as defined by a >10% decrease in end-systolic volume) had a higher initial SDI-16Q than nonresponders but in their small cohort this was not statistically significant.

Marsan et al. [4] investigated 60 patients meeting standard criteria for CRT. They performed 3D echocardiography before and within 48 h of CRT and calculated the SDI-16Q. They excluded dyskinetic segments from their analysis. All patients were in sinus rhythm and most patients were in NYHA class III; 62% of patients had ischemic cardiomyopathy. Three-dimensional echocardiography revealed severe LV dilation (mean LV end-diastolic volume 201 ± 48 ml), with depressed LV function (mean LVEF $28\pm6\%$). The SDI-16Q was significantly higher in responders, as compared with nonresponders ($9.7\pm4.1\%$ vs. $3.4\pm1.8\%$, p<0.0001). Moreover, responders demonstrated a significant reduction in SDI-16Q immediately after CRT (from $9.7\pm4.1\%$ to $3.6\pm1.8\%$, p<0.0001), whereas in nonresponders SDI-16Q remained unchanged (from $3.4\pm1.8\%$ to $3.1\pm1.1\%$, p=NS). In addition, the postero-lateral region (where the LV pacing lead is positioned) was activated latest in 74% of responders, as compared with 33% of nonresponders (p=NS). They performed receiver–operator characteristic to define a cut-off value of 5.6% for SDI-16Q, which had a sensitivity of 88% with a specificity of 86% to predict an acute reduction >15% of LV end-systolic volume (area under the curve =0.96, 95% CI 0.9–1.0, p<0.0001).

Van Dijk et al. [10] performed an acute study involving 17 patients who had severely impaired left ventricular function and NYHA class III or IV heart failure, but did not necessarily have a prolonged QRS duration. They investigated the utility of baseline SDI-17 to predict change in LV dp/dt due to biventricular pacing. They measured LV dp/dt invasively during intrinsic rhythm, and after sequentially pacing the RA appendage, postero-lateral branch of the coronary sinus and RV apex at a fixed AV delay of 100 ms to ensure no intrinsic conduction. The mean SDI-17 was $10.8\pm4.5\%$. They found that SDI-17 correlated better with change in LV dp/dt than QRS duration.

Soliman et al. [17] studied 39 patients (age 61 ± 12 years, 72% were male) with heart failure with LVEF<35%, QRS duration >120 ms and on optimal medical therapy who underwent CRT. At 12 months after CRT, 27 patients (69%) had more than 15% reduction in LVESV. These 27 volumetric responders had similar baseline characteristics except for a higher SDI-16Q compared with nonresponders ($16.3\pm3.3\%$ vs. $8.8\pm2.9\%$, p<0.001). The SDI-16Q was significantly improved in CRT responders, reaching almost normal values ($7.7\pm2.4\%$, p<0.001). Conversely, the

SDI-16Q worsened in nonresponders (8.8±2.9% to 11.7±3.8%, p<0.01). On the receiver operating characteristic curve, a value of SDI-16Q greater than 10% best predicted reverse LV remodeling after 12 months of CRT with a sensitivity of 93%, a specificity of 91%, and an area under the curve of 0.91.

The same group confirmed these findings in a similar cohort of 90 patients undergoing CRT [27]. After 12 months of CRT, 68 patients (76%) were responders. Responders had larger differences in LV end-diastolic volume (−21±7% vs. −11±18%, p<0.003), LV end-systolic volume (−33±8% vs. −12±25%, p<0.001), LVEF (43±13% vs. 5±9%, p<0.001), and 6-min walking distance (40±31% vs. 4±22%, p<0.001) compared with nonresponders. An SDI-16Q >10% predicted CRT response with good sensitivity (96%) and specificity (88%).

Miyazaki et al. [28] reported on a prospective single center study to evaluate modern echocardiographic dyssynchrony measures to predict response. They investigated M-mode, Doppler, tissue Doppler, 2D speckle as well as 3D dyssynchrony indices in 184 patients. Interestingly, they did not find that any echocardiographic modality was useful in the prediction of clinical response. However, their intra- and interobserver variability for SDI-16Q was over 23%, which was substantially higher than that reported by other groups, which may well explain the inability for SDI-16Q to predict response.

More recently, Kapetanakis et al. [29] investigated 187 patients from two institutions who were scheduled for CRT implant or upgrade to CRT from an existing pacemaker or defibrillator. After a mean of 7 months, they found that SDI-16 was a good predictor of echocardiographic and clinical response. Interestingly, in this cohort selected for CRT, QRS duration had no predictive ability to discriminate between responders and nonresponders. They proposed a SDI-16 cut-off of 10.4%, which identified over 90% of responders with a specificity of over 67%.

> SDI-16 seems to be a better predictor than QRS duration in determining acute response to CRT and long-term clinical outcomes.

These findings together suggest that SDI-16 may be a useful predictor of symptomatic benefit from CRT and that SDI-16 is a better predictor than QRS duration in determining acute response to CRT and long-term clinical outcomes. The cut-off value has varied between studies and between software used to determine CRT; further studies are warranted to confirm these findings in larger cohorts.

Recent guidelines on 3D echocardiography published jointly by the European Association of Echocardiography and the American Society of Echocardiography acknowledge the role of 3D echocardiography for patients undergoing CRT [1]. Three-dimensional echocardiographic assessment is recommended as the most accurate and reproducible method for assessment of LV volumes and EF and should therefore be used to assess response to CRT. While the authors note that 3D echocardiography-derived SDI is predictive of early, midterm, and late response to CRT and can also be used to identify optimal LV lead position, 3D assessment of dyssynchrony is not currently recommended for patient selection on the basis that the data is derived from single center, nonrandomized studies.

5.4   Dyssynchrony due to right ventricular pacing

Right ventricular (RV) pacing causes acute hemodynamic changes [30] as well as chronic detrimental effects [31]. Liu et al. [32] used 3D echocardiography to evaluate dyssynchrony in 35 patients with sick sinus syndrome who had had dual chamber pacemakers implanted in the last 3–128 months. They performed echocardiography when pacing the atrium, with intrinsic conduction, and when dual chamber pacing. With intrinsic conduction, the mean QRS duration was 90±14 ms, which was not significantly different from control patients. The ventricular lead was in the RV apex. They measured myocardial performance index, tissue Doppler imaging of 12 segments, and 3D echocardiography SDI-17.

The myocardial performance index was significantly higher with apical pacing (with pacing 0.42±0.18 vs. without pacing 0.31±0.14; p=0.004), and LVEF derived by 3D echocardiography was significantly lower with apical pacing (with pacing 54.4±7.7% vs. without pacing 56.7±7.9%; p=0.013), indicating a deterioration of left ventricular function with apical pacing. The mean change in LVEF with apical pacing in an individual patient was 4.1%. There was also more dyssynchrony associated with apical pacing (SDI-17 with pacing 7.00±2.54% vs. without pacing 5.36±2.17%; p=0.0003). Thus, right ventricular apical (RVA) pacing induced 30.6% change in SDI-17 from baseline without RVA pacing. However, the total pacing burden, or pacemaker programming of these patients is unknown, so it is unclear if there had been any chronic pacing-induced change in left ventricular mechanics after implantation.

Hong et al. [33] examined 19 patients with congenital heart block, and a further 9 patients with acquired heart block following congenital heart surgery. All had RV apical pacing. They found that SDI-16 was significantly higher in patients with heart block and congenital surgery (9.43±4.44%) compared to those with congenital heart block (6.68±2.44%) and to healthy controls (3.88±0.63%). Interestingly, they found that in patients with congenital complete heart block the peak displacement of lateral posterior and inferior segments were delayed, whereas in patients with congenital heart surgery and pacing the septal and inferior segments were delayed, although these patients were more frequently paced epicardially.

Fang et al. [34] studied 93 patients with sick sinus syndrome who had dual chamber pacemakers between 6 months and 13 years previously and who had a LV ejection fraction of greater than 50%. They performed 3D echocardiography during pacing and in intrinsic rhythm. The response to pacing was heterogeneous, and when significant dyssynchrony was defined as a value of SDI-16Q greater than two standard deviations above the mean of their normal population, they found that half the group developed significant dyssynchrony with RV pacing that was associated with an increase in left ventricular end-systolic volumes and a corresponding fall in LVEF. This group of patients was more likely to have a lower ejection fraction during intrinsic conduction, left ventricular hypertrophy and a greater proportion of ventricular pacing.

Wolber et al. [35] investigated 26 patients with RVA pacemakers and normal atrioventricular conduction and performed echocardiography during intrinsic conduction and sinus rhythm. During RVA pacing, a reversed apical-to-basal longitudinal contraction sequence was observed in 58% of all patients. RVA pacing was associated with increased left ventricular (LV) dyssynchrony (SDI increase from 4.4±2.2% to 6.3±2.4%, p=0.001) and reduced LVEF (decrease from 53±13% to 47±14%, p=0.05).

Two studies have looked at RV pacing in patients undergoing CRT implantation. Tanaka et al. [36] reported on a cohort of 308 patients undergoing CRT, 87 of whom were upgraded from RV pacemaker. They performed 3D speckle tracking in a subset of these patients (22 with RV pacing, 35 with left bundle branch block). Earliest mechanical activation was more likely to be at the apex or inferior septum with pacing compared with patients with LBBB, although the region of latest mechanical activation (usually the mid or basal portions of the posterior or lateral walls) was similar in both groups. Thebault et al. [20] compared RV pacing to optimized biventricular pacing in 60 patients. The RV lead had been targeted to the interventricular septum, although they did not report whether this was apical mid or basal septum. Using 3D speckle tracking, they report that biventricular pacing caused increased 3D longitudinal strain, reduced the dyssynchrony index calculated for 16 segments for each directional strain as well as for area strain, and also increased global peak 3D area strain.

5.5 Dyssynchrony in other situations

5.5.1 In children

Baker et al. [37] studied 18 children, 9 with left ventricular dysfunction and 9 controls. None of the patients had structural congenital heart disease, but had either dilated cardiomyopathy (n=7), tachycardia induced cardiomyopathy (n=1), or transplant rejection (n=1). The patients mean age was 14 years (range 4–18 years). The control children were matched for body surface area. The patients had more dilated ventricles and worse EF than controls. The median EF was 36%, as compared to that of controls, which was 60%. The children had more dyssynchronous hearts with a SDI-16Q of 4.37% (range 2.29–14.77%) as compared to 2.1% (range 0.71–2.78%) in control children (p=0.008). There was no significant difference in QRS duration between the two groups, and the longest QRS duration was 128 ms. They confirmed a strong negative correlation between SDI-16Q and EF.

Veeram Reddy et al. [38] reported on outcomes in children who had surgical repair of a ventricular septal defect in infancy. They reported normal left ventricular function in patients, but noted an increase in dyssynchrony compared to controls in the presence of right bundle branch block (SDI-16Q of 2.7 vs. 1.15).

5.5.2 In postsurgical correction of congenital heart disease

Raedle-Hurst et al. [39] investigated left ventricular dyssynchrony in a total of 30 consecutive patients with repaired congenital right heart disease and 30 sex- and age-matched healthy controls. Mean age was 14.8±6.3 years (range 6–31 years). Among the patients, 25 had a corrected tetralogy of Fallot, 2 had a corrected common arterial trunk, and 3 had a corrected pulmonary atresia. Mean follow-up time after corrective surgery was 149.4±72.2 months (range 53–297 months). One patient had had a dual-chamber pacemaker implanted after repair of tetralogy of Fallot due to postoperative complete atrioventricular block. All patients showed a right bundle branch block on the surface ECG with a mean QRS duration of 144.0±24.2 ms (range 110–210 ms). Of 30 patients, 14 (46.7%) did not have significant pressure or volume overload of the RV. Seven patients (23.3%) had an elevated RV systolic pressure that was primarily due to RV outflow tract obstruction. Nine patients (30%) had RV volume overload with moderate to severe pulmonary regurgitation and a mean gradient across the RV outflow tract of 21.9±14.0 mmHg. In 9 (30%) patients, a paradoxical septal movement was observed. Among healthy subjects, the mean SDI-16 was 3.1±1.2% and the mean SDI-17 3.7±1.2% and differed significantly to those found in the patient group (7.2±4.5% and 7.7±4.0%, p<0.001, respectively). Also, mean SDI-16 and SDI-17 were found to be significantly elevated in patients with a paradoxical septal movement (11.6±4.7% and 11.4±4.0%) as compared to those without it (5.3±3.0%, p=0.001 for SDI-16 and 6.2±2.8%, p=0.002 for SDI-17).

Ho et al. [40] reported on outcomes in 20 patients a mean of 18 years after Fontan procedure for tricuspid atresia. They performed 3D echocardiography as well as 2D speckle tracking. They found that patients had significantly greater volumes, lower EF, more dyssynchrony and lower values of strain than normal controls. SDI-16 in patients was 6.13±1.32% vs. 4.06±0.84% (p<0.001) in controls.

5.5.3 After acute myocardial infarction

Several groups have used 3D echocardiography to evaluate dyssynchrony after myocardial infarction (MI). Delgado et al. [7] studied 22 patients with acute ST elevation MI treated with primary percutaneous coronary intervention (PCI) within 4 h of pain with 3D echocardiography performed within 48 h. Eleven suffered an anterior MI and 11 an infero-posterior MI. None had bundle branch block. They found that the apical and mid regions of the wall that was affected by infarction were the latest to contract and that the mean SDI-16Q was 8.7±7.1%.

Subsequently, they have reported on a larger cohort of 193 patients with a first acute MI, in whom they performed 3D echocardiography 48 h after percutaneous coronary intervention and again after 6 months [41]. A total of 59 (40%) patients had an anterior acute MI. Mean LVEF was 47±8% and mean SDI-16 was 5.01±2.10%, respectively. As expected, at the 6-month follow-up, they noted a significant improvement in LVEF (50±9%, p<0.001) and SDI-16 (4.52±1.97%, p=0.003). However, they also found a strong correlation between LVEF change and SDI-16 change; and multivariate analysis identified SDI-16 change as an independent factor associated with changes in LVEF. This suggests that reduction in dyssynchrony independently influenced the recovery of LV function post myocardial infarction.

Yang et al. [42] also investigated 30 consecutive patients who presented with an acute MI. They excluded 6 patients because of poor images, 3 patients who were lost to follow-up, and 2 patients who died during the index admission. Yang et al. did not differentiate between ST elevation MI and non-ST elevation MI. All patients underwent echocardiography within 24 h of admission and after 3 months. In addition, all patients underwent coronary angiography within 36 h and where appropriate underwent revascularization. They divided the patients into those whose end-diastolic volume worsened by >10%, and those who did not. Those patients who did better seemed to have smaller MIs, as determined by the CK value, as well as whether or not they were initially thrombolyzed. The mean LVEF was 41% in both groups, and in neither group did it change on follow-up. Similarly, they found a baseline SDI-16 of 5.1±3.8% in the patients with adverse remodeling, 5.8±4.9% in those with favorable remodeling, and after 3 months this was 4.7±1.6%, and 5.1±2.6%, respectively. There were no significant differences in dyssynchrony between the groups at baseline or at follow-up.

Maruyama et al. [43] also reported on a cohort of 41 patients with acute MI. They performed echocardiography within 2 weeks and after 6 months of acute MI. Again, they found there was remodeling after 6 months, but multivariate analysis suggested that SDI-16 was not an independent predictor of change in LV ejection fraction. Instead, they described a novel parameter, the systolic dispersion index, which is the maximal difference between time to peak systolic contraction between any 2 of the 16 segments assessed. They found this marker to be an independent predictor of change in LVEF.

In summary several studies have indicated that dyssynchrony occurs after MI and while baseline dyssynchrony itself is not a good predictor of remodeling, change in dyssynchrony is an independent predictor of changes in LVEF.

5.5.4   In amyloidosis

Migrino et al. [44] investigated 10 consecutive patients with biopsy-proven amyloidosis, and compared them to 10 normal controls. Mean SDI-16Q in patients was 5.93±4.4%, whereas in controls it was 1.67±0.87% (p=0.003). In terms of patient characteristics, 8 patients were in NYHA class I, with 1 each presenting in class III and IV heart failure. LVEF was 62.4±0.6% in control subjects and 58.6±2.8% for patients with amyloidosis (p=NS). Patients had a thicker anteroseptum, increased left atrial volume index, and a tendency towards increased left ventricular mass index. Based on conventional evaluation of degree of diastolic dysfunction using mitral inflow and mitral annular velocity, 1 patient had normal diastolic function, 3 had mild (impaired relaxation pattern), 4 had moderate (pseudonormalization) and 2 had severe (restrictive) diastolic dysfunction.

5.6   Assessment of dyssynchrony after CRT

Porciani et al. [45] investigated 20 patients with CRT. These patients had been implanted with a St Jude CRT device that was capable of optimizing the delivery of CRT using an algorithm based upon intracardiac electrogram recordings. The patients underwent 3D echocardiography before and after optimization, using this method to assess dyssynchrony at a mean interval of 9 months after device implantation. After optimization, SDI-16Q and SDI-12Q significantly decreased from 8.1±4.9% to 4.2±4.0% (p<0.001) and from 6.0±5.7% to 3.0±3.7% (p=0.01), respectively, while SDI-6Q did not show significant change. This improvement in LV synchrony was associated with improved LV systolic function as indicated by the significant change in SV from 56±16 ml to 64±18 ml (p=0.01), and EF from 29.3±11.1% to 32.3±10.9% (p<0.001). EF improved in all but two patients; the mean increase was 3.0% from 29.3% to 32.3%. SV improved in all but 2 patients; the mean increase was 8 ml. Somewhat surprisingly, given the improvements in SV and EF, was that there were no significant changes in EDV or ESV.

> Optimization of LV lead position using 3D echocardiography might correlate with better clinical outcome of CRT.

Bertini et al. [46] performed an interesting investigation in 84 patients scheduled for CRT. They performed 3D echocardiography and 2D speckle tracking before, within 48 h of implantation, and after 6 months. They found that immediate improvements in EF and dyssynchrony predicted favorable outcomes at 6 months, defined as a 15% or greater fall in end-systolic volume associated with an improvement of 1 or more classes on the New York Heart Association heart failure scale. However, multivariate logistic regression pointed to improvements in subepicardial LV twist were the only parameter that was an independent predictor of favorable outcome, suggesting this is the cause of falling dyssynchrony.

Another factor in the delivery of CRT lies in the interplay between the latest contracting segment and LV lead position. Three-dimensional echocardiography can demonstrate which segment contracts latest. It is not yet clear if this is useful information, but a study by Becker et al. [47] suggests that when the LV pacing site is close to the latest contracting segment, then a patient is more likely to benefit from CRT. They demonstrated this by investigating 58 patients undergoing CRT and performed baseline echocardiography, and repeated echocardiography within a week and at 12 months after CRT. They determined the latest segment to reach minimum systolic volume (segment A), and they also determined the segment with the largest temporal difference between pre- and postoperative minimum systolic volume (segment B). They suggest that segment B was where the LV lead tip was placed, and this did correlate well with lead position as determined by fluoroscopy. In those patients in whom segment B and segment A were the same or in close proximity (optimal patients), the outcome from CRT was better than when these segments were widely separated (nonoptimal patients). Their outcome measures were echocardiographic volumes, EF and that of peak oxygen consumption on bicycle exercise which was performed at baseline and after 12 months.

For example the improvement in EF in optimal patients was 10±2%, whereas in nonoptimal patients, the improvement was 6±3% (p<0.01), and in VO$_2$max the increase was 2.4±0.3 ml/kg/min, as compared to 1.5±0.4 ml/kg/min (p<0.01). There was

1 patient with an optimal LV lead position and 3 patients with a nonoptimal LV lead who were categorized as inadequate responders based on clinical information with no subjective clinical benefit and based on echocardiographic information with a decrease in LV end-systolic volume of <15%. This suggests that optimal LV lead position does identify a population of patients who might do better than nonoptimal lead position, but that the population of patients with nonoptimal lead position do still obtain some benefit from CRT.

5.7   Conclusion

Three-dimensional echocardiography has shown promise in its ability to assess intraventricular dyssynchrony across a range of cardiac disease. Feasibility of measurements has been demonstrated, normal values defined, and our understanding of the pathophysiology of dyssynchrony has been advanced. Several studies suggest it can be used to predict benefit from CRT. Larger studies are needed to see how generalizable these findings are among different echocardiography laboratories, whether dyssynchrony assessments by 3D echocardiography can help improve CRT delivery, and identify a group of patients without conventional criteria for CRT who might benefit from this novel therapy.

References

1. Lang RM, Badano LP, Tsang W et al (2012) EAE/ASE Recommendations for Image Acquisition and Display Using Three-Dimensional Echocardiography. Eur Heart J Cardiovasc Imaging 13:1–46
2. van Dijk J, Dijkmans PA, Götte MJW et al (2008) Evaluation of global left ventricular function and mechanical dyssynchrony in patients with an asymptomatic left bundle branch block: a real-time 3D echocardiography study. Eur J Echocardiogr 940–46
3. Gimenes VML, Vieira MLC, Andrade MM et al (2008) Standard values for real-time transthoracic three-dimensional echocardiographic dyssynchrony indexes in a normal population. J Am Soc Echocardiogr 21:1229–1235
4. Marsan NA, Bleeker GB, Ypenburg C et al (2008) Real-time three-dimensional echocardiography permits quantification of left ventricular mechanical dyssynchrony and predicts acute response to cardiac resynchronization therapy. J Cardiovasc Electrophysiol 19:392–399
5. Kapetanakis S, Kearney MT, Siva A et al (2005) Real-time three-dimensional echocardiography: a novel technique to quantify global left ventricular mechanical dyssynchrony. Circulation 112:992–1000
6. Cerqueira MD, Weissman NJ, Dilsizian V et al (2002) Standardized myocardial segmentation and nomenclature for tomographic imaging of the heart: a statement for healthcare professionals from the Cardiac Imaging Committee of the Council on Clinical Cardiology of the American Heart Association. Circulation 105:539–452
7. Delgado V, Sitges M, Vidal B et al (2008) Assessment of left ventricular dyssynchrony by real-time three-dimensional echocardiography. Revista Española de Cardiología (Internet) 61:825–834
8. Takeuchi M, Jacobs A, Sugeng L et al (2007) Assessment of left ventricular dyssynchrony with real-time 3-dimensional echocardiography: comparison with Doppler tissue imaging. J Am Soc Echocardiogr 20:1321–1329
9. Burgess MI, Jenkins C, Chan J, Marwick TH (2007) Measurement of left ventricular dyssynchrony in patients with ischaemic cardiomyopathy: a comparison of real-time three-dimensional and tissue Doppler echocardiography. Heart 93:1191–1196
10. van Dijk J, Knaapen P, Russel IK et al (2008) Mechanical dyssynchrony by 3D echo correlates with acute haemodynamic response to biventricular pacing in heart failure patients. Europace 10:63–68
11. Nesser H, Sugeng L, Corsi C et al (2007) Volumetric analysis of regional left ventricular function with real-time three-dimensional echocardiography: validation by magnetic resonance and clinical utility testing. Heart 93:572–578
12. Marsan NA, Henneman MM, Chen J et al (2008) Real-time three-dimensional echocardiography as a novel approach to quantify left ventricular dyssynchrony: a comparison study with phase analysis of gated myocardial perfusion single photon emission computed tomography. J Am Soc Echocardiogr 21:801–807
13. Pérez de Isla L, Balcones DV, Fernández-Golfín C et al (2009) Three-dimensional-wall motion tracking: a new and faster tool for myocardial strain assessment: comparison with two-dimensional-wall motion tracking. J Am Soc Echocardiogr 22:325–330
14. Seo Y, Ishizu T, Enomoto Y et al (2011) Endocardial surface area tracking for assessment of regional LV wall deformation with 3D speckle tracking imaging. JACC Cardiovasc Imaging 4:358–635
15. Kleijn SA, Aly MFA, Terwee CB et al (2011) Three-dimensional speckle tracking echocardiography for automatic assessment of global and regional left ventricular function based on area ttrain. J Am Soc Echocardiogr 24:314–321
16. Chung ES, Leon AR, Tavazzi L et al (2008) Results of the predictors of response to CRT (PROSPECT) trial. Circulation 117:2608–2616
17. Soliman OII, van Dalen BM, Nemes A et al (2009) Quantification of left ventricular systolic dyssynchrony by real-time three-dimensional echocardiography. J Am Soc Echocardiogr 22:232–239
18. Conca C, Faletra FF, Miyazaki C et al (2009) Echocardiographic parameters of mechanical synchrony in healthy individuals. Am J Cardiol 103:136–142
19. Tanaka H, Hara H, Saba S, Gorcsan J (2010) Usefulness of three-dimensional speckle tracking strain to quantify dyssynchrony and the site of latest mechanical activation. Am J Cardiol 105:235–242
20. Thebault C, Donal E, Bernard A et al (2011) Real-time three-dimensional speckle tracking echocardiography: a novel technique to quantify global left ventricular mechanical dyssynchrony. Eur J Echocardiogr 12:26–32
21. Harkel ten ADJ, van Osch-Gevers M, Helbing WA (2009) Real-time transsthoracic three dimensional echocardiography: normal reference data for left ventricular dyssynchrony in adolescents. J Am Soc Echocardiogr 22:933–938
22. Cui W, Gambetta K, Zimmerman F et al (2010) Real-time three-dimensional echocardiographic assessment of left ventricular systolic dyssynchrony in healthy children. J Am Soc Echocardiogr 23:1153–1159
23. de Castro S, Faletra F, Di Angelantonio E et al (2008) Tomographic left ventricular volumetric emptying analysis by real-time 3-dimensional echocardiography: influence of left ventricular dysfunction with and without electrical dyssynchrony. Circulation: Cardiovascular Imaging 1:41–49
24. Zeng X, Shu X-H, Pan C-Z et al (2006) Assessment of left ventricular systolic synchronicity by real-time three-dimensional echocardiography in patients with dilated cardiomyopathy. Chin Med J 119:919–924
25. Cheung YF, Hong WJ, Chan GCF et al (2010) Left ventricular myocardial deformation and mechanical dyssynchrony in children with normal ventricular shortening fraction after anthracycline therapy. Heart 96:1137–1141
26. Bax JJ, Abraham T, Barold SS et al (2005) Cardiac resynchronization therapy: Part 1--issues before device implantation. J Am Coll Cardiol 46:2153–2167
27. Soliman OII, Geleijnse ML, Theuns DAMJ et al (2009) Usefulness of left ventricular systolic dyssynchrony by real-time three-dimensional echocardiography to predict long-term response to cardiac resynchronization therapy. Am J Cardiol 103:1586–1591
28. Miyazaki C, Redfield MM, Powell BD et al (2010) Dyssynchrony indices to predict response to cardiac resynchronization therapy: a comprehensive prospective single-center study. Circulation: Heart Failure 3:565–573
29. Kapetanakis S, Bhan A, Murgatroyd F et al (2011) Real-time 3D echo in patient selection for cardiac resynchronization therapy. JACC Cardiovasc Imaging 4:16–26

30. Lieberman R, Padeletti L, Schreuder J et al (2006)Ventricular pacing lead location alters systemic hemodynamics and left ventricular function in patients with and without reduced ejection fraction. Journal of the American College of Cardiology 48:1634–1641

31. Karpawich PP, Rabah R, Haas JE (1999) Altered cardiac histology following apical right ventricular pacing in patients with congenital atrioventricular block. Pacing Clin Electrophysiol 22:1372–1377

32. Liu W-H, Chen M-C, Chen Y-L et al (2008) Right ventricular apical pacing acutely impairs left ventricular function and induces mechanical dyssynchrony in patients with sick sinus syndrome: a real-time three-dimensional echocardiographic study. J Am Soc Echocardiogr 21:224–229

33. Hong WJ, Yung T, Lun K et al (2009) Impact of right ventricular pacing on three-dimensional global left ventricular dyssynchrony in children and young adults with congenital and acquired heart block associated with congenital heart disease. Am J Cardiol 104:700–706

34. Fang F, Chan JY-S, Yip GW-K et al (2010) Prevalence and determinants of left ventricular systolic dyssynchrony in patients with normal ejection fraction received right ventricular apical pacing: a real-time three-dimensional echocardiographic study. Eur J Echocardiogr 11:109–118

35. Wolber T, Haegeli L, Huerlimann D et al (2010) Altered left ventricular contraction pattern during right ventricular pacing: assessment using realtime three-dimensional echocardiography. Pacing and Clinical Electrophysiology 34:76–81

36. Tanaka H, Hara H, Adelstein EC et al (2010) Comparative mechanical activation mapping of RV pacing to LBBB by 2D and 3D speckle tracking and association with response to resynchronization therapy. JACC Cardiovasc Imaging 3:461–471

37. Baker GH, Hlavacek AM, Chessa KS et al (2008) Left ventricular dysfunction is associated with intraventricular dyssynchrony by 3-dimensional echocardiography in children. J Am Soc Echocardiogr 21:230–233

38. Veeram Reddy SR, Du W, Zilberman MV (2009) Left ventricular mechanical synchrony and global systolic function in pediatric patients late after ventricular septal defect patch closure: a three-dimensional echocardiographic study. Congenital Heart Disease 4:454–458

39. Raedle-Hurst TM, Mueller M, Rentzsch A et al (2009) Assessment of left ventricular dyssynchrony and function using real-time 3-dimensional echocardiography in patients with congenital right heart disease. Am Heart J 157:791–798

40. Ho P-K, Lai CTM, Wong SJ, Cheung Y-F (2012) Three-dimensional mechanical dyssynchrony and myocardial deformation of the left ventricle in patients with tricuspid atresia after Fontan procedure. J Am Soc Echocardiogr 25:393–400

41. Nucifora G, Bertini M, Marsan NA et al (2012) Temporal evolution of left ventricular dyssynchrony after myocardial infarction: relation with changes in left ventricular systolic function. Eur Heart J Cardiovasc Imaging 13:1040–1046

42. Yang N-I, Hung M-J, Cherng W-J et al (2008) Analysis of left ventricular changes after acute myocardial infarction using transthoracic real-time three-dimensional echocardiography. Angiology 59:688–694

43. Maruyama Y, Masaki N, Yoshimoto N (2009) Dyssynchrony during acute phase determined by real-time three-dimensional echocardiography predicts reverse cardiac remodeling and improved cardiac function after reperfusion therapy. J Cardiol 54:432–440

44. Migrino RQ, Harmann L, Woods T et al (2008) Intraventricular dyssynchrony in light chain amyloidosis: a new mechanism of systolic dysfunction assessed by 3-dimensional echocardiography. Cardiovasc Ultrasound 6:40

45. Porciani MC, Rao CM, Mochi M et al (2008) A real-time three-dimensional echocardiographic validation of an intracardiac electrogram-based method for optimizing cardiac resynchronization therapy. Pacing Clin Electrophysiol 31:56–63

46. Bertini M, Delgado V, Nucifora G et al (2010) Effect of cardiac resynchronization therapy on subendo- and subepicardial left ventricular twist mechanics and relation to favorable outcome. Am J Cardiol 106:682–687

47. Becker M, Hoffmann R, Schmitz F et al (2007) Relation of optimal lead positioning as defined by three-dimensional echocardiography to long-term benefit of cardiac resynchronization. Am J Cardiol 100:1671–1676

48. Brunekreeft JA, Graauw M, de Milliano PAR, Keijer JT (2007) Influence of left bundle branch block on left ventricular volumes, ejection fraction and regional wall motion. Netherlands heart journal : monthly journal of the Netherlands Society of Cardiology and the Netherlands Heart Foundation 15:89–94v

The right ventricle

Stephan von Bardeleben, Thomas Buck, Andreas Franke

T. Buck et al. (Hrsg.), *Three-dimensional Echocardiography*,
DOI 10.1007/978-3-642-36799-1_6, © Springer-Verlag Berlin Heidelberg 2014

Because the right ventricle (RV) has a much more complex geometry compared to the left ventricle, assessment of its volume and function is more challenging using two-dimensional (2D) echocardiographic image planes. This is due to the fact that no simple three-dimensional (3D) geometric model accurately represents this chamber even in the absence of disease. Although these conditions would clearly favor a 3D analysis, it is challenging to find an adequate acoustic window because of the retrosternal location of the RV.

Besides geometry, the contraction pattern of the RV is also complex. In the first contraction phase, there is a combination of radial shortening of the short minor axis of the RV inflow tract with long-axis shortening, which draws the tricuspid annulus toward the apex. Under normal hemodynamic conditions, the low pulmonary vascular resistance allows for a significant change in volume and, thus, sufficient stroke volume with rather small degrees in myocardial shortening. In the last phase of the ejection process, there is a contraction pulse in the RV outflow tract with smaller volume displacement.

Pressure or volume overload significantly change the shape of the right ventricle. This results in changes in the interventricular septal wall, including variable or constant flattening as well as increases in the size of the chamber geometry, volumes, and wall thickness. These changes may be due to left heart systolic functional impairment, valvular heart disease, pulmonary vascular disease, or congenital or ischemic heart disease, including interventricular or interatrial shunts.

> ❯ **Real-time 3D echocardiography has been demonstrated to provide accurate and reproducible RV volumes and ejection fractions.**

Recently, real-time three-dimensional echocardiography (RT-3DE) has been demonstrated to provide an anatomically realistic representation of the right ventricle (❒ Fig. 6.1 and ❒ Fig. 6.2). Views of the RV by RT3DE provide the cardiologist for the first time detailed insight and understanding of the complex anatomy of the RV with clear visualization of the three compartments: the inlet with tricuspid valve, the highly trabeculated apical region, and the outlet [1]. Because of the asymmetric geometry of the RV, on the one hand, and the ability of unlimited orientation of cut planes in a 3D dataset, multiple viewing planes of the RV can be obtained. Different useful views of the RV are presented in ❒ Fig. 6.1, ❒ Fig. 6.2, and ❒ Fig. 6.3 and have also recently been recommended [2].

Beyond the advantages of improved anatomic assessment, RT3DE has been demonstrated to provide accurate and reproducible data on RV volumes and ejection fraction with good correlation to reference standards such as magnetic resonance

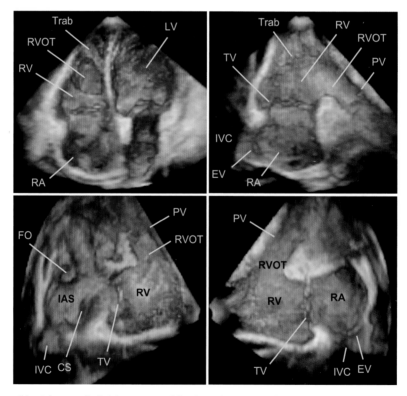

❒ **Fig. 6.1** Anatomic 3D views of the right ventricle (*RV*) from a RT3DE full volume dataset. *Top left* Standard 4-chamber view encompassing the entire RV. A direct perspective to the right ventricular outflow tract (*RVOT*) is provided in this view. Note the marked trabeculation (*Trab*) in the apical region of the RV. *Top right* Coronal view obtained by a long-axial 90° clockwise rotation providing a perspective to the RV free wall. The view shows the characteristic anatomy of the RV existing of the inflow tract, the trabeculated apical region and the outflow tract. Note the detection of a remnant Eustachian valve (*EV*) at the entrance of the inferior vena cava (*IVC*) in this patient. *Bottom right* Anatomic alignment of the top right view by 90° counterclockwise rotation. *Bottom left* Counterpart of the bottom right view providing the perspective towards the interatrial septum (*IAS*) and the interventricular septum. The thin interatrial septum at the fossa ovalis (*FO*) appears translucent as a result of a dropout. Note the detection of the entrance of the coronary sinus (*CS*). *RA* right atrium, *LV* left ventricle, *TV* tricuspid valve, *PV* pulmonary valve. [→Videos 6.1A–D]

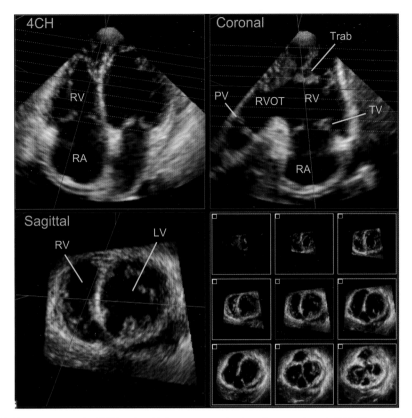

Fig. 6.2 RV analysis using multiplane representation (*MPR*) and multislice representation based on transthoracic RT3DE in a patient with right heart burden due to postinfarct ventricular septal defect (*VSD*; same patient as in ▶ Fig. 12.10A–C in Chapter 12). The right ventricle (*RV*) is shown in his three main cutplanes reconstructed from the RT3DE dataset: 4-chamber plane (*4CH; top left*), coronal plane (*top right*), and sagittal plane (*bottom left*). Multislice representation provides nine short-axis slices along the RV long-axis from the apex to the base for qualitative analysis of RV shape, size, and function, as well as motion pattern of the interventricular septum (*bottom right*). *RA* right atrium, *PV* pulmonary valve, *RVOT* right ventricular outflow tract, *Trab* trabeculation, *TV* tricuspid valve, *LV* left ventricle. [→Videos 6.2A,B]

imaging (MRI) [3][4][5][6][7][8]. Similar to left ventricular analysis, slight but significant underestimation of MRI-derived RV volumes by 3D echocardiographic methods was found in several studies, while ejection fraction agreed very well. For example, using dedicated RT3DE RV analysis software, Leibundgut et al. [4] found slightly lower RV volumes with RT3DE compared to MRI (EDV: 124.0±34.4 ml vs. 134.2±39.2 ml, p<0.001; ESV: 65.2±23.5 ml vs. 69.7±25.5 ml, p=0.02), while no significant difference was observed for ejection fraction (47.8±8.5% vs. 48.2±10.8%, p=0.57). RT3DE is also able to enhance our understanding of impaired RV function, thus, overcoming some of the limitations and assumptions of 2D echocardiography. However, image quality remains a major concern in the assessment of RV and atrial structures with RT3DE when used by a transthoracic approach. In patients with only minor calcification in the area of the aortic valve, the use of transesophageal 3D imaging either in transgastric or transesophageal views might add new imaging options for a precise and more detailed description of the right-sided chambers (▶ Fig. 6.3) [9].

6.1 Assessment of right ventricular volumes and function

Due to the complex RV morphology, assessment of size, shape, and function so far has been mostly qualitative in clinical practice. Nevertheless, the quantification of RV size and function has been shown to be of diagnostic and prognostic importance [10][11][12][13]. However, quantitative 2D echocardiography permits only rough estimates of the true volume in an apical 4-chamber view comparing cavity areas of the right in relation to the left ventricle [14][15][16]. Due to missing landmarks and the variable geometry of the RV compared to the more symmetric shape of the left ventricle, these estimations have been shown to bear a rather high degree of test–retest variability [17]. This, in principle, should complicate especially normal shaped RVs, while the geometry in right ventricular enlargement leads to a more distinct predominance of the inflow chamber resulting in a more ellipsoid morphology. However, in clinical practice, some studies reported increasing underestimation of RV volumes with increasing RV size [7][9], which is most likely related to incomplete capture of dilated RVs due to the limited acoustic window.

> Initial studies using RT3DE for RV analysis were based on the use of software dedicated for the left ventricle.

6

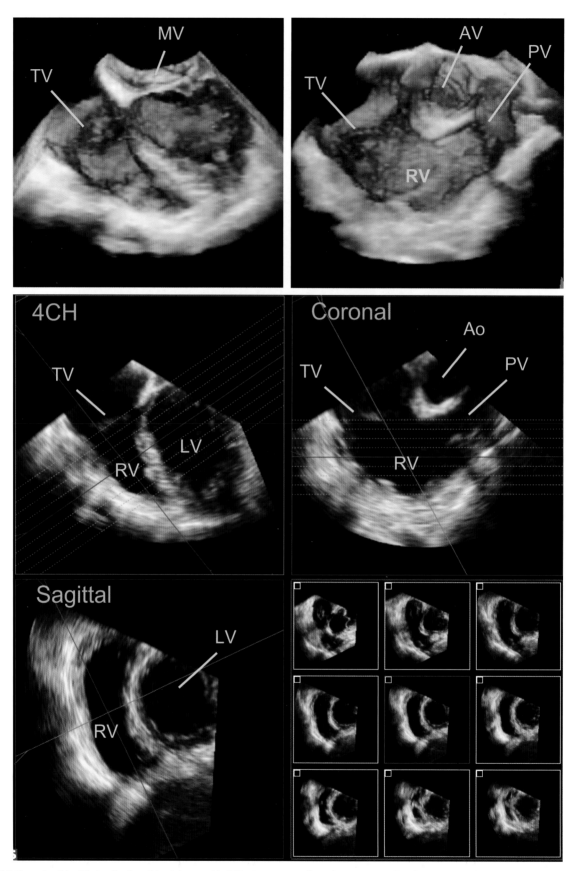

Fig. 6.3 Example of the 3D visualization of the right ventricle (*RV*) using transesophageal RT3DE in a 4-chamber view (*top left*) and coronal view (*top right*) in a normal subject. Compared to standard 2D views, RT3DE imaging enables anatomic realistic understanding of RV morphology and surrounding structures. Multiplane and multislice representation are useful for qualitative RV analysis (Fig. 6.2). The multislice representation shows the RV in nine short-axis slices from the base to the apex (*bottom right*). *TV* tricuspid valve, *MV* mitral valve, *AV* aortic valve, *PV* pulmonary valve, *LV* left ventricle, *Ao* aorta. [→Videos 6.3A–D]

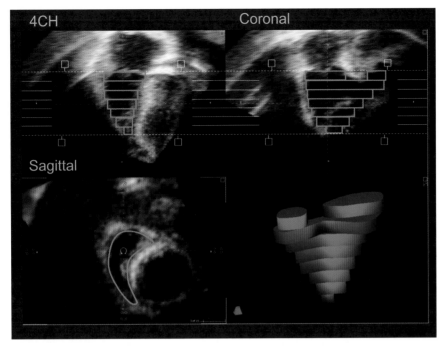

◘ Fig. 6.4 Example of right ventricular (RV) volume analysis using 3D summation-of-disk method (EchoView© version 5.4, TomTec, Unterschleissheim, Germany). Note the relatively coarse reconstruction of the RV shape particularly in the basal inflow and outflow region potentially causing measurement errors

More pronounced trabeculation in the apical region of the RV compared to the LV is another source of error both for manual tracing and for automated endocardial delineation (◘ Fig. 6.1 and ◘ Fig. 6.2). Unlike the missing geometric model in 2D echocardiography, anatomically realistic 3D representation of the chamber can be achieved using RT3DE. This has been shown to lead to a more precise approach to quantitate RV volumes and function. However, there have been significantly fewer investigations into the use of RT3DE for evaluation of the RV than the left ventricle. Early studies using reconstructive 3D echocardiography and 3D disk method or 3D surfacing algorithms for RV volume analysis already demonstrated the usefulness of 3D RV analysis with superior accuracy compared to 2D echocardiographic methods [19][20][21]. Initial studies using RT3DE imaging were based on the use of software dedicated for the left ventricle [17]. However, the use of software based on apical rotation and disk summation algorithms can only be regarded as provisional, because Simpson's rule assumes an elliptic symmetry present in the left, but not the RV, as stated by Jiang et al. [22].

In principle, two practical approaches exist to quantitate RV volumes using either a 3D summation-of-disk method based on manual tracing of six to ten parallel cross-sectional RV planes (◘ Fig. 6.4) [6][7][9][23][24] or dedicated commercially available RV analysis software (◘ Fig. 6.5, ◘ Fig. 6.6, ◘ Fig. 6.7), both having been validated in experimental studies [21][25][26][27][28]. The RV analysis software solution is based on semiautomated contour finding algorithms using endocardial border delineation in the three main cut planes at end-diastole and end-systole (◘ Fig. 6.5). The RV endocardial border is followed throughout systole and a 3D model is created providing RV end-diastolic and end-systolic volumes, dynamic RV volume–time curves, and

ejection fraction (◘ Fig. 6.6 and ◘ Fig. 6.7) [3][29][30]. Several clinical studies validated this semiautomated RV analysis software for determination of RV volumes and function to independent reference methods such as MRI [3][4][8][31]. In a recent meta-analysis of 23 studies using 3D echocardiography for quantification of RV volumes and function in comparison to MRI, Shimada et al. [32] reported systematic underestimation of RV volumes and ejection fraction (EF), where larger volumes and EF were associated with larger underestimation.

> Today, dedicated 3D RV analysis software is available providing improved accuracy and faster analysis time.

Studies that directly compared the 3D disk method and 3D RV surface reconstruction against true volumes or MRI for reference could demonstrate improved accuracy and reproducibility and faster analysis time for semiautomated 3D RV surface reconstruction [7][27]. The disk summation method is fundamentally limited due to its inability to accurately determine RV boundaries in the basal slices, since the tricuspid valve and the RV outflow tract are often not in one plane (◘ Fig. 6.4). Tamborini et al. [30] applied this RV analysis to RT3DE datasets in a large series of normal subjects and determined normal reference values with mean RV end-diastolic and end-systolic volumes of $49\pm10\,\mathrm{ml/m^2}$ and $16\pm6\,\mathrm{ml/m^2}$, respectively, and mean RV ejection fraction of $67\pm8\%$. Other studies demonstrated the value of RT3DE assessment of RV volumes and function in patients with RV enlargement or dysfunction due to congenital heart disease [3][7][8]33] [34] as well as in patients with cardiac diseases, including ischemic heart disease, various cardiomyopathies, valvular heart disease, and congenital or idiopathic diseases associated with pulmonary hypertension [4][29][35][36][37][38].

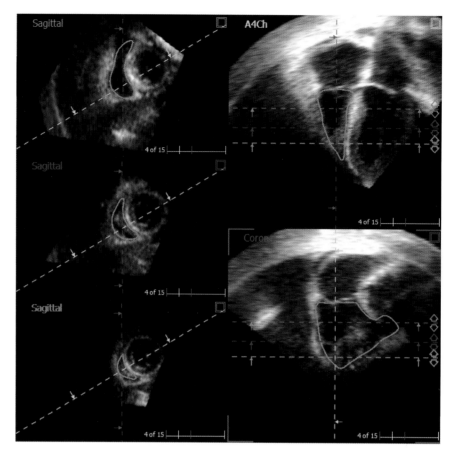

◘ Fig. 6.5 Semiautomated contour definition of the right ventricle (*RV*) in three sagittal short-axis planes (*left*), 4-chamber view (*4CH; top right*), and coronal plane (*bottom right*) for RV volume reconstruction (4D RV-Function©, TomTec, Unterschleissheim, Germany)

6.2   New aspects of 3D right ventricular analysis

Beyond measurements of RV volumes and ejection fraction, 3D RV analysis offers more realistic 3D insight into contraction disorders in ischemic regional wall motion, in myocardial structural disease or valve disease than 1D surrogates of the ejection fraction, e.g., tricuspid valve annular motion during systole (TAPSE) [23, 29]. As a further potential improvement of RV analysis based on 3D volume reconstruction, additional definition of the three compartments, inflow tract, apex, and outflow tract, has recently been introduced (◘ Fig. 6.8). This allows separate analysis of absolute volumes and volume changes of the three compartments. Based on this, characteristic changes of the three compartments could be used for identification of different RV diseases and different grades of severity.

Recently, RV analysis based on RT3DE datasets was directly compared to cardiac computed tomography (cCT) and cardiac MRI using the same dedicated RV surface reconstruction software [27]. In this study, which eliminates potential errors from using different analysis software, RT3DE and cCT were demonstrated to have similar limits of agreement compared to cardiac MRI used for reference, with a lower variability of RT3DE measurements compared to cardiac MRI.

Compared to quantitative left ventricular analysis, RV analysis is still in a relatively early stage. This is mainly because quantitative analysis of RV function was considered to be less clinically important for a long time, the RV is more difficult to image, and analysis of RV function was more difficult due to the complex geometry. However, recently dedicated 3D RV analysis software was demonstrated to provide accurate assessment of RV volumes and function. Based on this, more advanced 3D RV analysis, including regional function, segmental timing, and deformation, is likely to become available in the future.

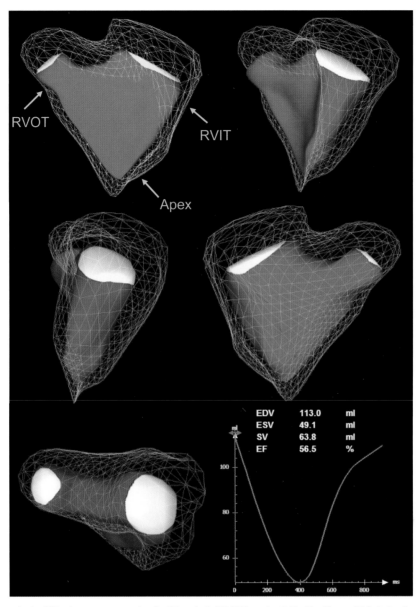

Fig. 6.6 Result of right ventricular (*RV*) volume reconstruction for RV analysis (4D RV-Function©, TomTec, Unterschleissheim, Germany) in a normal subject (same subject as shown in Fig. 6.5). The surface model is presented in different perspectives by rotation to provide better understanding of the complex RV geometry. Quantitative analysis of RV function is represented by a volume–time curve. RV ejection fraction (*EF*) was measured to be 56.5%. *RVOT* right ventricular outflow tract, *RVIT* right ventricular inflow tract. [→Videos 6.6A–D]

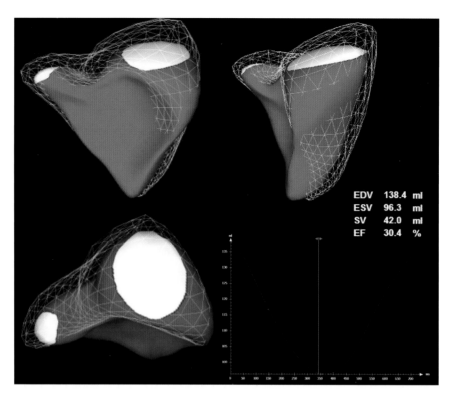

EDV	138.4	ml
ESV	96.3	ml
SV	42.0	ml
EF	30.4	%

Fig. 6.7 RV analysis using RV volume reconstruction (4D RV-Function©, TomTec, Unterschleissheim, Germany) in the same patient with right heart burden due to postinfarct ventricular septal defect (*VSD*) shown in Fig. 6.1 and Fig. 6.2. Compared to the normal RV shown in Fig. 6.6, the RV shown here is significantly dilated, volumes are larger, especially the end-systolic volume (96.3 ml), and ejection fraction (*EF*) is significantly reduced (30.4%). [→Videos 6.7A,B]

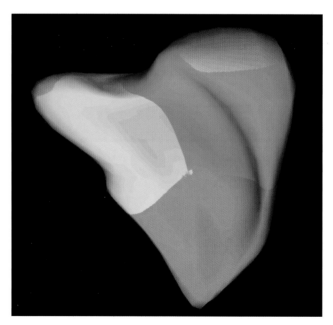

Fig. 6.8 Example of advanced RV model visualization with definition of the three RV compartments – inflow tract (*green*), apex (*red*), outflow tract (*yellow*) – in different colors

References

1. Mangion JR (2010) Right ventricular imaging by two-dimensional and three-dimensional echocardiography. Curr Opin Cardiol 25:423–429

2. Lang RM, Badano LP, Tsang W et al (2012) EAE/ASE recommendations for image acquisition and display using three-dimensional echocardiography. Eur Heart J Cardiovasc Imaging 13:1–46

3. Niemann PS, Pinho L, Balbach T et al (2007) Anatomically oriented right ventricular volume measurements with dynamic three-dimensional echocardiography validated by 3-Tesla magnetic resonance imaging. J Am Coll Cardiol 50:1668–1676

4. Leibundgut G, Rohner A, Grize L et al (2010) Dynamic assessment of right ventricular volumes and function by real-time three-dimensional echocardiography: a comparison study with magnetic resonance imaging in 100 adult patients. J Am Soc Echocardiogr 23:116–126

5. Shiota T (2009) 3D echocardiography: evaluation of the right ventricle. Curr Opin Cardiol 24:410–414

6. Gopal AS, Chukwu EO, Iwuchukwu CJ et al (2007) Normal values of right ventricular size and function by real-time 3-dimensional echocardiography: comparison with cardiac magnetic resonance imaging. J Am Soc Echocardiogr 20:445–455

7. Khoo NS, Young A, Occleshaw C et al (2009) Assessments of right ventricular volume and function using three-dimensional echocardiography in older children and adults with congenital heart disease: comparison with cardiac magnetic resonance imaging. J Am Soc Echocardiogr 22:1279–1288

8. Grewal J, Majdalany D, Syed I et al (2010) Three-dimensional echocardiographic assessment of right ventricular volume and function in adult patients with congenital heart disease: comparison with magnetic resonance imaging. J Am Soc Echocardiogr 23:127–133

9. Nesser HJ, Tkalec W, Patel AR et al (2006) Quantitation of right ventricular volumes and ejection fraction by three-dimensional echocardiography in patients: comparison with magnetic resonance imaging and radionuclide ventriculography. Echocardiography 23:666–680

10. de Groote P, Millaire A, Foucher-Hossein C et al (1998) Right ventricular ejection fraction is an independent predictor of survival in patients with moderate heart failure. J Am Coll Cardiol 32:948–954

11. Pfisterer M, Emmenegger H, Soler M, Burkart F (1986) Prognostic significance of right ventricular ejection fraction for persistent complex ventricular arrhythmias and/or sudden cardiac death after first myocardial infarction: relation to infarct location, size and left ventricular function. Eur Heart J 7:289–298

12. Ghio S, Klersy C, Magrini G et al (2010) Prognostic relevance of the echocardiographic assessment of right ventricular function in patients with idiopathic pulmonary arterial hypertension. Int J Cardiol 140: 272–278

13. Gavazzi A, Berzuini C, Campana C et al (1997) Value of right ventricular ejection fraction in predicting short-term prognosis of patients with severe chronic heart failure. J Heart Lung Transplant 16:774–785

14. Bleeker GB, Steendijk P, Holman ER et al (2006) Assessing right ventricular function: the role of echocardiography and complementary technologies. Heart 92 (Suppl 1):i19–i26

15. Lang RM, Bierig M, Devereux RB et al (2005) Recommendations for chamber quantification: a report from the American Society of Echocardiography's Guidelines and Standards Committee and the Chamber Quantification Writing Group, developed in conjunction with the European Association of Echocardiography, a branch of the European Society of Cardiology. J Am Soc Echocardiogr 18:1440–1463

16. Kaul S, Tei C, Hopkins JM, Shah PM (1984) Assessment of right ventricular function using two-dimensional echocardiography. Am Heart J 107: 526–531

17. Jenkins C, Chan J, Bricknell K et al (2007) Reproducibility of right ventricular volumes and ejection fraction using real-time three-dimensional echocardiography: comparison with cardiac MRI. Chest 131:1844–1851

18. Jiang L, Handschumacher MD, Hibberd MG et al (1994) Three-dimensional echocardiographic reconstruction of right ventricular volume: in vitro comparison with two-dimensional methods. J Am Soc Echocardiogr 7:150–158

19. Jiang L, Siu SC, Handschumacher MD et al (1994) Three-dimensional echocardiography. In vivo validation for right ventricular volume and function. Circulation 89:2342–2350

20. Fujimoto S, Mizuno R, Nakagawa Y et al (1998) Estimation of the right ventricular volume and ejection fraction by transthoracic three-dimensional echocardiography. A validation study using magnetic resonance imaging. Int J Card Imaging 14:385–390

21. Schindera ST, Mehwald PS, Sahn DJ, Kececioglu D (2002) Accuracy of real-time three-dimensional echocardiography for quantifying right ventricular volume: static and pulsatile flow studies in an anatomic in vitro model. J Ultrasound Med 21:1069–1075

22. Jiang L, Levine RA, Weyman AE (1997) Echocardiographic assessment of right ventricular volume and function. Echocardiography 14:189–206

23. Kjaergaard J, Petersen CL, Kjaer A et al (2006) Evaluation of right ventricular volume and function by 2D and 3D echocardiography compared to MRI. Eur J Echocardiogr 7:430–438

24. Chua S, Levine RA, Yosefy C et al (2009) Assessment of right ventricular function by real-time three-dimensional echocardiography improves accuracy and decreases interobserver variability compared with conventional two-dimensional views. Eur J Echocardiogr 10:619–624

25. Shiota T, Jones M, Chikada M et al (1998) Real-time three-dimensional echocardiography for determining right ventricular stroke volume in an animal model of chronic right ventricular volume overload. Circulation 97:1897–1900

26. Chen G, Sun K, Huang G (2006) In vitro validation of right ventricular volume and mass measurement by real-time three-dimensional echocardiography. Echocardiography 23:395–399

27. Sugeng L, Mor-Avi V, Weinert L et al (2010) Multimodality comparison of quantitative volumetric analysis of the right ventricle. JACC Cardiovasc Imaging 3:10–18

28. Hoch M, Vasilyev NV, Soriano B et al (2007) Variables influencing the accuracy of right ventricular volume assessment by real-time 3-dimensional echocardiography: an in vitro validation study. J Am Soc Echocardiogr 20:456–461

29. Tamborini G, Brusoni D, Torres Molina JE et al (2008) Feasibility of a new generation three-dimensional echocardiography for right ventricular volumetric and functional measurements. Am J Cardiol 102:499–505

30. Tamborini G, Marsan NA, Gripari P, et al (2010) Reference values for right ventricular volumes and ejection fraction with real-time three-dimensional echocardiography: evaluation in a large series of normal subjects. J Am Soc Echocardiogr 23:109–115

31. Ostenfeld E, Carlsson M, Shahgaldi K et al (2012) Manual correction of semi-automatic three-dimensional echocardiography is needed for right ventricular assessment in adults; validation with cardiac magnetic resonance. Cardiovasc Ultrasound 10:1

32. Shimada YJ, Shiota M, Siegel RJ, Shiota T (2010) Accuracy of right ventricular volumes and function determined by three-dimensional echocardiography in comparison with magnetic resonance imaging: a meta-analysis study. J Am Soc Echocardiogr 23:943–953

33. van der Hulst AE, Roest AA, Holman ER et al (2011) Real-time three-dimensional echocardiography: segmental analysis of the right ventricle in patients with repaired tetralogy of fallot. J Am Soc Echocardiogr 24:1183–1190

34. Vitarelli A, Sardella G, Roma AD et al (2012) Assessment of right ventricular function by three-dimensional echocardiography and myocardial strain imaging in adult atrial septal defect before and after percutaneous closure. Int J Cardiovasc Imaging 28:1905–1916

35. Prakasa KR, Dalal D, Wang J et al (2006) Feasibility and variability of three dimensional echocardiography in arrhythmogenic right ventricular dysplasia/cardiomyopathy. Am J Cardiol 97:703–709

36. Bello, V, Conte L, Delle Donne MG et al (2013) Advantages of real time three-dimensional echocardiography in the assessment of right ventricular volumes and function in patients with pulmonary hypertension compared with conventional two-dimensional echocardiography. Echocardiography 30:820–828

37. Grapsa J, Gibbs JS, Dawson D et al (2012) Morphologic and functional remodeling of the right ventricle in pulmonary hypertension by real time three dimensional echocardiography. Am J Cardiol 109:906–913

38. Kong D, Shu X, Dong L et al (2013) Right ventricular regional systolic function and dyssynchrony in patients with pulmonary hypertension evaluated by three-dimensional echocardiography. J Am Soc Echocardiogr 26:649–65

Valvular heart disease – insufficiencies

Thomas Buck

T. Buck et al. (Hrsg.), *Three-dimensional Echocardiography*,
DOI 10.1007/978-3-642-36799-1_7, © Springer-Verlag Berlin Heidelberg 2014

Valvular insufficiencies are among the most frequent heart diseases [1][2]. Valvular flow regurgitation causes a burden of volume overload to the heart which ultimately leads to progressive heart failure [3][4][5][6]. Improved understanding of the mechanism of valvular regurgitation is of critical importance for diagnostic and therapeutic patient management [7][8]. In addition, accurate estimation of the severity of regurgitation was demonstrated to be of significant importance for patient management and prognosis [4][9] and consequently has been widely recognized in recent guidelines [7][8][10][11]. However, evaluation of both the mechanism and severity of regurgitation can be potentially difficult with the largest challenges presenting in cases of mitral regurgitation [12].

Recently, three-dimensional (3D) echocardiography has been demonstrated to add important diagnostic information about the valve morphology, mechanism, and severity of valvular regurgitation, thus, overcoming inherent limitations of two-dimensional (2D) echocardiography and potentially improving patient management [13][14][15][16][17][18][19]. Besides accurate, anatomically realistic representation of valve morphology from en face views, particularly by the use of transesophageal 3D imaging, accurate and rapid quantitative analysis by implemented 3D analysis software has opened the door to a far more detailed and accurate description of valve diseases.

7.1   Mitral regurgitation

Mitral regurgitation (MR) is the most common valve disease with a prevalence of 2–3% of significant regurgitation (moderate to severe and severe) in the general population [1]. MR is caused by a spectrum of different etiologies and correct identification of the underlying mechanism, including functional MR, mitral valve prolapse, flail leaflet due to chordal rupture, degeneration, or destruction due to endocarditis, is of critical importance for making therapeutic decisions [7, 20][21][22][23][24].

While 2D imaging only provides a planar cross-sectional view through the mitral valve, a direct en face view from either the left atrium (surgeon's view) or the left ventricle to the nonplanar surface of the mitral valve is provided by 3D echocardiography (◘ Fig. 7.1) [16][17][19]. Three-dimensional imaging of the mitral valve can be obtained using both transthoracic echocardiography (TTE) and transesophageal echocardiography (TEE); however, the transesophageal approach provides significantly better image quality in most patients (◘ Fig. 7.2). The superior image quality of TEE is not only because of the closer contact of the probe to the heart but also because the mitral valve in TEE is more in the transducer near field where the line density is higher, whereas in TTE the mitral valve is more in the far field where the line density became lower due to increased scan line divergence (▶ Fig. 2.18).

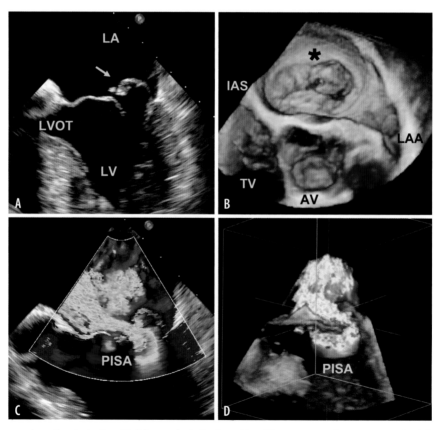

◘ **Fig. 7.1** Side-by-side comparison of a mitral valve with flail posterior leaflet (*arrow*) in a 2D cross-sectional representation (*top left*) and the RT3DE en face view from the left atrium to the mitral leaflet surface (*top right*). While the 2D cross-sectional view provides information on leaflet thickness and height of leaflet separation, the RT3DE image shows the size of the affected leaflet with flail of the P2/P1 segments (*) in relation to the total valve area as well as neighboring anatomic structures, e.g., the aortic valve (*AV*), left atrial appendage (*LAA*), interatrial septum (*IAS*), and tricuspid valve (*TV*). The 2D color Doppler shows the eccentric jet of severe mitral regurgitation with a beautiful PISA zone (*bottom left*). In a RT3DE image that is turned by 45° (see coordinate lines), color Doppler shows an asymmetric PISA zone along the commissure (*bottom right*). *LA* left atrium, *LVOT* left ventricular outflow tract, *LV* left ventricle, *PISA* proximal isovelocity surface area. [→Videos 7.1A–D]

TTE full volume 31 Hz   TTE live 3D zoom 9 Hz

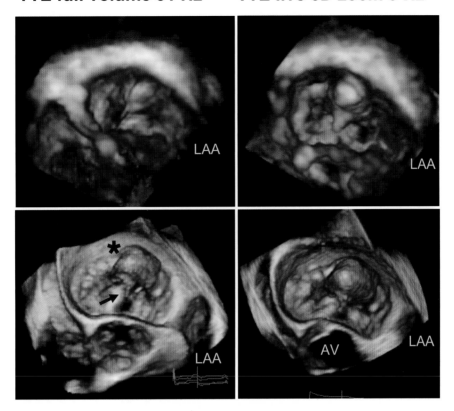

TEE full volume 30 Hz   TEE live 3D zoom 12 Hz

■ **Fig. 7.2** Comparison of 3D transthoracic (*TTE, top row*) versus 3D transesophageal (*TEE, bottom row*) visualization of a mitral valve with flail leaflet of the P2 segment (*) with a ruptured chord (*arrow*). Although the 3D TTE representation is of good quality in this example, 3D TEE generally provides significantly better image quality. Importantly, 3D full volume datasets (*left*) provide higher temporal resolution with 31 Hz and 30 Hz in this example compared to 9 Hz and 12 Hz of live 3D zoom datasets (*right*), whereas live 3D zoom datasets often provide better image quality. *LAA* left atrial appendage, *AV* aortic valve. [→Videos 7.2A–D]

> ❯ Real-time 3D echocardiography provides a direct en face view of the nonplanar surface of the mitral valve.

7.1.1 Morphologic evaluation of mitral valve insufficiency

For accurate evaluation of mitral valve disease using 3D echocardiography, a protocol of standard 3D views is recommended. Such a protocol of standard 3D views including 3D color Doppler is presented in ► Chapter 2 (► Fig. 2.25). Similar protocols have recently been published by Salcedo et al. [25] and also have been recognized in current recommendations [26]. Two principal orientations of the mitral valve are commonly used (■ Fig. 7.3):
- the **surgical orientation** representing the viewing direction of the surgeon towards the mitral valve during operation, and
- the **anatomic orientation** of the heart in the patient's body where anterior (patient's chest or ascending aorta) is oriented towards the examiner.

Although recent recommendations for image acquisition and display recommended the surgical perspective as the standard display [26], there seem to be situations where the anatomic orientation of the mitral valve provides an easier and more intuitive anatomic understanding of mitral valve disease with the relationship to neighboring cardiac structures and other cardiac disease. For example, viewing towards the curtain of regurgitant flow along the commissure in typical functional MR is more intuitive in anatomic orientation. Also, guiding a MitraClip towards the mitral leaflets is commonly performed in anatomic orientation. However, in cases where the mitral valve is evaluated in the context of a direct comparison with surgical exploration, the surgical perspective towards the mitral valve is used.

For an even increased spatial understanding of mitral valve disease a 3D dual-view mode provides simultaneous viewing from the left atrium to the mitral valve as well as from the left ventricle to the mitral valve (■ Fig. 7.4).

> ❯ For accurate evaluation of mitral valve disease using 3D echocardiography, a protocol of standard views is recommended.

Three aspects are important for a systematic evaluation of the mitral valve morphology:
- spatial orientation,
- anatomic definition of the mitral valve apparatus, and
- anatomic definition of the mitral leaflets.

Surgical perspective   ## Anatomic orientation

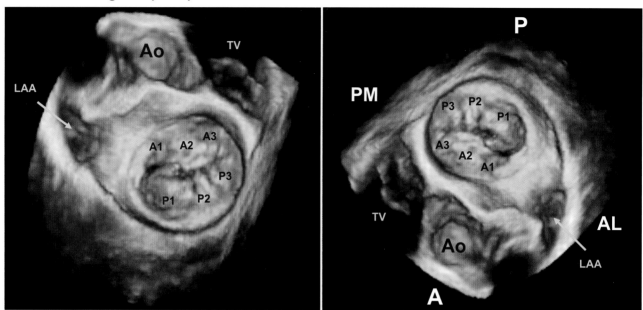

□ **Fig. 7.3** Demonstration of the surgical perspective of the mitral valve compared to the anatomic orientation of the mitral valve in the patient with P1 flail leaflet shown in □ Fig. 7.1. Note that the surgical orientation is simply a 160° clockwise rotation of the anatomic orientation. For further evaluation, leaflet segments of the mitral valve (*P1–3* and *A1–3*) are indicated (see also □ Fig. 7.6). *A* anterior, *P* posterior, *PM* postero-medial, *AL* antero-lateral, *Ao* aorta, *TV* tricuspid valve, *LAA* left atrial appendage. [→Videos 7.3A,B]

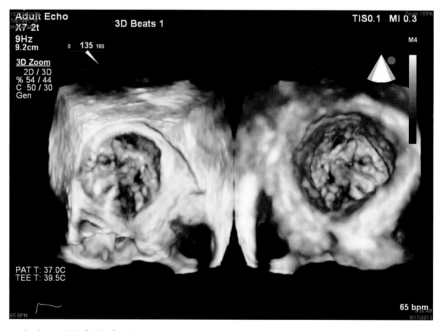

□ **Fig. 7.4** Example of a mitral valve with P2 flail leaflet shown in 3D dual-view mode. The 3D dual-view mode presents the same 3D dataset simultaneously in a perspective from the left atrium to the mitral valve (*left*) and from the left ventricle to the mitral valve (*right*). [→Video 7.4]

For orientation it is important to identify anterior, posterior, lateral and medial – and, of course, superior, and inferior. The importance of anatomic structures to identify the spatial orientation is illustrated in □ Fig. 7.3: the aortic valve is located anterior; thus, the opposite side of the mitral valve is posterior; the left atrial appendage is located antero-lateral; and the opposite side of the mitral valve is postero-medial. The majority of mitral valve disease causing insufficiency are not limited to the mitral leaflets, but involve other parts of the mitral valve apparatus as well, existing of the saddle-shaped mitral annulus, the two leaflets, and the chordae tendineae (tendinous cords) connecting the leaflets to the papillary muscles [27]. The anatomy of the leaflets is commonly divided into three leaflet segments of the posterior leaflet (P1–3) and three segments of the anterior leaflet (A1–3) according to the classification of Carpentier et al. [28].

◘ Tab. 7.1 Synopsis of functional classification of mitral valve insufficiency modified from Carpentier et al. [29] and Al-Radi et al. [30] and morphologic classification

Functional classification		Morphologic classification			
Type	Leaflet motion	Valve pathology	Prolapse or flail	Leaflet thickening	Functional or organic MR
Ia	Normal	Annular dilatation			Functional or organic
Ib		Leaflet defect			Organic
IIa	Increased	Chordal elongation	Prolapse	Not thickened (FED or thickened (Barlow)	
IIb		Chordal rupture	Flail leaflet		
IIc		Papillary muscle elongation	Prolapse		
IId		Papillary muscle rupture	Flail leaflet		
IIIa	Restricted	Commissural or chordal fusion or shortening			
IIIb		Leaflet tethering by LV dilatation			Functional

LV left ventricle, *FED* fibroelastic deficiency, *MR* mitral regurgitation

7.1.2 Classification of mitral valve insufficiency

For correct interpretation and communication of 3D images of insufficient mitral valves, the understanding of the different existing classifications of mitral valve disease causing regurgitation is important. Beside the definition of mitral valve insufficiency based on morphology and etiology, Carpentier et al. [29] introduced a functional classification mainly based on leaflet motion which was modified later by Al-Radi et al. [30] for further differentiation (◘ Tab. 7.1). In principle, etiology of mitral regurgitation can be divided into either functional or organic mitral valve disease. In functional mitral regurgitation, mitral leaflets are normal and regurgitation is mainly caused by incomplete mitral leaflet closure due to annular dilatation and/or leaflet tethering, while organic mitral valve disease is caused by malformation of the mitral leaflets or subvalvular apparatus, including mitral valve prolapse, flail leaflet due to chordal rupture, leaflet degeneration, leaflet perforation, and papillary muscle rupture. Within this spectrum, a more differentiated description of mitral valve prolapse is based on either billowing or prolapsing of one or both leaflets [31] and thickening of mitral leaflets of less than 5 mm (nonclassic prolapse) or 5 mm and more (classic prolapse) [32]. Etiologies of mitral valve prolapse are differentiated into fibroelastic deficiency (FED) with or without chordal rupture or myxoid degeneration present in Barlow's disease, which includes leaflet thickening, large redundant leaflets, chordal elongation or rupture, and annular dilatation [33]. A finding of mild-to-moderate mitral valve degeneration between a normal valve and true myxomatous degeneration is described as a forme fruste of myxomatous Barlow's disease [33]. Flail leaflet refers to the condition of mitral valve prolapse with chordal rupture causing significant displacement of one or more segments of either the posterior or anterior leaflet towards the left atrium combined with severe eccentric mitral regurgitation (◘ Fig. 7.1) [34].

Beside the common malformations of the mitral leaflets associated with organic mitral valve insufficiency as described above, recently 3D TEE brought the presence of deep indentations or deep slits between posterior or anterior leaflet segments to our attention. These deep slits are extreme expressions of the indentations particularly common between P1/P2 and P2/P3 and reach from the commissure line up to the mitral annulus (◘ Fig. 7.5) [26][35]. According to a recent study by Ring et al. [36] deep slits are frequent findings in patients with mitral valve prolapse or flail and are predominantly found in the posterior leaflet but can also be present in the anterior leaflet. Two deep slits are frequently found in the posterior leaflet but mitral valves with up to five slits and more have been reported [36].

Compared to morphology-based classification, functional classification by Carpentier differentiates mitral valve disease according to normal (type I), increased (type II), or restricted leaflet motion (type III) [29]. The complexity of criteria is illustrated in ◘ Tab. 7.1, which provides a synopsis of the different classifications of mitral valve insufficiency. For simplification and consistency, the morphologic classification of mitral valve insufficiency has been primarily used in this chapter.

7.1.3 Mitral valve prolapse, flail, and Barlow's disease

Based on current diagnostic criteria, the prevalence of mitral valve prolapse (MVP), including the subgroups of flail leaflet or Barlow's disease, is estimated at 2–3% [32]. While mitral valve prolapse or flail of the posterior or anterior leaflet can be easily detected by 2D echocardiography, accurate assessment of size and location of the affected leaflet segments using a systematic examination protocol (◘ Fig. 7.6) is difficult and allows only mental reconstruction of the 3D valve pathology [37].

> ❯ Accurate assessment of size and location of mitral valve prolapse or flail using 2D echocardiography is difficult and requires mental reconstruction of the 3D valve pathology.

Compared to 2D echocardiography, real-time 3D echocardiography (RT3DE) provides rapid visual representation by direct viewing of the valve surface which allows for intuitive spatial recognition of affected leaflet segments and accurate detection of size and location of the prolapsing leaflet segments in relation to the leaflet segment classification by Carpentier (◻ Fig. 7.7) [16] [19][25][28][35][38][39] . While initial transthoracic application already demonstrated the benefit of 3D visualization of the mitral valve [15][18][40][41], morphologic assessment of the mitral valve improved dramatically with the availability of real-time 3D TEE [17][38][39], particularly in complex cases with pathologies of multiple leaflet segments (◻ Fig. 7.8).

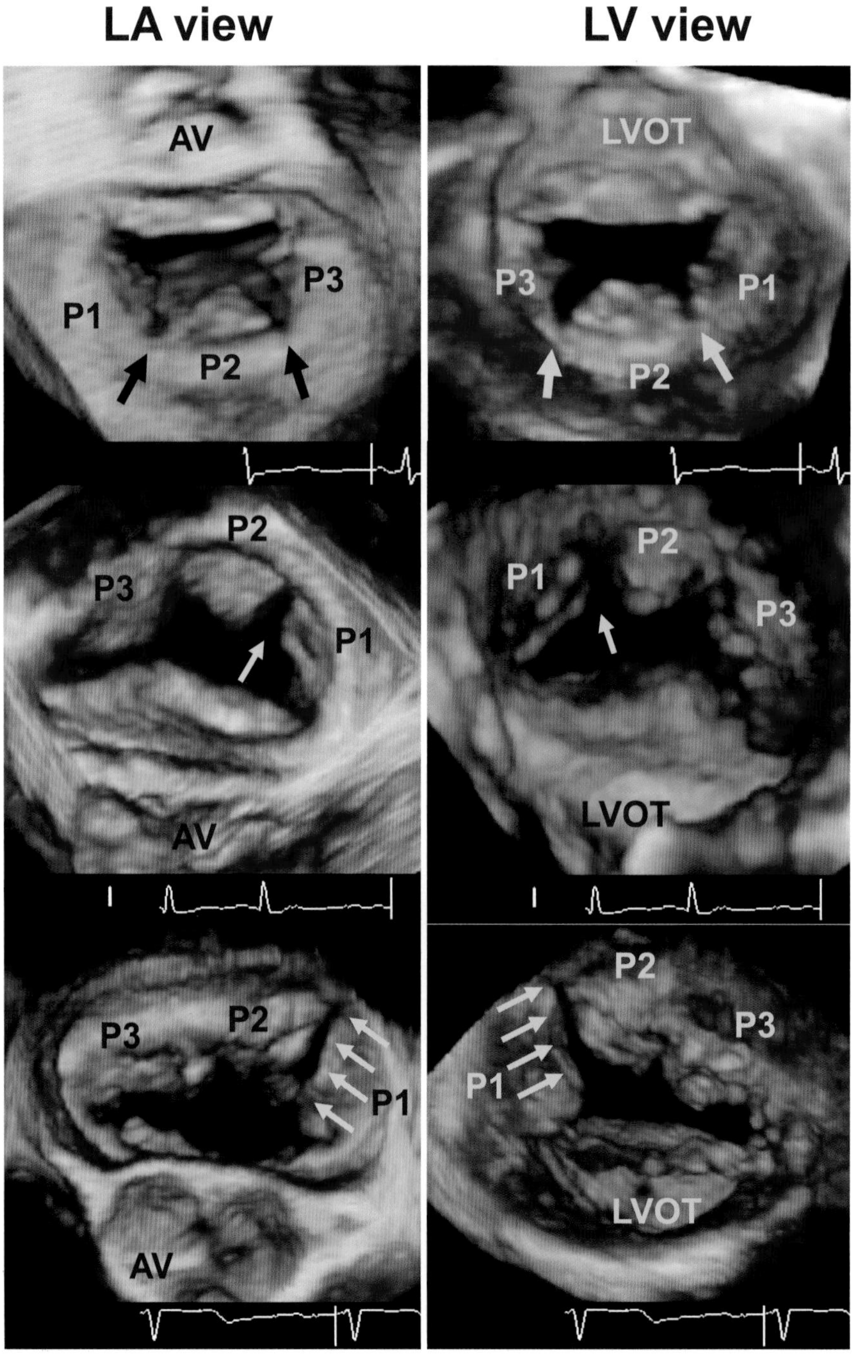

LA view   **LV view**

◻ **Fig. 7.5** Examples of deep slits in mitral valve leaflets in three different patients where each mitral valve is shown in an en face view from the left atrium (*LA*; *left*) and from the left ventricle (*LV*; *right*). *Top* Two typical deep slits (*arrows*) in the posterior leaflet separating P1 and P2 and P2 and P3 are shown and reach up to the posterior mitral annulus. *Middle* One deep slit (*arrow*) between P1 and P2 reaching up to the mitral annulus in a patient with P3 flail is shown (→ Video). *Bottom* A deep slit between P1 and P2 in a patient with severe prolapse of the posterior leaflet with another deep slit between P2 and P3 is shown (→Video). *AV* aortic valve, *LVOT* left ventricular outflow tract. [→Videos 7.5A–F]

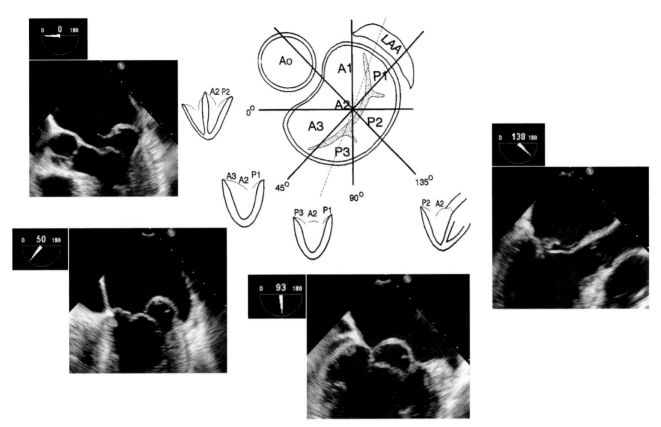

Fig. 7.6 Example of systematic 2D transesophageal image acquisition by axial image plane rotation in a patient with P2 flail leaflet and representation of image plane position in a schematic of the mitral valve with leaflets segments. According to the 2D view orientation, the schematic represents the mitral valve in a view from the left ventricle towards the mitral valve. Source [37]; Copyright Elsevier. [→Videos 7.6A–D]

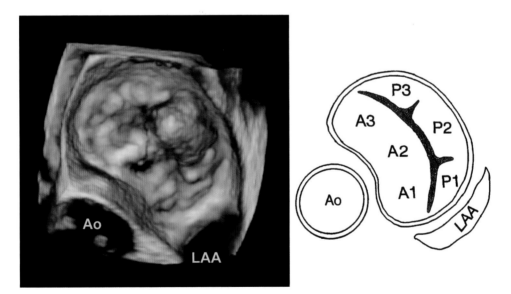

Fig. 7.7 Side-by-side representation of a RT3DE en face view (surgeon's view) from the left atrium to the mitral valve in the same patient shown in Fig. 7.6 (*left*) and the schematic of anterior (*A1–3*) and posterior (*P1–3*) mitral leaflet segments by Carpentier in the same orientation (*right;* source [28]; Copyright Elsevier). The RT3DE image in live 3D zoom mode clearly shows a flail leaflet of the P2 segment with a ruptured chord. *Ao* aortic root, *LAA* left atrial appendage. [→Video 7.7]

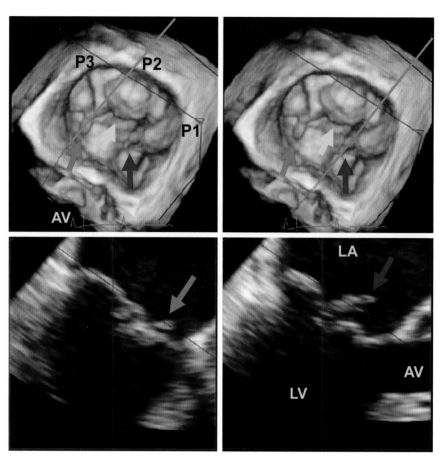

Fig. 7.8 Example of a complex pathology of a mitral valve with severe MR and a ruptured chord at P1 segment of the posterior leaflet (*blue arrow*), another ruptured chord at P3 segment (*red arrow*) and a prolapsing P2 segment (*yellow arrow*) in between. The *green* planes cutting through the 3D dataset in the *upper left* and *right panel* show the ruptured chord at P3 in the *lower left panel* (*red arrow*) and the ruptured chord at P1 in the *lower right panel* (*blue arrow*). The complexity of this pathology could not be anticipated from the conventional 2D TEE examination. *AV* aortic valve, *LA* left atrium, *LV* left ventricle. [→Video 7.8]

In Barlow's disease, RT3DE allows rapid recognition of the typical hyperelastic prolapse motion towards the left atrium of the entire mitral valve including the dilated mitral annulus. Conventional 2D echocardiographic cross-sectional imaging of the valve leaflets, however, provides important additional information of leaflet thickness and structure (■ Fig. 7.9 and ■ Fig. 7.10) which is of particular importance in the detection of Barlow's disease with characteristic myxomatous leaflet thickening [42][43]. The importance of leaflet thickness and structure in the differential diagnosis of fibroelastic deficiency (FED) and Barlow's disease emphasizes the complementary nature of 2D echocardiography and RT3DE: RT3DE provides important information beyond 2D echocardiography, but at the same time 2D echocardiographic cross-sectional views add indispensable information to RT3DE. Differentiation between FED and Barlow's disease is important for the surgical procedure because mitral valve repair is more difficult and might be less successful in Barlow's disease [33][44].

In contrast to Barlow's disease, FED is characterized by normal or near-normal valve size, no excess tissue, thin leaflets and thin chordae, eventual chordal rupture, and typically single segment prolapse, most commonly of the P2 segment, or single leaflet prolapse (■ Fig. 7.10) [19][33]. In a recent study Chandra et al. [45] demonstrated the usefulness of RT3DE to reliably differentiate FED from Barlow's disease using multiple parameters of mitral valve geometry. In Barlow's disease, the frequency of bileaflet prolapse and posterior leaflet prolapse were found to be nearly in histopathologic studies, whereas in FED posterior leaflet prolapse was dominant and bileaflet prolapse very rare. Isolated anterior leaflet prolapse was rare in both FED and Barlow's disease [46].

> RT3DE provides important information beyond 2D echocardiography, but at the same time 2D echocardiographic cross-sectional views add indispensable information to RT3DE.

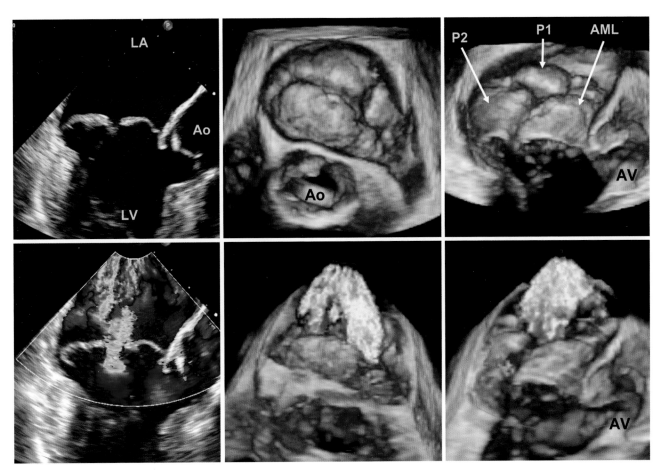

◻ **Fig. 7.9** Example of patient with Barlow's disease with typical distinct prolapse motion of the entire mitral valve towards the left atrium. The 2D cross-sectional image of the mitral valve shows typical myxomatous thickening of mitral valve leaflets (*top left*). RT3DE en face view to the mitral valve shows prolapsing of all leaflet segments toward the left atrium (*top middle*). RT3DE side view to the mitral valve apparatus demonstrates the extent of the prolapse motion (*top right*). However, the typical prolapse motion with tilting of the mitral annulus toward the left atrium is most obvious in the videos. The 2D color Doppler shows moderate-to-severe mitral regurgitation due to malcoaptation of the prolapsing leaflets (*bottom left*). RT3DE color Doppler view in the same perspective as the image above shows two regurgitant jets at the antero-lateral and postero-medial intersection of the posterior leaflet (*bottom middle*). RT3DE color Doppler side view in the same perspective as the image above shows the regurgitant jet at the antero-lateral intersection between the anterior mitral leaflet (*AML*), P1, and P2 (*bottom right*). *LA* left atrium, *LV* left ventricle, *Ao* aortic root, *AV* aortic valve. [→Videos 7.9A–F]

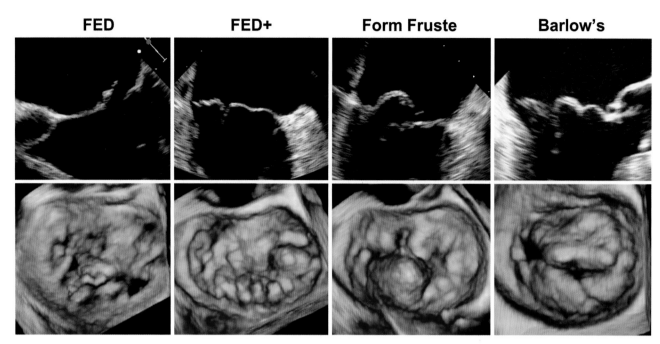

FED   **FED+**   **Form Fruste**   **Barlow's**

■ **Fig. 7.10** Live 3D en face visualization compared to 2D cross-sectional views in four examples of degenerative type II mitral valve insufficiency (3D views oriented in surgical perspective): fibroelastic deficiency (*FED*) with a ruptured chord and A2 flail leaflet, fibroelastic deficiency with increased excess of tissue (*FED+)* but still thin leaflets, forme fruste of Barlow's disease with focal excess of tissue, mild-to-moderate leaflet thickening and a ruptured chord (P2 segment), and typical Barlow's disease with severe excess of tissue of both leaflets and true myxomatous leaflet thickening. [→Videos 7.10A–H]

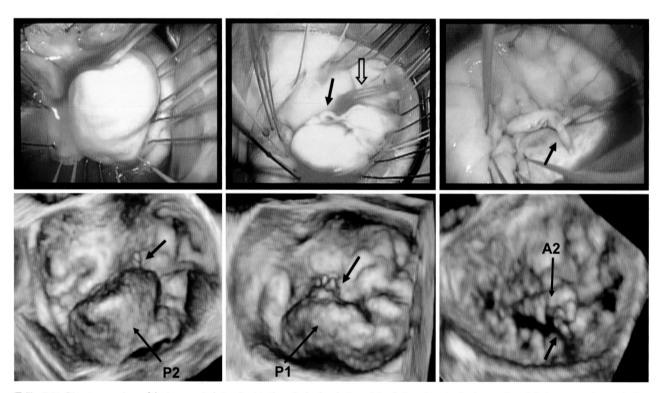

■ **Fig. 7.11** Direct comparison of the true surgical view (*top*) to the mitral valve during minimally invasive mitral valve repair and the intraoperative surgical view of the mitral valve using RT3D TEE. *Left* A large P2 fail leaflet is shown. RT3DE (*bottom left*) clearly depicts a ruptured chord (*bold arrow*) which is not detected in the intraoperative aspect of the flail. *Middle* A large P1 flail leaflet is shown. Both the surgical (*top middle*) and the RT3DE (*bottom middle*) representations depict a ruptured chord (*bold arrow*). In the surgical view, a regurgitant water jet is captured during water testing (*white arrow*). *Right* Typical FED with A2 flail leaflet with a ruptured chord (*bold arrow*) is shown. The three examples demonstrate that there is usually no perfect agreement between representation of the mitral valve pathology in the surgical view during operation and RT3DE representation. [→Videos 7.11A–C]

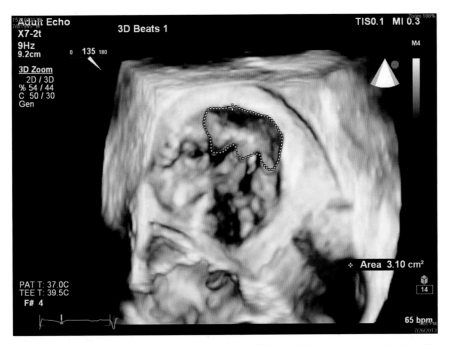

Fig. 7.12 Illustration of direct 3D measurement of the area of a flail P2 segment in a 3D image (3D measurement on the glass). The image shows the direct planimetry (*dotted line*) of the area of the flail leaflet segment indicated as 3.10 cm² in the *lower right*. [→Video 7.12]

Direct comparison between intraoperative findings of mitral valve pathologies from the surgeon's view and RT3DE representation demonstrated high agreement with the advantage that RT3DE shows the valve in physiologic motion and under pressure conditions (■ Fig. 7.11; see ► Chapter 12) [16][45][47].

7.1.4 Mitral valve quantification

Quantification of mitral valve anatomy and pathologies is challenging because of the complex geometry of the mitral apparatus including the saddle-shaped annulus and often asymmetric leaflet prolapse or tenting. Thus, quantification of mitral valve morphology by distances and areas in planar cut views using multiplanar reconstruction (MPR; see ► Fig. 2.38) is very limited. New 3D software allows direct 3D measurements of distances and areas on 3D images (■ Fig. 7.12), where measurements are made like on a translucent plane of glass with the 3D mitral valve anatomy shown behind (see ► Chapter 2.5). This makes 3D measurements much easier and faster, but might not provide true 3D dimensions and is limited by foreshortening errors. Beyond visual assessment of mitral valve pathology, graphical 3D analysis software has recently been realized for advanced 3D quantitative analysis and graphic reconstruction of the entire mitral apparatus (■ Fig. 7.13) [19][25][26][38][45][48], thus, opening the door for detailed quantitative analysis of the mitral apparatus before and after mitral valve surgery and interventions with potential implications on patient and procedure selection [45]. This mitral valve quantification (MVQ) application provides a wide spectrum of 1D, 2D, and 3D parameters of the mitral valve (■ Fig. 7.14, ■ Fig. 7.15, ■ Fig. 7.16) that could not be obtained by conventional 2D echocardiography. Moreover, MVQ is a promising approach to overcome the limitation that measurements until now could not be performed directly in 3D images (► Chapter 2). Potentially important parameters derived by RT3DE before mitral valve repair in type II disease include the antero-posterior diameter (DAP) and anterolateral–posteromedial diameter (DAlPm) of the mitral ring, the 3D curvilinear length of the posterior and anterior leaflet, the exposed area of leaflets (A3DE), the minimal area of leaflets within the saddle-shaped annulus (A3Dmin), the volume of leaflet prolapse (VProl), the maximal prolapse height (HProl) and the length of antero-lateral and postero-medial chordae tendinae. Recently, mitral valve quantification based on RT3D TEE has been validated to accurately predict the length of artificial chordae required for mitral valve repair which shortened cardiopulmonary bypass time and aortic cross-clamp time while improving the results of mitral valve repair [49]. Based on these parameters, the ratio of A3DE to A3Dmin as a measure of excess tissue and the ratio of exposed prolapse area to leaflet area as a measure of leaflet displacement may also improve planning of mitral valve repair and prediction of outcome as described below [45][48]. Recent studies even demonstrated the possibility of direct measurement of the anatomic regurgitant orifice using 3D mitral valve quantification software [50][51].

> Mitral valve quantification (MVQ) provides a wide spectrum of 1D, 2D, and 3D parameters of the mitral valve.

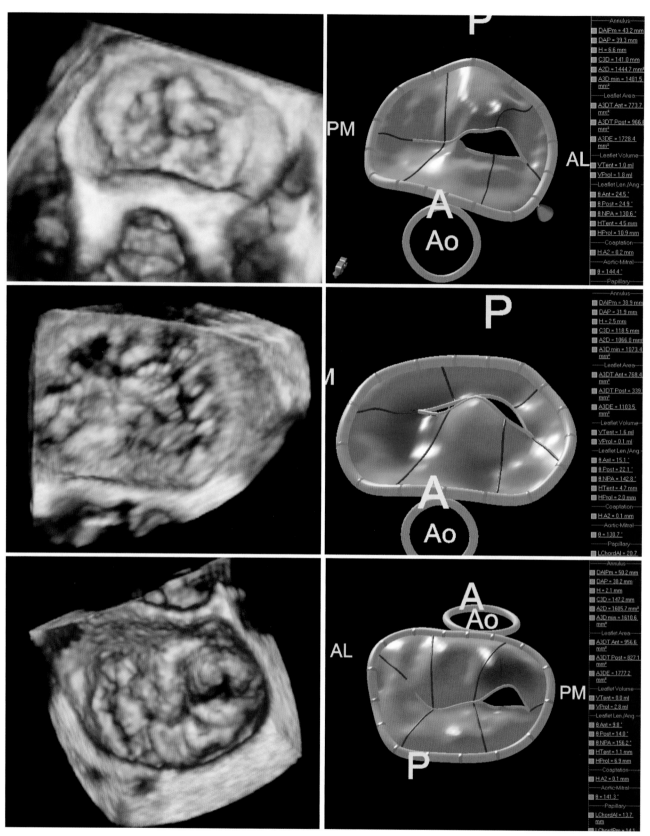

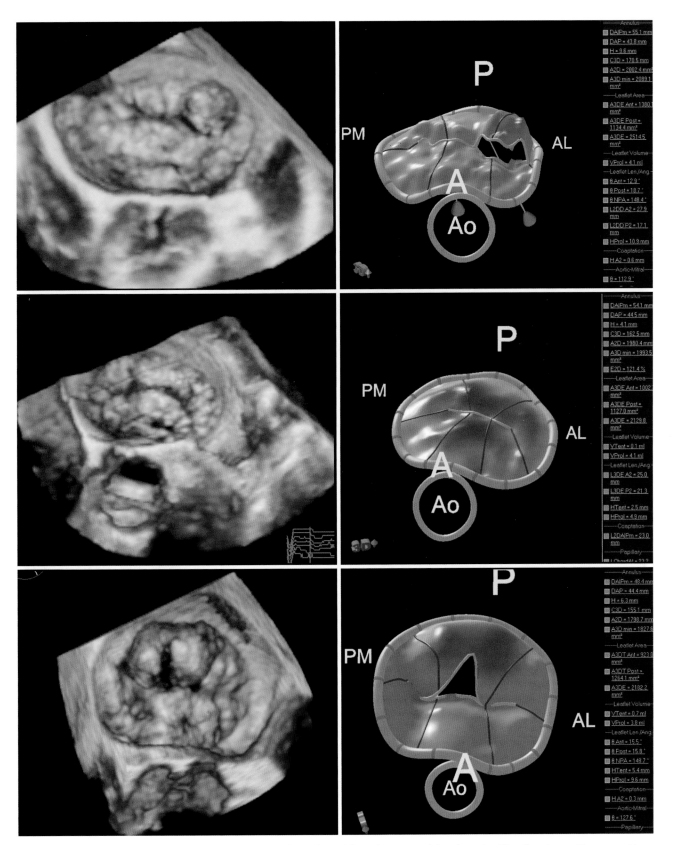

Fig. 7.13 (continued) Different cases of mitral valve prolapse or flail leaflet at different locations and sizes shown in a 3D en face view and in a parametric visualization from MVQ v7.0 analysis. *Top* (previous page) Flail leaflet of the P2 segment with three or four stumps of ruptured chords. *Middle* (previous page) Small flail leaflet of the A2 segment with single ruptured chord. *Bottom* (previous page) Flail leaflet of the A3 segment with no ruptured chord visible. *Top* Flail leaflet of the P1 segment with single ruptured chord. *Middle* Prolapse of all segments of both leaflets (=bileaflet billowing) like in a patient with Barlow's disease; however, in this patient, the leaflets were relatively thin indicating FED+. *Bottom* Prolapse of the P2 segment with a rare cleft-like incision of the leaflet segment. *PM* postero-medial, *AL* antero-lateral, *A* anterior, *P* posterior, *Ao* aortic root. [→Videos 7.13A–F]

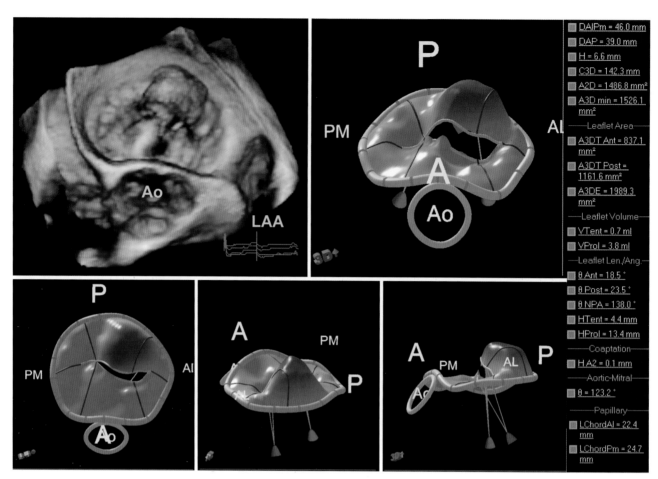

■ **Fig. 7.14** Example of mitral valve quantification using MVQ analysis software (v7.0) in the case of flail leaflet of the P2 segment shown in ■ Fig. 7.2, ■ Fig. 7.6, and ■ Fig. 7.7. The *two top panels* show side-by-side the RT3DE en face view to the mitral valve (*top left*) and the parametric visualization of the mitral valve as the result of MVQ analysis where the color spectrum from red to blue encodes the height of the leaflet surface to the mitral annulus level on both sides of the surface (*top right*). The measurement parameters on the right border represent a list of valve dimensions represented individually in ■ Fig. 7.16. *Bottom* Three different perspectives of the mitral valve reconstruction are presented. *Ao* aortic root, *LAA* left atrial appendage *PM* postero-medial, *AL* antero-lateral, *A* anterior, *P* posterior. [→Video 7.14]

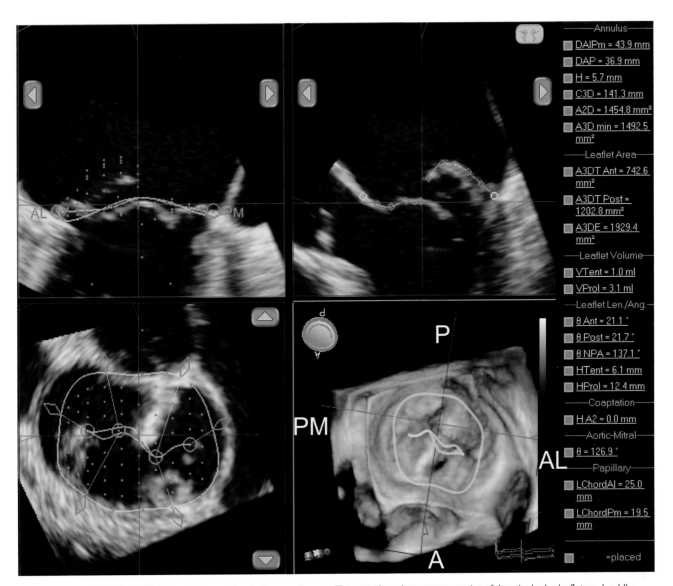

Fig. 7.15 Example of the MVQ v7.0 analysis procedure in the case shown in ▫ Fig. 7.14 based on accurate tracing of the mitral valve leaflets and saddle-shaped mitral annulus within tomographic planes through the 3D dataset. *Top left* A side view to the mitral valve through the 3D dataset with the mitral annulus and the leaflet surface points. *Top right* A single tomographic plane with a cross-sectional view through the mitral leaflets with leaflet tracing points is shown. *Bottom left* An en face view to the mitral valve with the mitral annulus and the leaflet surface points along ten tomographic slices is depicted. *Bottom right* A 3D en face view to the mitral valve provides a view of the P2 flail segment, the mitral annulus, and the commissure line. *PM* postero-medial, *AL* antero-lateral, *A* anterior, *P* posterior

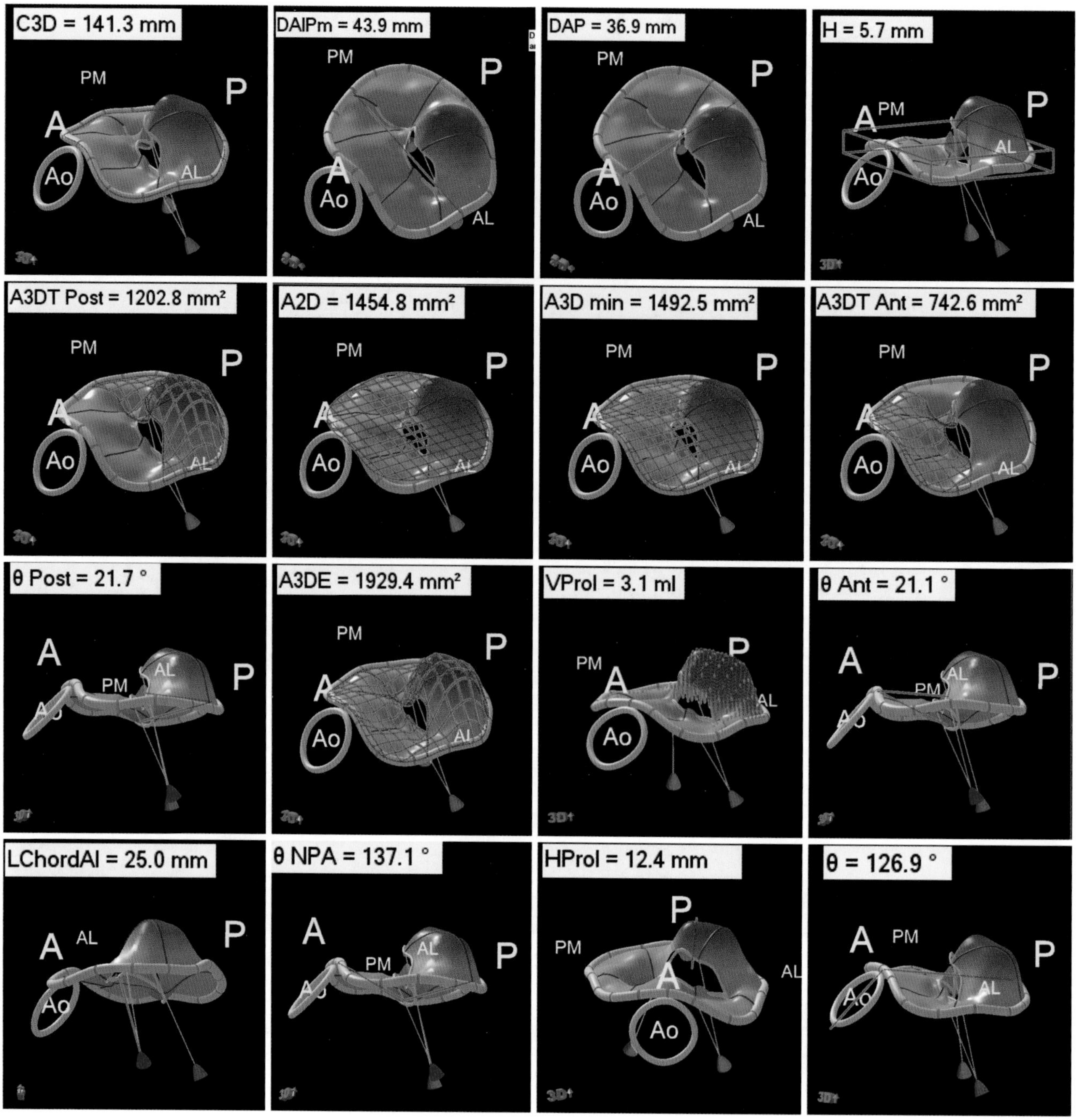

■ **Fig. 7.16** Examples of quantitative measurements of the mitral valve apparatus obtained from the MVQ v7.0 analysis. The individual measurements are indicated (*green*). *Left to right and top to bottom: DAIPm* anterolateral–posteromedial diameter of annulus, *DAP* anterior to posterior diameter of annulus, *H* annulus height (due to saddle shape), *C3D* perimeter of annulus, *A2D* area of annulus in the projection plane, *A3Dmin* area of minimal surface spanning annulus, *A3DT Ant* total area of anterior leaflet, *A3DT Post* total area of posterior leaflet, *A3DE* exposed area of leaflets, *VProl* volume of leaflet prolapse, *θ Ant* angle of anterior leaflet, *θ Post* angle of posterior leaflet, *θ NPA* nonplanar angle of leaflets, *HProl* maximal prolapse height, *θ* aortic orifice to mitral plane angle, *LChordAl* length of antero-lateral chordae tendinae

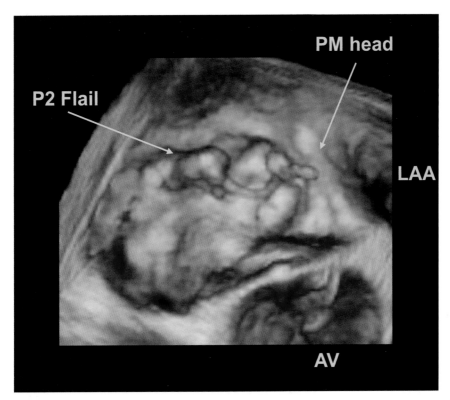

◻ Fig. 7.17 Live 3D Zoom TEE en face view of a mitral valve with P2 flail due to rupture of only one of the multiple heads of the antero-lateral papillary muscle. The thickened chord connecting the papillary muscle head (*PM head*) and P2 segment can be clearly identified. *AV* aortic valve, *LAA* left atrial appendage. [→Video 7.17]

7.1.5 Papillary muscle rupture

Acute papillary muscle rupture, a rare complication of myocardial infarction with an incidence of about 1% of autopsied cases, usually occurs 3–5 days after infarction. Rupture of the postero-medial papillary muscle is about 6–12 times more frequent than rupture of the antero-lateral papillary muscle [52]. Complete rupture of the papillary muscle at the common trunk results in severe MR with flail leaflet and the mobile papillary muscle attached to the chordae tendinae prolapsing into the left atrium in systole. Less severe deterioration with rupture of only one of the multiple heads of the papillary muscle or rupture of chordae tendinae is more frequent but can be more difficult to recognize (◻ Fig. 7.17). Whereas identification of the degree of rupture and location might be difficult using 2D echocardiography, RT3D TEE provides unlimited visualization of the left ventricle and the two papillary muscles with detailed information of the ruptured structures (◻ Fig. 7.18). This information is of potential importance for planning surgical repair.

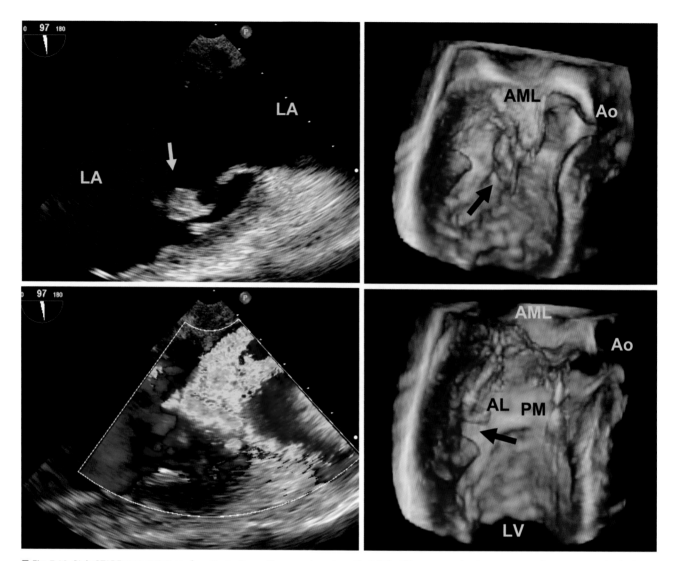

Fig. 7.18 *Right* RT3DE representation of a patient with papillary muscle rupture. *Top left* The 2D representation in a transgastric long-axis view clearly shows the ruptured papillary muscle at the anterior LV wall with the free floating papillary muscle head (*arrow*) connected by chordae tendinae to the anterior leaflet. However, spatial orientation of the anatomy is difficult. *Bottom left* The 2D color Doppler image with the same orientation shows severe mitral regurgitation. *Top right* The RT3DE representation shows the ruptured head (*arrow*) of the antero-lateral (*AL*) papillary muscle hanging on the anterior mitral leaflet (*AML*) in a diastolic phase. *Bottom right* RT3DE representation clearly shows the ruptured AL papillary muscle (*arrow*) opposite the intact postero-medial (*PM*) papillary muscle in a systolic phase with the left ventricular outflow tract and the aortic root in the upper right back. *LV* left ventricle, *LA* left atrium. [→Videos 7.18A–C]

7.1.6 Functional mitral regurgitation

Functional mitral regurgitation (MR) is frequently found as regurgitation due to incomplete mitral leaflet closure caused predominantly by geometric distortion of the mitral apparatus, but not by organic changes of the mitral valve [53]. Characteristic findings by 2D echocardiography are tenting of the mitral leaflets due to leaflet tethering towards the displaced papillary muscles and central mitral regurgitation along the commissural line [14][54]. Common parameters of functional mitral regurgitation by 2D echocardiography are mitral valve diameter (MVD), tenting area, which is defined as the area between the two leaflets and the mitral annulus level, coaptation height or depth (CH) [11][55], which is defined as the length between the annular line and coaptation point of the two leaflets, coaptation length (CL), which is defined as the length of coaptation of the two leaflets between the coaptation point of the leaflets and the leaflet tips, and coaptation length index (CLI), which is defined as the quotient of CL and MVD [56]. Functional MR is typically characterized by increased MVD, increased CH, reduced CL, and reduced CLI. Calafiore et al. [55] proposed a preoperative CH of 10 mm or less to be a prognostic parameter for successful mitral valve repair and a preoperative CH of 11 mm or higher to implicate mitral

valve replacement. Yamauchi et al. [56] measured a restored CL of 11.6±4.6 mm after successful mitral valve repair. Recent studies, however, have shown that leaflet tenting is asymmetric and that the magnitude and pattern of asymmetry vary with infarct anatomy [51][57]. These data suggest that isolated single-plane indexes of leaflet tenting as measured in either a parasternal long-axis or apical 4-chamber view are potentially inaccurate, inconsistent, and inadequate to describe the pathologic anatomy and mechanics. RT3DE, however, provides visual assessment as well as 3D quantitative analysis of the geometry of the entire mitral apparatus (◘ Fig. 7.19 and ◘ Fig. 7.20). Initial quantitative analysis by Otsuji et al. [53] showed that mitral regurgitant volume and orifice area did not correlate with LV ejection fraction and dP/dt but did correlate with changes in the tethering distance from the papillary muscles to the anterior annulus derived from 3D reconstructions, especially papillary muscle shifts in the posterior and mediolateral directions, as well as with annular area (p<0.0005).

❯ RT3DE provides advanced 3D quantitative analysis of the geometry of the entire mitral valve apparatus in patients with functional MR.

Beyond this, tenting volume below tethered leaflets can be determined from 3D echocardiographic datasets, which is potentially

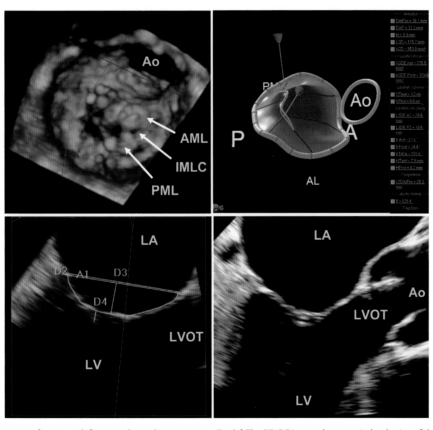

◘ **Fig. 7.19** RT3DE representation of a case with functional mitral regurgitation. *Top left* The RT3DE image shows typical tethering of the anterior and posterior mitral leaflet (*AML, PML*) toward the LV lateral wall with incomplete mitral leaflet closure (*IMLC*) along the commissure. The video clip of the image makes the incomplete mitral leaflet closure more impressive. *Top right* Parametric visualization using MVQ analysis shows the leaflets tethered towards the LV (*blue*). The green cross-plane through the 3D dataset in the antero-posterior direction (*top and bottom left*) shows the basic 2D parameters of functional MR: tenting area (*A1*=2.55 cm²), anterior to posterior diameter of annulus (*D2*=3.59 cm), tenting or coaptation height (*D3*=0.98 cm), coaptation length (*D4*=0.32 cm; *bottom left*). The 2D image and video provide cross-sectional information of leaflet tethering and tenting and poor coaptation (*bottom right*). *Ao* aorta, *A* anterior, *P* posterior, *AL* antero-lateral, *PM* postero-medial, *LA* left atrium, *LV* left ventricle, *LVOT* left ventricular outflow tract. [→Videos 7.19A,B]

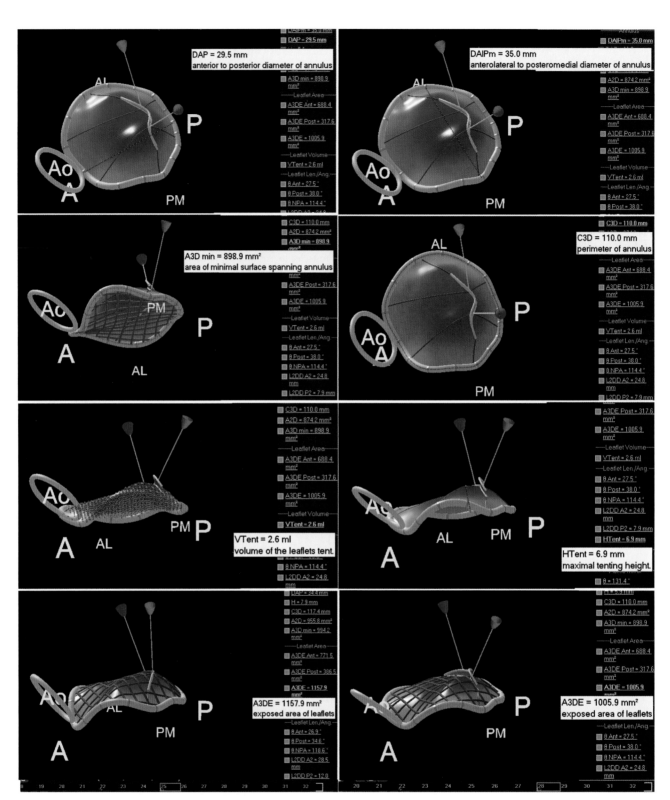

◘ **Fig. 7.20** Quantitative 3D parameters for the analysis of the mitral apparatus in patients with functional MR. Antero-posterior annulus diameter (*DAP; top left*); anterolateral–posteromedial annulus diameter (*DAIPm; top right*); mitral annulus area (*A3Dmin; 2nd row left*); annulus circumference (*C3D; 2nd row right*); tenting volume (*VTent; 3rd row left*); tenting height (*HTent; 3rd row right*). The difference between 3D tenting surface area (*A3DE*) at the onset of MV closure (*bottom left*) and 3D tenting surface area at the maximum MV closure (*bottom right*) divided by 3D tenting surface area at the onset of MV closure yields a coaptation index of 1.13. The mitral valve tenting volume (*3rd row left*) over mitral annulus area (*2nd row left*) yields a tenting index of 2.89. *Ao* aorta, *A* anterior, *P* posterior, *AL* antero-lateral, *PM* postero-medial

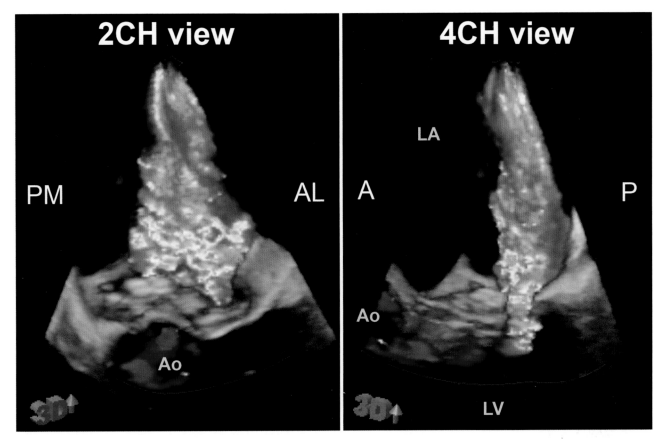

Fig. 7.21 RT3DE representation of the typical color Doppler finding of regurgitant flow in functional MR with a narrow jet in the 4-chamber (*4CH*) view (*right*) and a broad jet in 2-chamber (*2CH*) view (*left*) because of flow along the commissural line due to incomplete leaflet closure. *Ao* aorta, *A* anterior, *P* posterior, *AL* antero-lateral, *PM* postero-medial, *LAA* left atrial appendage, *LA* left atrium, *LV* left ventricle. [→Videos 7.21A,B]

more accurate compared to 2D tenting area, because the 2D tenting area is dependent on the location of the cross-sectional view through the mitral valve and, therefore, prone to underestimation [51][58][59][60]. The mitral valve tenting index, which is defined as the mitral valve tenting volume divided by the mitral annulus area, has also been proposed to provide a quantitative description of leaflet tenting that is independent of mitral annular dilation (◼ Fig. 7.20) [61]. As another promising parameter obtained by RT3DE, the mitral leaflet coaptation index has been demonstrated to provide a superior measure of the extent of coaptation compared to 2D coaptation length, the coaptation index being defined as the difference between 3D tenting surface area at the onset of MV closure and 3D tenting surface area at the maximum MV closure divided by 3D tenting surface area at the onset of MV closure (◼ Fig. 7.20) [62].

Thus, for planning surgical mitral valve reconstruction by ring implantation, potentially important 3D parameters include the antero-posterior annulus diameter (DAP), anterolateral-posteromedial annulus diameter (DAlPm), mitral annulus area and circumference, mitral valve area, tenting volume, tenting volume index, tenting height, and coaptation length index (◼ Fig. 7.20).

In patients with functional MR, RT3DE with color Doppler provides improved understanding of the characteristic jet geometry with a broad jet along the commissure in the 2-chamber view, while the jet appears narrow in the 4-chamber view (◼ Fig. 7.21). Color Doppler information from RT3DE datasets also allows improved assessment of effective regurgitant orifice area (EROA) for evaluation of MR severity (► Section 7.1.11) [14]. Alternatively, 3D mitral valve quantification software allows for direct measurement of the anatomic regurgitant orifice [50] [51]. Beyond this, RT3DE provides important information before and during interventional mitral valve reconstruction using a percutaneous annuloplasty device (Viacor) or percutaneous mitral valve clipping (see ► Chapter 12).

⊗ RT3DE color Doppler datasets allow improved assessment of effective regurgitant orifice area for evaluation of MR severity.

7.1.7 Endocarditis

Endocarditis can cause MR by destruction of one or both leaflets, by destruction of the commissural leaflet edges, or by destruction of the chords leading to flail leaflet [63]. RT3DE provides anatomically realistic visualization of valve pathology that is potentially important for planning mitral valve surgery (◼ Fig. 7.22). Visual assessment of location, size, and mobility of vegetations might assist in estimating the risk of embolization (see ► Chapter 11).

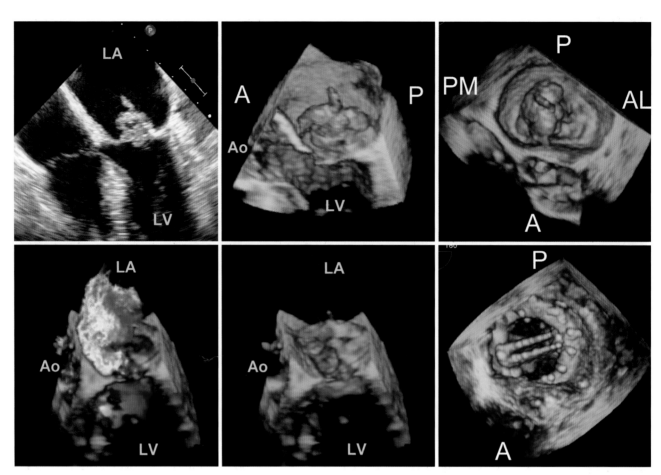

🔲 **Fig. 7.22** Example of severe endocarditis of the mitral valve with a large solid vegetation on the posterior mitral leaflet and a smaller soft and mobile mass on top which could also be thrombus. *Top left* The 2D 4-chamber view. *Top middle* Live 3D view showing the size, shape, and surface structure of the solid vegetation on the posterior leaflet. *Top right* Live 3D en face view to the mitral valve from the LA showing the extent of the vegetation growth on the posterior leaflet. *Bottom left and middle* Same live 3D color Doppler dataset represented with color Doppler (*left*) and color Doppler suppressed (*middle*) showing severe eccentric MR towards the anterior LA wall due to destruction of the posterior leaflet. *Bottom right* Live 3D en face view of the bileaflet mechanical prosthesis after mitral valve surgery. *Ao* aorta, *A* anterior, *P* posterior, *AL* antero-lateral, *PM* postero-medial, *LA* left atrium, *LV* left ventricle. [→Videos 7.22A–F]

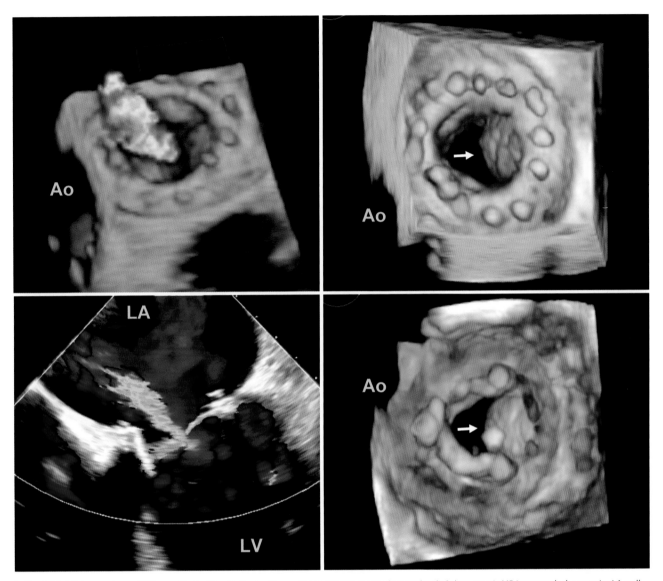

Fig. 7.23 Mild to moderate MR in a patient with mitral valve bioprosthesis. The 2D image depicts the slightly eccentric MR jet towards the anterior LA wall (*bottom left*). The 3D color Doppler image provides better understanding of the direction and central location of the MR jet (*top left*). The true mechanism becomes first obvious from the live 3D en face view of the prosthesis from the LA (*top right*) and LV (*bottom right*) clearly showing an immobile posterior leaflet (*arrow*) causing the eccentric MR jet directed anteriorly. *Ao* aorta, *LA* left atrium, *LV* left ventricle. [→Videos 7.23A–D]

7.1.8 Mitral valve prosthesis

In patients with mitral valve prostheses, MR can occur as paravalvular or valvular leakage. Valvular leakage is usually a result of the valve construction or leaflet geometry and is only of mild degree (◘ Fig. 7.23). Compared to this, paravalvular leakage is either a result of mechanical dehiscence due to one or more torn out stitches or focal endocarditis. Using 2D echocardiography, paravalvular leakages are usually detected by the origin of color Doppler regurgitant jets with TEE providing much more detailed information. However, both 2D TTE and TEE can potentially miss smaller paravalvular leakages (◘ Fig. 7.24). RT3DE, com-

pared to 2D echocardiography, minimizes the risk of overlooking paravalvular leakages, because it provides an unlimited overview of the mitral valve prosthesis in the surface mode only or with color Doppler (◘ Fig. 7.24 and ◘ Fig. 7.25). RT3DE also provides accurate information on the size, shape, and exact location of the leakage, which is of utmost importance for planning interventional device closure (see ▶ Chapter 12) [47].

> ❯ RT3DE provides an unlimited overview of mitral valve prostheses, thereby minimizing the risk of overlooking paravalvular leakages.

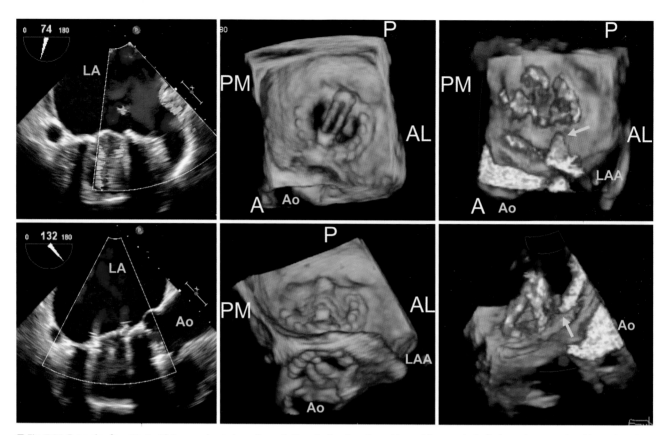

◨ Fig. 7.24 Example of a patient with two mechanical prostheses in the mitral and aortic positions with paravalvular leakage that was missed in routine 2D color Doppler TEE. Standard 2D TEE views in 0°, 40°, 74° (*top left*), and 132° (*bottom left*) revealed normal findings without signs of paravalvular leakage. The live 3D en face view (*top middle*) of the mitral valve prosthesis and the view from the aortic root to the aortic valve prosthesis (*bottom middle*) also showed normal findings. Acquisition of 3D color Doppler, however, unexpectedly revealed a paravalvular leak (*arrow*) in the anterior to antero-lateral location (*top right,* en face view to mitral valve prosthesis). The 3D color Doppler image from a postero-medial position (*bottom right*) shows the two typical regurgitant jets of mechanical prostheses and the paravalvular leak (*arrow*). *Ao* aorta, *A* anterior, *P* posterior, *AL* antero-lateral, *PM* postero-medial, *LAA* left atrial appendage, *LA* left atrium. [→Videos 7.24A–F]

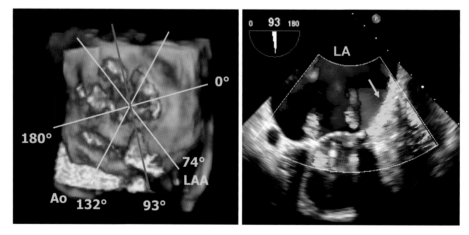

◨ Fig. 7.25 The 3D color Doppler en face view of the mitral valve prosthesis in the same patient as in ◨ Fig. 7.24 showing the location of the paravalvular leak between the left atrial appendage (*LAA*) and aorta (*Ao*) in relation to the 2D color Doppler view planes at 74° and 132° that missed the leak (*left*) as well as to the view plane at 93° (*red*) where the leak was depicted afterwards in 2D color Doppler (*right*). *LA* left atrium. [→Video 7.25]

7.1.9　Mitral valve repair

Today, mitral valve repair (MVR) is the method of first choice in most patients with type II mitral regurgitation; however, literature reports failure of reconstruction with at least moderate MR in 6–8% of patients [64][65][66]. The aim of mitral valve reconstruction is to restore a sufficient leaflet coaptation with a coaptation length of 7 mm or more. Coaptation length of less than 5 mm frequently causes incomplete closure and MR remains (◼ Fig. 7.26). Potential reasons for failure of MVR are paravalvular leakage due to endocarditis or stitch dehiscence (◼ Fig. 7.27 and ◼ Fig. 7.28) or malcoaptation of the leaflets due to leaflet distortion or degenerated leaflet edges. Mechanical dehiscence of annular sutures in extreme cases can lead to subtotal rupture of the mitral annuloplasty ring (◼ Fig. 7.29) [67]. RT3DE has been demonstrated to be an important method to describe the mechanism of mitral regurgitation in patients after MVR [47][67] and provides accurate measurement of leakage size (◼ Fig. 7.28). Intraoperatively RT3DE also provides superior assessment of the success of MVR compared to standard water testing by the surgeon (see ▶ Chapter 12). Moreover, RT3DE might be useful to predict the success of MVR in patients with organic mitral valve disease based on characteristics of mitral valve geometry as recently proposed by Chandra et al. [45]. Comparing preoperative 2D and 3D echocardiographic findings with intraoperative surgical mitral valve assessment they identified a billowing or prolapsing volume of >1.15 ml as a characteristic parameter to differentiate between FED and Barlow's disease and to anticipate the complexity of MVR. In another study, Chikwe et al. [48] compared 3D echocardiographic quantitative parameters of mitral valve geometry with the complexity of repair technique required to achieve a satisfactory result and identified prolapsing height, multisegment involvement, bileaflet prolapse and anterior leaflet surface area are strong predictors of repair complexity. Maffessanti et al. [68] demonstrated the usefulness of intraoperative RT3D TEE for quantitative evaluation of the mitral valve apparatus in patients with FED and Barlow's disease before and after mitral valve repair.

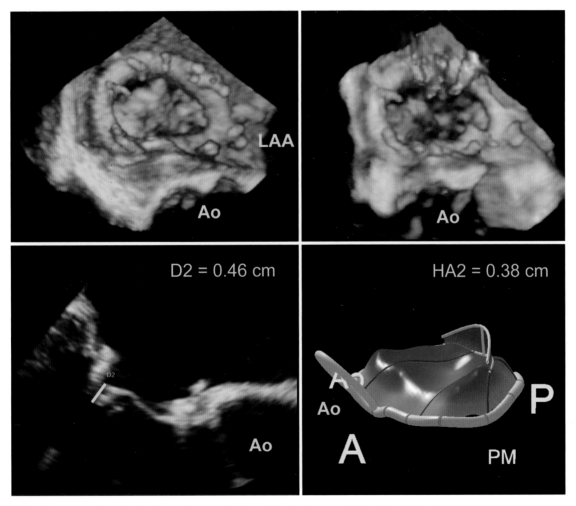

◼ **Fig. 7.26** Live 3D representation of a mitral valve after reconstruction with mitral ring implantation (*top left*). The 3D color Doppler image shows a satisfactory result with three small jets along the commissure indicating mild MR (*top right*). The 2D TEE image demonstrates a moderate coaptation length of 0.46 cm as a potential reason for the mild regurgitation (*bottom left*). MVQ analysis provides 3D graphic visualization of the mitral valve with the coaptation length at segment A2 (*HA2*) of 0.38 cm indicated (*bottom right*). *Ao* aorta, *LAA* left atrial appendage, *LA* left atrium, *A* anterior, *P* posterior, *PM* postero-medial. [→Videos 7.26A,B]

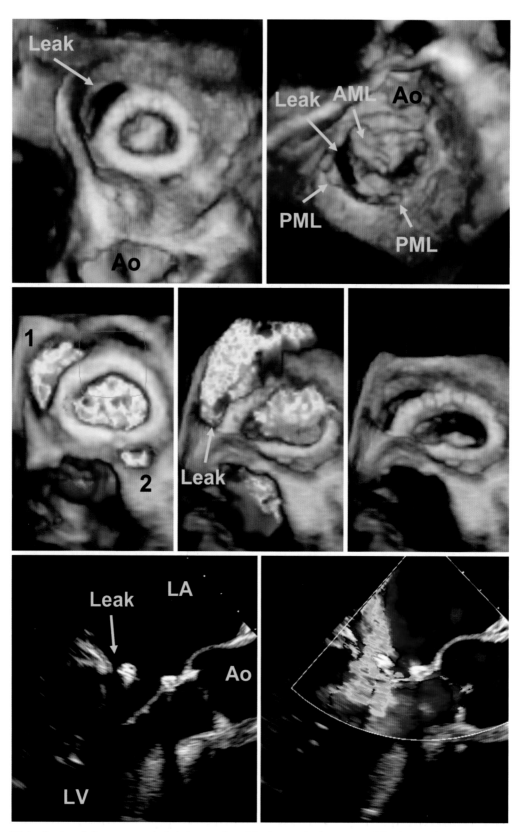

◼ **Fig. 7.27** The 3D visualization of a large paraannular leak due to endocarditis after mitral valve repair: 3D full volume en face view from the LA to the mitral valve (*top left*); 3D en face view from the LV to the mitral valve shows the posterior mitral leaflet (*PML*) on the other side of the displaced ring (*top right*); the 3D color Doppler en face view cropped to the valve level revealed mitral regurgitation through the large paraannular leak (*1*), through an additional smaller paraannular leak (*2*), plus severe valvular regurgitation (*middle left*); the uncropped 3D color Doppler dataset shows the large regurgitant jet through the large paraannular leak but not the small leak (*middle center*); the same 3D color Doppler dataset with color off mode (*middle right*); the 2D cross-sectional view shows the dehiscence between the ring and posterior annulus (*bottom left*); the same 2D cross-sectional view with color Doppler (*bottom right*). *Ao* aorta, *AML* anterior mitral leaflet, *LA* left atrium, *LV* left ventricle. [→Videos 7.27A–F]

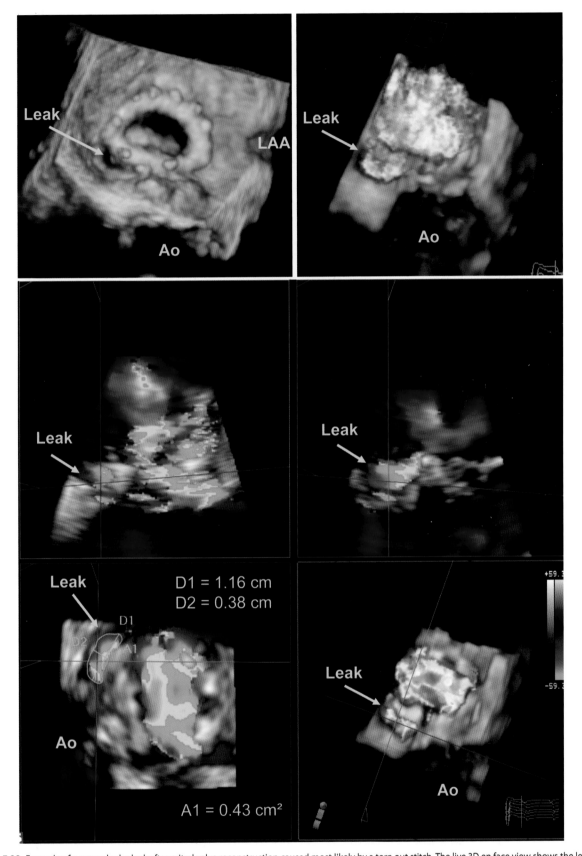

Fig. 7.28 Example of a paravalvular leak after mitral valve reconstruction caused most likely by a torn out stitch. The live 3D en face view shows the leak adjacent to the knot of the stitch (*top left*). Three-dimensional color Doppler demonstrates the regurgitant flow through the leak, but moreover, severe valvular mitral regurgitation (*top right*) making the patient unsuitable for interventional occluder device implantation. Quantitative assessment of leakage size using 3D analysis software (Qlab, Philips) demonstrates an asymmetric orifice of 0.43 cm² corresponding to moderate-to-severe MR (*four bottom panels*). *Ao* aorta, *LAA* left atrial appendage. [→Videos 7.28A,B]

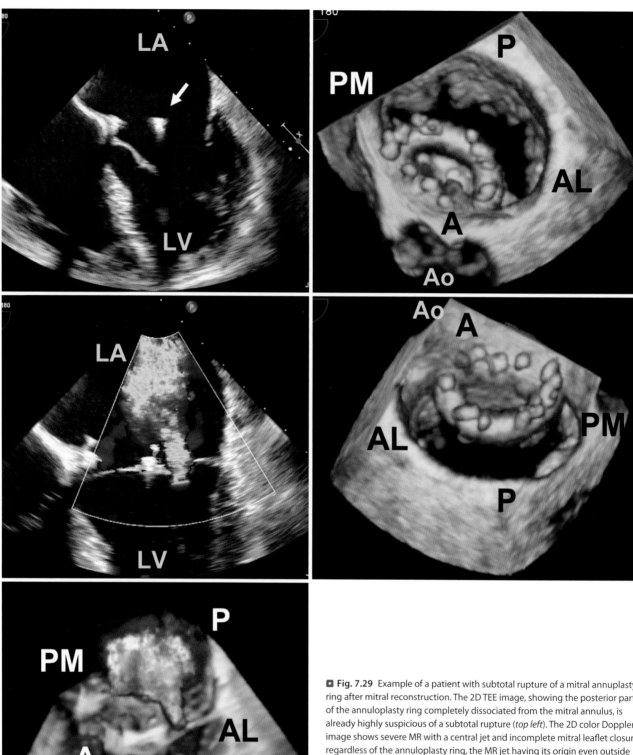

■ **Fig. 7.29** Example of a patient with subtotal rupture of a mitral annuplasty ring after mitral reconstruction. The 2D TEE image, showing the posterior part of the annuloplasty ring completely dissociated from the mitral annulus, is already highly suspicious of a subtotal rupture (*top left*). The 2D color Doppler image shows severe MR with a central jet and incomplete mitral leaflet closure regardless of the annuloplasty ring, the MR jet having its origin even outside the ring and the anterior leaflet hitting against the free ring (*middle left*). Only by means of live 3D views is the full extent of the rupture visible, which is more than half of the ring circumference (*top right and middle right*). The live 3D images also depict a huge discrepancy between the size of the dilated mitral annulus and the ring. The curved curtain of regurgitant flow jet located at the outer curvature of the annuloplasty ring can be observed using 3D color Doppler (*bottom left*). *Ao* aorta, *A* anterior, *P* posterior *AL* antero-lateral, *PM* postero-medial, *LA* left atrium, *LV* left ventricle. [→Videos 7.29A–E]

7.1.10 Rare etiologies

Mitral regurgitation can also be present in cases with rare and difficult-to-define mitral valve disease that are challenging to detect by 2D echocardiography. In the two cases shown in ◘ Fig. 7.30 and ◘ Fig. 7.31 (one representing an isolated cleft mitral valve [69][70] and the other representing a double orifice mitral valve [71]), the true pathology causing mitral regurgitation was missed by 2D echocardiography, while it was clearly shown by RT3DE. Both cases represent examples where complete understanding of the complex mitral valve pathology was only possible using RT3DE (see ▶ Chapter 9).

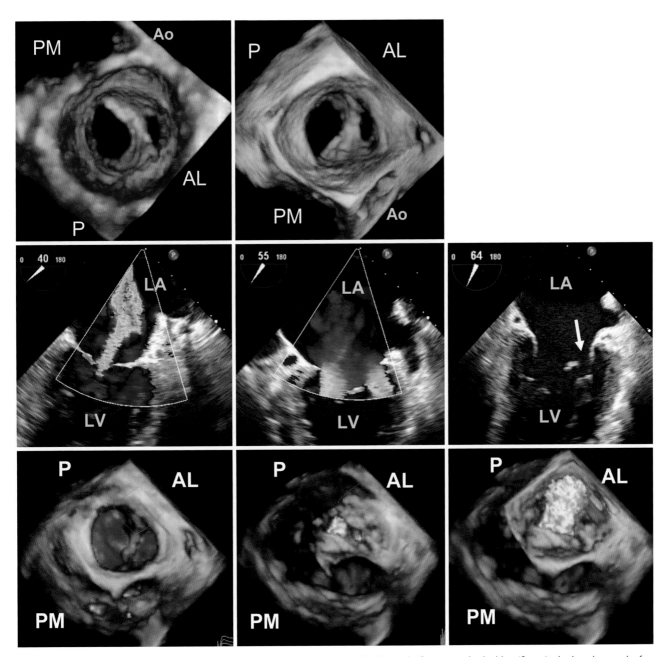

◘ **Fig. 7.30** Case of a 30-year-old woman with known moderate MR for many years. RT3DE was the first to reveal a double orifice mitral valve where each of the two orifices seems to work as a unicuspid valve independent of each other (*top left* view from the LV toward the MV; *top right* view from the LA toward the MV). Standard 2D echocardiography showed moderate central MR (*middle left*). Careful 2D re-examination after RT3DE revealed double orifice inflow (*middle center*) and a gap (*arrow*) in the anterior leaflet (*middle right*) which were previously described as part of the commissure. RT3DE color Doppler demonstrated filling flow in diastole (*bottom left*) as well as mitral regurgitation (*bottom center*) through each of the two mitral orifices with a confluence of MR flow forming one jet (*bottom right*). *Ao* aorta, *P* posterior, *AL* antero-lateral, *PM* postero-medial, *LA* left atrium, *LV* left ventricle. [→Videos 7.30A–G]

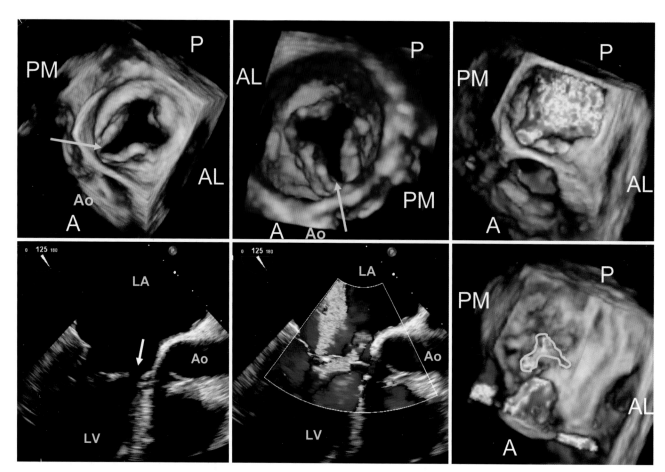

■ **Fig. 7.31** Rare case of an isolated cleft mitral valve in a 72-year-old woman with known moderate MR for many years and with no evidence of congenital heart disease. RT3DE clearly shows the coaptation pattern between the three leaflets with insertion of chordae tendinae to all three leaflet edges (*top left* view from the LA toward the MV; *top middle* view from the LV toward the MV). The cleft (*arrow*) is oriented towards the aorta. RT3DE color Doppler in the same LA perspective as in *top left* shows severe MR through all parts of the tricuspid mitral valve (*top right*) with the shape and size of the vena contracta shown in the *bottom right image*. Standard 2D echocardiography showed a gap in the AML (*arrow; bottom left*) with regurgitant flow passing through the gap (*bottom middle*) which was suspicious of being an AML defect. *Ao* aorta, *A* anterior, *P* posterior, *AL* antero-lateral, *PM* postero-medial, *LA* left atrium, *LV* left ventricle, *AML* anterior mitral leaflet. [→Videos 7.31A–E]

way of assessment	Jet size	<4.0 cm², <20% LA (1)	4.0-8.0 cm², 20-40% LA (2)	>8.0 cm², >40% LA (3)	increase of diagnostic accuracy
	Jet direction	central (1)		eccentric (2)	
	LA size	≤4.0 cm ≤36 ml/m² (1)		>4.0 cm >36 ml/m² (2)	
	Vena contracta width	<0.3 cm (1)	0.3-0.69 cm (3)	≥0.7 cm (5) or >0.8 cm for biplane*	

Score (sum of scoring points)	4–5	6	7–8	9	10–12
Severity	**I**	**(I-II)**	**II**	**(II-III)**	**III**

Fig. 7.32 Scoring system for estimation of the severity of mitral regurgitation based on current international recommendations (modified from [72]; Copyright Urban & Vogel). Note that in patients with asymmetric vena contracta shape, a biplane measurement in a 2- and 4-chamber view with a biplane vena contracta width of >0.8 cm has been proposed [14] and recently recommended to define severe MR [8][11]

7.1.11 Assessment of severity of mitral regurgitation

Today, 2D echocardiography with color Doppler is the standard method for routine assessment of MR severity. Recent guidelines recommended an integrative approach of different semiquantitative and quantitative 2D and color Doppler parameters for estimation of MR severity [7][8][10][11]. This integrative approach can be practically applied in clinical routine for grading MR severity by using a standardized scoring system (**Fig. 7.32** and **Fig. 7.33**) [72].

As a practical approach to effective regurgitant orifice area (EROA), which corresponds hemodynamically to the cross-sectional area of the vena contracta (VC) as the narrowest portion of the proximal regurgitant jet [73][74][75], the VC width (VCW) of a color Doppler jet has become an accepted semiquantitative parameter for estimating MR severity [10][11][12][76][77][78]. However, this simplified assumption only holds when the EROA is nearly circular, and recent studies have indicated that the EROA is noncircular in most patients [78][79][80], particularly when the VCW at the same time appears narrow in the 4-chamber view and broad in the 2-chamber view as in most cases of functional MR due to incomplete mitral leaflet closure (**Fig. 7.34**, **Fig. 7.35**, **Fig. 7.36**, **Fig. 7.37**) [53].

2D   **RT3DE**

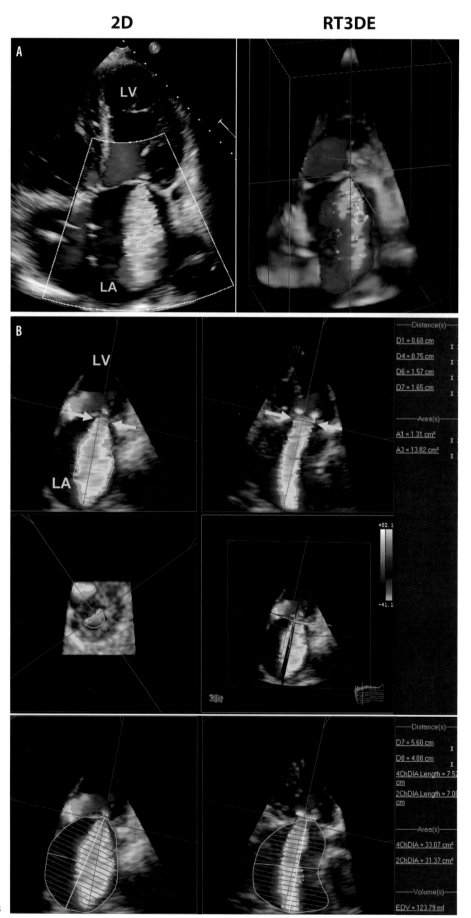

■ Fig. 7.33

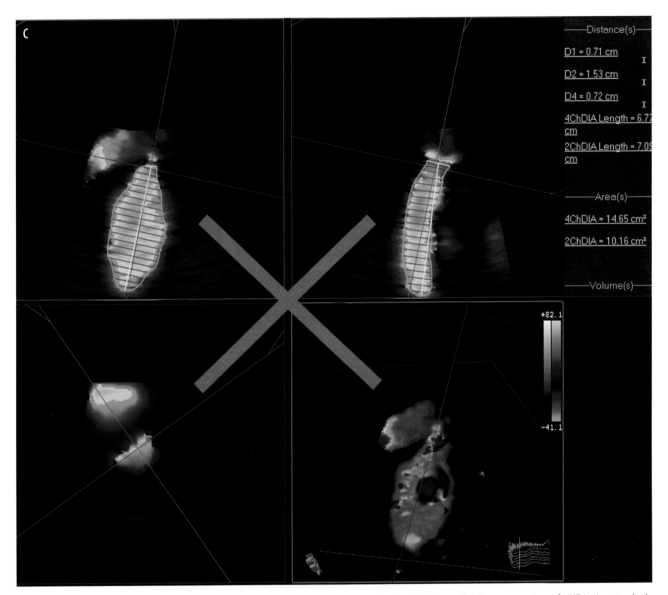

C

Distance(s)

D1 = 0.71 cm

D2 = 1.53 cm

D4 = 0.72 cm

4ChDIA Length = 6.7?
cm

2ChDIA Length = 7.09
cm

Area(s)

4ChDIA = 14.65 cm²

2ChDIA = 10.16 cm²

Volume(s)

+82. 1

−41. 1

◼ **Fig. 7.33** (continued) Example of the application of MR scoring to a transthoracic 3D color Doppler dataset. **A** A direct comparison of a MR jet in a standard 2D apical 4-chamber view (*left*) with a 3D 4-chamber view (*right*) in the same patient is shown. **B** The measurement of all parameters of MR severity within the 3D color Doppler dataset shown in **A** is demonstrated: vena contracta width and jet area in 4-chamber view (*top left*); biplane LA diameter and volume (*bottom left and right*). Measurement of vena contracta width in 2-chamber view (*top right*) and vena contracta area (*middle left*) are optional in patients with asymmetric vena contracta area (*see below*). **C** The measurement of regurgitant jet volume in the views with a *red cross* indicates the wrongness of this measurement because the MR jet volume does not correlate with MR severity because the jet volume is mainly determined by the jet momentum which is determined by LV contractility [112]. *LA* left atrium, *LV* left ventricle. [→Videos 7.33A(a,b)]

En face view   4-chamber view   2-chamber view

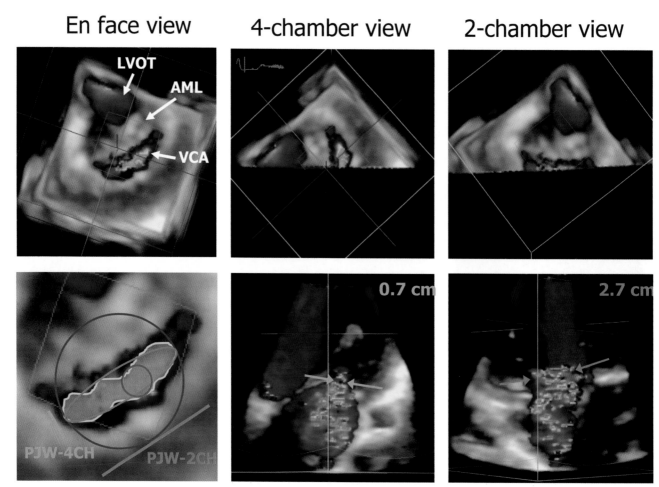

◘ **Fig. 7.34** Quantitative assessment of vena contracta (*VC*) shape and size in a transthoracic RT3DE color Doppler dataset in a patient with functional MR. The 3D en face view from the left ventricle toward the mitral valve and a cross-section of the VC (*top left*) shows a typical asymmetric vena contracta area (*VCA*) along the commissural line. The *blue* Doppler signal above indicates LV outflow. The RT3DE dataset cropped along the 4-chamber dimension of the VCA shown in a 3D en face view (*top middle*) and, by tilting 90° upwards, in a 4-chamber view (*bottom middle*) shows a typical narrow VCW. The RT3DE dataset cropped along the 2-chamber dimension of the VCA shown in a 3D en face view (*top right*) and, by tilting 90° upwards, in a 2-chamber view (*bottom right*) shows a typical broad VCW. Quantitative assessment of VCA dimensions (*bottom left*): *yellow*=manual planimetry of VCA (1.68 cm²; ◘ Fig. 7.2); *turquoise*=VCW-4CH (0.68 cm); *purple*=VCW-2CH (2.71 cm); *red*=VCA-4CH (0.4 cm²); *blue*=VCA-2CH (5.7 cm²); *green*=biplane VCA (1.5 cm²). *LVOT* left ventricular outflow tract, *AML* anterior mitral leaflet, *PJW-4CH* 4-chamber proximal jet width, *PJW-2CH* 2-chamber proximal jet width (*VCW* and *PJW* are used as synonyms). Source [14]; Copyright American Society of Echocardiography

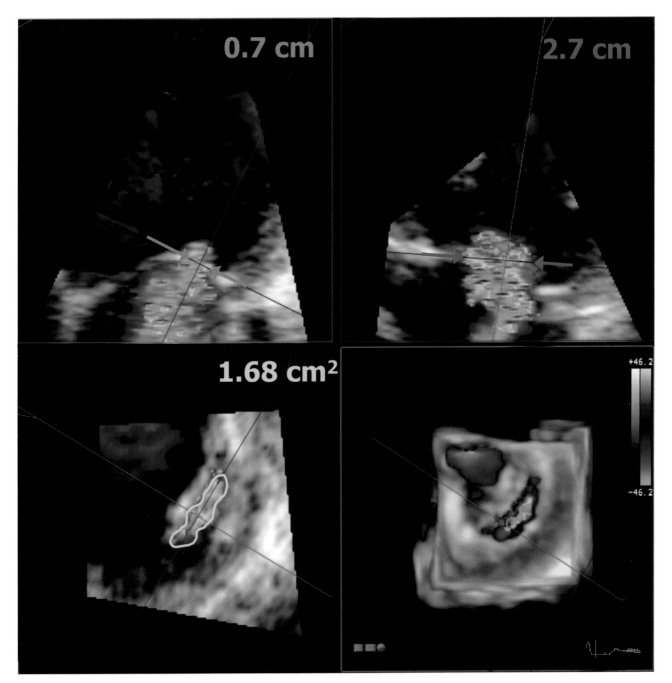

Fig. 7.35 Demonstration of measurement of vena contracta dimensions in the same 3D color Doppler dataset as in ▢Fig. 7.34 using 3D analysis software (QLAB, Philips Medical Systems). *Top left* The 4-chamber view with measurement of a narrow 3D vena contracta width (*green arrows*). *Top right* The 2-chamber view with measurement of a broad 3D vena contracta width (*red arrows*). *Bottom left* The 3D en face view to asymmetric vena contracta area of 1.68 cm² and with an asymmetry index of 3.79. Source [14]; Copyright American Society of Echocardiography

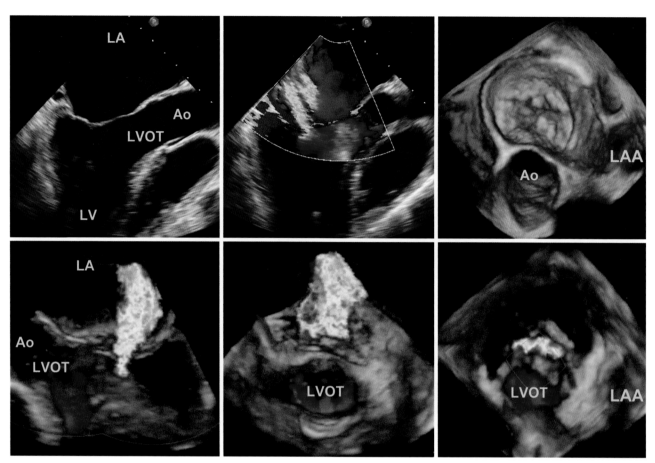

⬛ **Fig. 7.36** Example of 3D assessment of functional MR by 3D TEE. The 2D cross-sectional views show mitral leaflet tethering and tenting with poor leaflet coaptation (*top left*) causing significant mitral regurgitation (*top middle*). RT3DE view to the mitral valve shows only moderate focal nodular degeneration of mitral leaflet (*top right*). Cropping of a 3D color Doppler dataset reveals a vena contracta area which is narrow in the 4-chamber view (*bottom left*), broad in the 2-chamber view (*bottom middle*), and asymmetric along the commissural line in an en face view of the mitral valve (*bottom right*). *Ao* aorta, *LA* left atrium, *LV* left ventricle, *LVOT* left ventricular outflow tract, *LAA* left atrial appendage. [→Videos 7.36A–E]

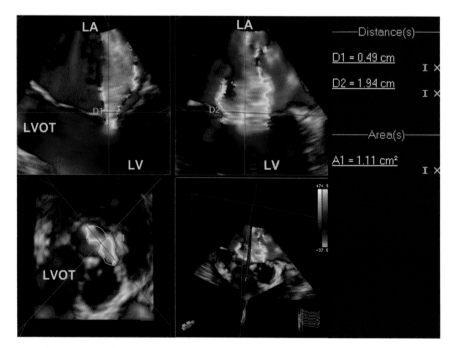

⬛ **Fig. 7.37** Measurement of vena contracta dimensions in the same 3D TEE color Doppler dataset as in ⬛ Fig. 7.36 using 3D analysis software (QLAB, Philips Medical Systems). *Top left* The 4-chamber view with measurement of a narrow 3D vena contracta width. *Top right* The 2-chamber view with measurement of a broad 3D vena contracta width. *Bottom left* The 3D en face view to asymmetric vena contracta area of 1.11 cm² and asymmetry index of 3.96. *LVOT* left ventricular outflow tract, *LV* left ventricle, *LA* left atrium

Recently, color Doppler RT3DE was demonstrated in clinical studies to provide improved understanding and assessment of the asymmetric geometry of mitral regurgitant flow [81]. Khanna et al. [80] initially demonstrated color Doppler RT3DE as a feasible method to provide direct visualization and planimetry of vena contracta area (VCA) of a regurgitant jet. Kahlert et al. [14] showed that RT3DE overcomes the limitations of 2D measurements of vena contracta width (VCW) by direct assessment of the size and shape of the VCA and demonstrated the differences in VCA asymmetry among different etiologies of MR (◘ Fig. 7.38). In the majority of patients with functional MR, RT3DE showed typical elongation of the VCA along the semilunar-shaped line of incomplete mitral leaflet closure due to leaflet tethering (◘ Fig. 7.34, ◘ Fig. 7.35, ◘ Fig. 7.36, ◘ Fig. 7.37). Subsequent studies pro-

vided further validation of RT3DE assessment of the asymmetric VCA by comparison against independent methods [82] and the proof of superiority of 3D VCA measurements compared to 2D VCA measurement in both central and eccentric jets [83] as well as in multiple jets [84]. The overwhelming variability of shape, size, and number of VCAs in a spectrum of patients with both functional and organic MR is shown in ◘ Fig. 7.39. An overview of current studies in which 3D VCA measurement has been compared with other methods of MR quantification [12][85] is shown in ◘ Tab. 7.2. In all studies, the correlation between direct 3D measurement of VCA and 2D methods was good, but 2D methods, particularly 2D VCW and hemispherical PISA, systematically underestimated true effective regurgitant orifice area the more elliptic or asymmetric it was [14][82][83][84][86][87][88][89].

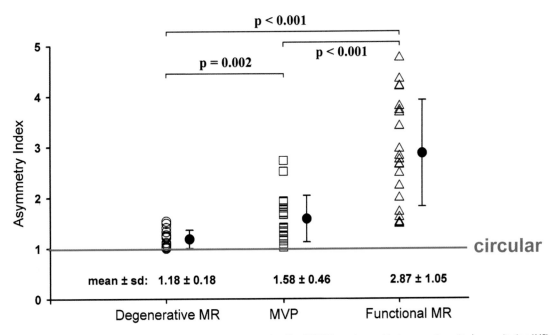

◘ Fig. 7.38 Differences in the asymmetry of the vena contracta area as visualized by RT3DE in patients with degenerative mitral regurgitation (*MR*), mitral valve prolapse (*MVP*), and functional MR. Source [14]; Copyright American Society of Echocardiography

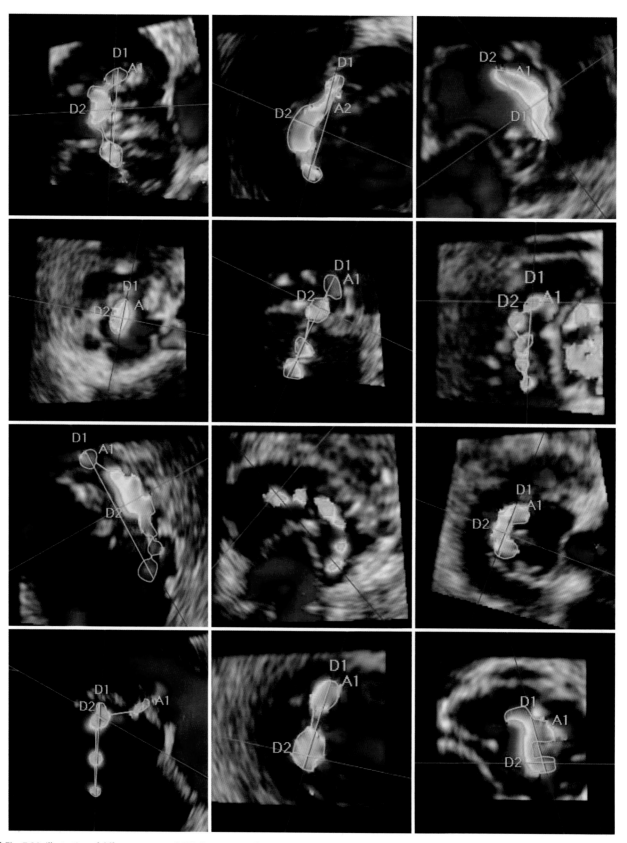

◨ **Fig. 7.39** Illustration of different pattern of VCA shape, size and number along the commissural line of mitral leaflets. RT3D TEE images show VCA traced as A1 as well as long and short VC width (*D1*, *D2*) for determination of asymmetry index (*AI*), both indicated below. Etiologies presented are as follows: (*1*) FED with bileaflet billowing (VCA 1.33 cm², AI 4.01), (*2*) functional MR (1.09 cm², 4.80), (*3*) functional MR (1.03 cm², 4.15), (*4*) degenerative mitral valve disease (*DMVD*) with leaflet thickening (0.74 cm², 2.00), (*5*) Barlow's disease (0.90 cm², 5.49), (*6*) DMVD with thickening of leaflet tips (0.40 cm², 6.97), (*7*) AML prolapse (0.77 cm², 6.80), (*8*) DMVD with AML billowing and thickening of leaflet tips (0.86 cm², 6.65), (*9*) A2 flail (1.42 cm², 3.73), (*10*) functional MR (0.30 cm², 6.24), (*11*) DMVD with leaflet thickening (1.19 cm², 3.10), (*12*) DMVD with leaflet thickening (0.57 cm², 1.92)

◻ Tab. 7.2 Studies validating 3D vena contract area (*VCA*) measurement in vivo against 2D methods or independent reference methods

Study	Patients (n)	3D method	Etiology	Comparison method	Agreement	Interobserver/intra-observer variability
Khanna et al. [80]	44	TTE	not reported	Ventriculographic grading	r=0.88; limits of agreement not reported	r^2=0.99; r^2=0.97
Iwakura et al. [86]	109	TTE	FMR: 63%	EROA by 2D PISA; EROA by 2D QD	r=0.93 with 2D PISA r=0.91 with 2D QD (limits of agreement ±0.2 cm^2)	8.6%/9.0%
Kahlert et al. [14]	57	TTE	FMR: 36%	EROA by 2D PISA	r=0.96 with hemielliptic PISA (limits of agreement ±0.14 cm^2) r=0.93 with hemispheric PISA (limits of agreement ±0.20 cm^2	0.04 cm^2/ –
Little et al. [82]	61	TTE	FMR: 44%	EROA by 2D QD	r=0.85; limits of agreement not reported	0.03/0.05 cm^2
Yosefy et al. [83]	49	TTE	FMR: 58%	EROA by 2D QD	r^2=0.86 with hemielliptic PISA (limits of agreement ±0.06 cm^2)	0.03/0.02 cm^2
Marsan et al. [87]	64	TTE	FMR: 100%	RVol by CMR	r=0.94 (limits of agreement ±7.7 ml)	0.06/0.04 cm^2
Shanks et al. [88]	30	TEE	FMR: 53%	RVol by CMR	r not reported; 63.2±41.3 ml (3DE) vs. 65.1±42.7 ml (CMR)	0.01/0.01 cm^2
Zeng et al. [89]	83	TTE	FMR: 47%	integrated 2DE methods	r=0.88; limits of agreement not reported	0.03/0.04 cm^2
Hyodo et al. [84]	60	TEE	FMR: 100%	EROA from 3D left ventricular volume and thermodilution data	r=0.90 (limits of agreement ±0.06 cm^2)	0.06/0.05 cm^2

FMR functional mitral regurgitation, *QD* quantitative Doppler, *RVol* regurgitant volume, *CMR* cardiac magnetic resonance, *EROA* effective regurgitant orifice area, *2DE* two-dimensional echocardiography, *3DE* three-dimensional echocardiography, *PISA* proximal isovelocity surface area.

Based on the VC measurements obtained by RT3DE, Kahlert et al. [14] proposed a larger cutoff value of 0.6 cm^2 for the VCA compared to 0.4 cm^2 for 2D-derived effective regurgitant orifice area (EROA) and accordingly 0.8 cm for mean VCW (4- and 2-chamber views) instead of 0.7 cm for 4-chamber-based VCW for severe MR for all etiologies, including functional MR. This concept of the asymmetric VCA with new cut-off values was recently adopted by the European guidelines [8][11]. Differently, Zeng et al. [89] proposed a cut-off value of 0.41 cm^2 for differentiation of moderate from severe MR that can be applied in all etiologies and orifice shapes. As a potential explanation for the two different cut-off values, Kahlert et al. derived their 3D cut-off value of 0.6 cm^2 by correcting the prior 2D-based cut-off value for the underestimation of the true asymmetric VCA by 2D methods [14]. Compared to this, Zeng et al. [89] derived their 3D VCA cut-off value of 0.41 cm^2 from MR grading based on an integration of conventional 2D methods including 2D PISA, 2D

VCW and 2D jet area, which is a potential explanation why the 0.41 cm^2 were so much closer to the previously proposed 2D cut-off value of 0.4 cm^2 [7][8][9][10][11].

❯ Color Doppler RT3DE provides direct assessment of the size and shape of the vena contracta area.

Visualization of the VCA in a 3D en face view can be obtained by cropping a 3D dataset by an image plane that is manually adjusted to be perpendicular to the jet direction. The cropping plane is then moved along the jet direction until the smallest jet cross-sectional area at the level of the VC is visualized (◻ Fig. 7.34 and ◻ Fig. 7.36). The VCA can then be measured by manual planimetry of the color Doppler flow signal (◻ Fig. 7.35 and ◻ Fig. 7.37). A practical alternative approach to the assessment of the vena contracta is described in ◻ Fig. 7.40 applying the iSlice tool for more accurate identification of the level of the vena contracta.

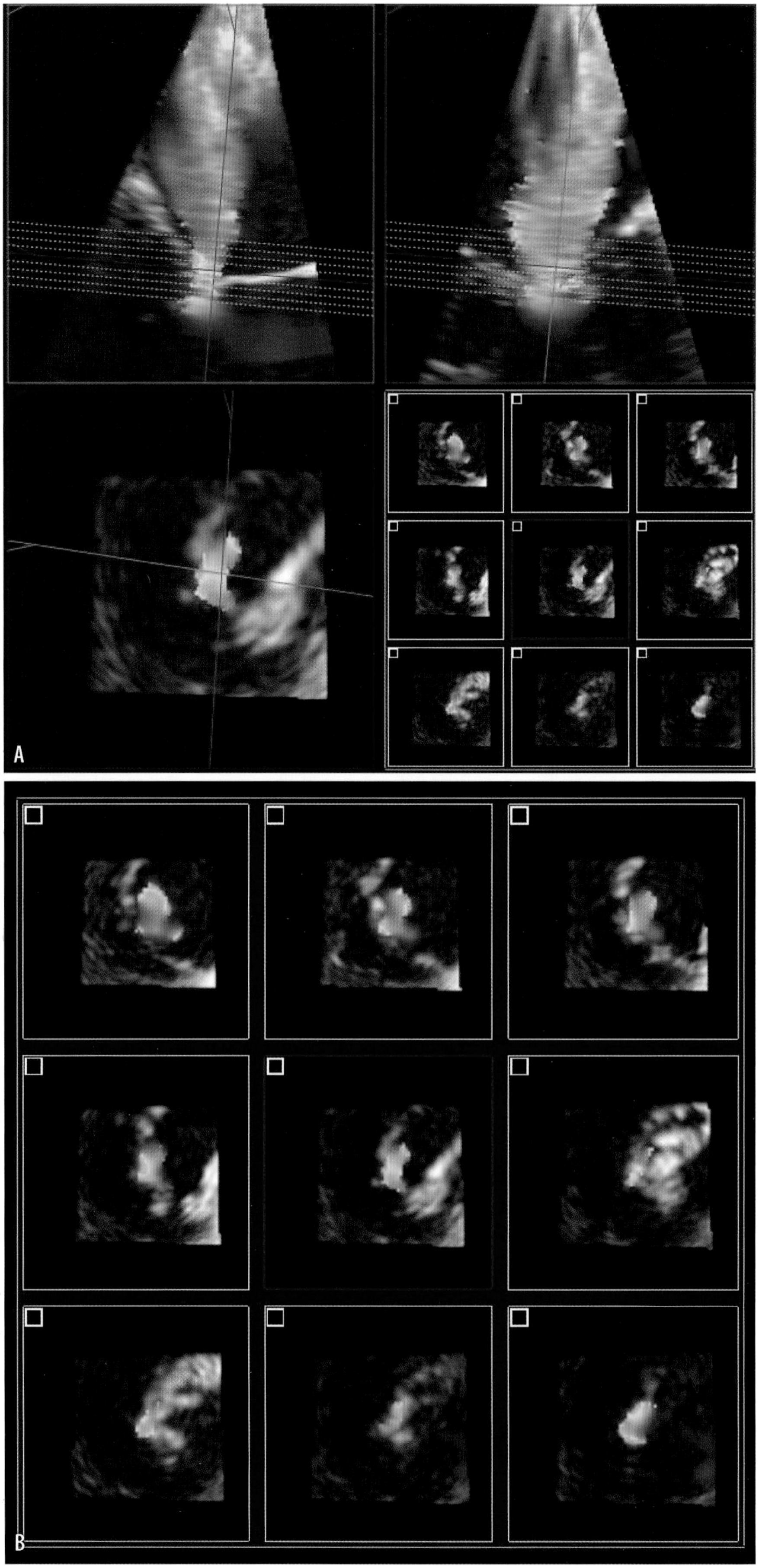

■ Fig. 7.40

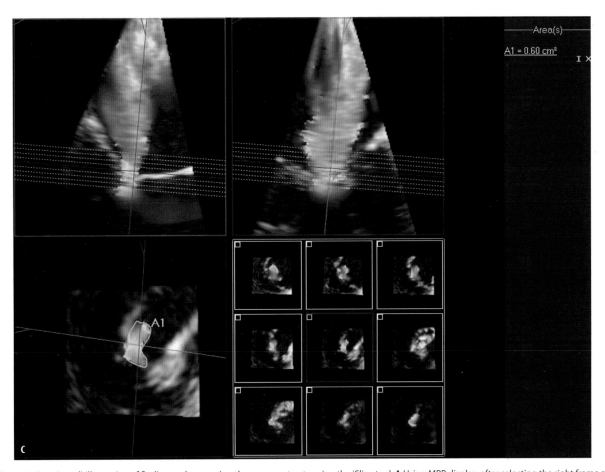

◻ Fig. 7.40 (continued) Illustration of finding and measuring the vena contracta using the iSlice tool. **A** Using MPR display, after selecting the right frame and aligning the *two upper images* (*red* and *green plane*) to the jet and placing the lower left (*blue plane*) to the origin of the jet, the iSlice tool is activated which brings up 9 parallel short-axis planes (4 above the *blue plane* and 4 below). These nine tomographic slices are displayed as short-axis planes through the jet (*lower right*). **B** Displaying the iSlice view in one big image allows more accurate identification and selection of the level of the vena contracta. In this example the center plane represented the vena contracta best. The plane to the *right* (located more towards the jet) already showed a blurred jet cross-section, whereas the plane to the *left* (located more towards the orifice) showed strong leaflet tissue signals diminishing the color Doppler signal. **C** The plane that represents the vena contracta best, in this case the central one, after being selected (marked by *blue frame*) is then shown in the *lower left panel* where the vena contracta area can be traced (0.60 cm²)

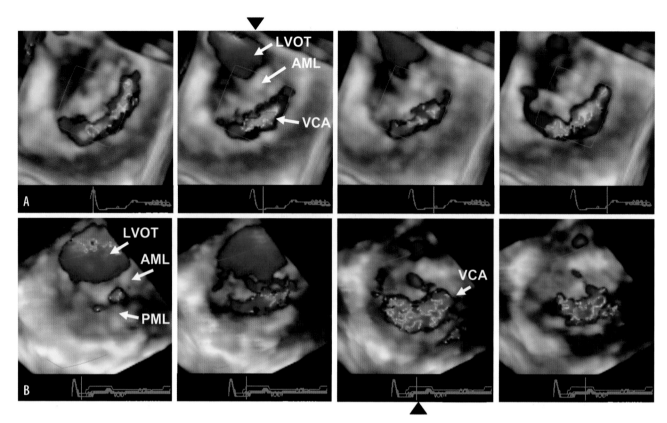

◘ Fig. 7.41 Demonstration of temporal resolution of dynamic 3D color Doppler representation of vena contracta area (*VCA*) throughout systole in a patient with functional MR (**A**, *top*) and a patient with MVP of the entire posterior leaflet (**B**, *bottom*). Although temporal resolution of RT3DE was low (*top*: 10 Hz; *bottom*: 12 Hz), the four systolic frames available in the two examples provided sufficient representation of the dynamic changes of the VCA to select the frame that best represented the hemodynamically relevant lesion size: in **A** with typical mid systolic decrease of EROA the 2nd frame (*arrow*) was selected, VCA in the 3rd frame being too small for accurate measurement; in **B** the 3rd frame (*arrow*) showing typical late systolic maximum of EROA in MVP was selected. *LVOT* left ventricular outflow tract, *AML* anterior mitral leaflet, *PML* posterior mitral leaflet, *LVOT* left ventricular outflow tract. Source [14]; Copyright American Society of Echocardiography

Because MR flow is in most cases dynamic throughout systole [79][90], a frame in systole that represents the hemodynamically relevant lesion size should be selected for measurement of the VC dimensions: (1) in functional MR, where the EROA is usually smaller in mid systole, a mid systolic frame with a VCW large enough to be measured should be selected, (2) in organic MR, where the EROA is more constant throughout systole, a mid systolic frame should be selected, and (3) in MVP, a frame in the second half of systole, where the EROA is usually largest, is selected (◘ Fig. 7.41) [14].

> **❯** RT3DE allows accurate calculation of regurgitant flow volume from the VCA times the velocity–time integral of regurgitant flow.

As regurgitant flow is determined by the multiplication of EROA and flow velocity, direct measurement of the VCA by RT3DE offers important future perspectives for improving quantitation of regurgitant flow volume. Recently, Marsan et al. [87] calculated regurgitant flow volume from the VCA by multiplying RT3DE and the velocity–time integral of regurgitant flow by continuous wave Doppler. In this study, mitral regurgitant volume measured by RT3DE showed excellent correlation with regurgitant volume measured by velocity-encoded cardiac magnetic resonance (VE-CMR; r=0.94) used for reference, without a significant difference between these techniques (mean difference=–0.08 ml/beat). In comparison, 2D echocardiographic assessment of regurgitant volume using vena contracta width in the 4-chamber view significantly underestimated regurgitant volume (p=0.006) as compared with cardiac MRI (mean difference=2.9 ml/beat).

As a promising alternative approach, Plicht et al. [91] demonstrated that multiple color Doppler aliasing of regurgitant flow at the VCA from a RT3DE color Doppler dataset can be unmasked by de-aliasing to accurately calculate absolute regurgitant flow. Alternatively, Skaug et al. [92] described a new method based on multiple-beam HPRF (high pulse repetition frequency) color Doppler analysis using 3D color Doppler for accurate automated identification of the VCA and calculation of regurgitant flow.

Understanding of VCA asymmetry as visualized by RT3DE is also relevant for the proximal isovelocity surface area (PISA) method which is based on the hemodynamic assumption of a hemispheric shape of isovelocities in the proximal flow field that only holds for a circular regurgitant lesion in unconfined flow [93][94]. As a result the hemispheric PISA method has been demonstrated to underestimate regurgitant flow and the EROA in noncircular regurgitant lesions [86][95][96][97]. Kahlert et al. [14] found significant underestimation of the EROA determined using the conventional hemispheric PISA method compared to the EROA measured by hemielliptic PISA, particularly in patients with MVP and functional MR. Hemielliptic PISA can be obtained from RT3DE datasets using PISA width, length, and radius for the calculation of the hemielliptic PISA surface by a hemielliptic formula (◘ Fig. 7.42). The EROA from hemielliptic

PISA can then be calculated as EROA = PISA(HE) times Nyquist velocity divided by MR flow velocity as measured by continuous wave Doppler echocardiography. To overcome the limitations of 2D analysis of PISA shape and size, several research groups either validated estimates of the 3D PISA shape by manual measurements of three perpendicular PISA diameters [14][96][98], more diameters [97][99], PISA surface [100][101][102] or investigated computer simulations for semi-automated 3D reconstruction of PISA [103] and found significantly improved accuracy of 3D

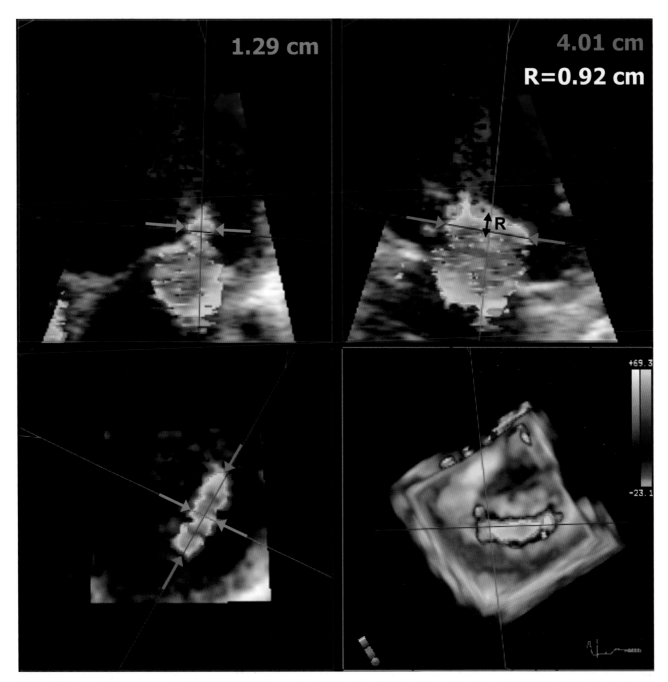

◘ **Fig. 7.42** Example of measurement of hemielliptic 3D PISA in a patient with functional MR using 3D analysis software (QLAB, Philips Medical Systems). *Top left* Narrow 3D PISA width (*green arrows*) in the 4-chamber view. *Top right* Broad 3D PISA length (*red arrows*) in the 2-chamber view. R=PISA radius. *Bottom left* Horizontal cross-sectional plane through the 3D PISA showing PISA width and length. *Bottom right* The 3D en face view of the hemielliptic 3D PISA. Nyquist velocity=23.1 cm/s. Source [14]; Copyright American Society of Echocardiography

PISA estimates of EROA and regurgitant flow. Recently, a commercially available method for 3D quantification of PISA without geometric assumptions using single-beam RT3DE color Doppler datasets was described to be feasible in a clinical setting and to be more accurate compared to the hemispheric 2D PISA method [104][105][106]. However, potential limitations of the existing automated 3D methods being subject of future research include underestimation of convergent flow velocities near the base of the PISA where velocity vectors are almost perpendicular to the vector of the ultrasound beam, dynamic changes of regurgitant flow rate and PISA size during systole combined with dynamic axial translation of the center of the regurgitant orifice.

7.2   Aortic regurgitation

Aortic regurgitation (AR) is the second most common valve disease [1] in the general population, whereas it ranked behind aortic stenosis and mitral regurgitation in a hospital-based patient population [2], thus, indicating AR commonly to be less symptomatic. The predominant etiology of AR is degeneration of the native valve, including prolapse, which is followed by functional AR, rheumatic and congenital diseases, and endocarditis (◻ Fig. 7.43, ◻ Fig. 7.44, ◻ Fig. 7.45, ◻ Fig. 7.46) [2]. AR is frequently present in combination with degenerative aortic stenosis (◻ Fig. 7.43 and ◻ Fig. 7.44).

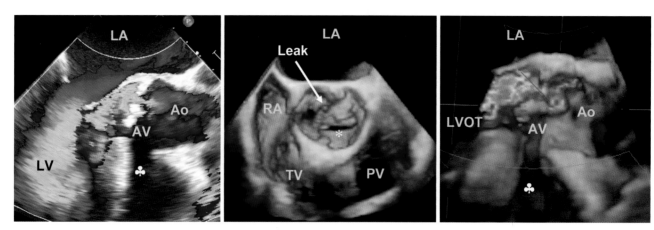

◻ **Fig. 7.43** Example of significant eccentric aortic regurgitation in a patient with a severely degenerated bicuspid aortic valve. The 2D color Doppler cross-sectional image shows eccentric regurgitant flow towards the anterior mitral leaflet with severely calcified and thickened aortic valve cusps with significant shadowing (*cloverleaf; left*). The diastolic RT3DE en face view from the aorta to the aortic valve depicts the location of the leak between the two leaflets with a severely degenerated and thickened left coronary cusp causing a dropout artifact (*asterisk; middle*). RT3DE color Doppler volume with the long-axis view of the aortic regurgitant flow (*right*). *Ao* aorta, *LA* left atrium, *LV* left ventricle, *AV* aortic valve, *RA* right atrium, *TV* tricuspid valve, *PV* pulmonary valve, *LVOT* LV outflow tract. [→Videos 7.43A–C]

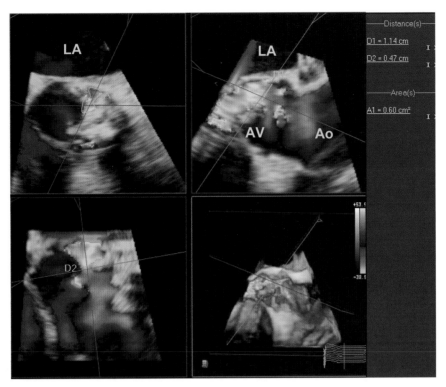

Fig. 7.44 Quantitative 3D assessment of vena contracta size and shape in the same patient with aortic regurgitation shown in **❏** Fig. 7.43. *Top left* The asymmetric vena contracta area of 0.60 cm² indicates severe AR. The two diameters of the vena contracta are shown: D1=1.14 cm (*top right*) and D2=0.47 cm (*bottom left*). *LA* left atrium, *Ao* aorta, *AV* aortic valve

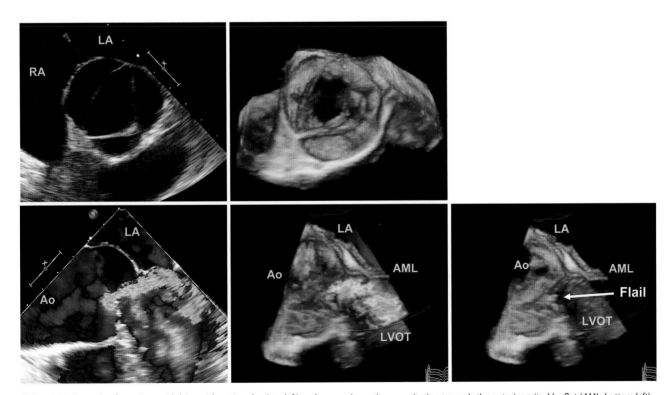

Fig. 7.45 Example of a patient with bicuspid aortic valve (*top left*) and eccentric aortic regurgitation towards the anterior mitral leaflet (*AML; bottom left*). Aortic cusps are very thin causing severe dropout artifacts in the live 3D en face view of the AV cusps (*top middle*). The 3D color Doppler volume with color (*bottom middle*) and with color suppressed (*bottom right*) reveals a small flail segment of the left coronary cusps as the cause of the eccentric regurgitant jet. *Ao* aorta, *LA* left atrium, *RA* right atrium, *LVOT* left ventricular outflow tract. [→Videos 7.45A–E]

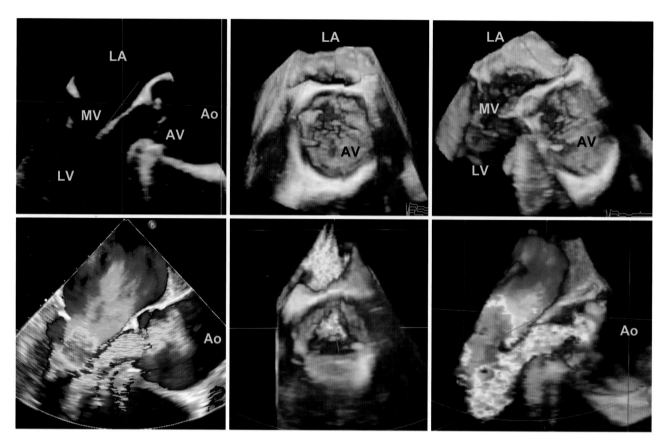

◘ Fig. 7.46 Example of severe aortic regurgitation after endocarditis. The long-axis 2D and color Doppler TEE views show a thickened and shortened non-coronary cusp (*top left*) and severe central regurgitation (*bottom left*) but do not clarify the underlying mechanism. The 3D en face view from the aorta to the aortic valve reveals central destruction of the noncoronary cusp with a large defect (*top middle* and *top right*). The 3D color Doppler view to the vena contracta in the short-axis view (*bottom middle*) represents the shape, size, and location of the vena contracta. *Bottom right* Long-axis 3D color Doppler view of the aortic regurgitant flow. *Ao* aorta, *LA* left atrium, *LV* left ventricle, *MV* mitral valve, *AV* aortic valve. [→Videos 7.46A–F]

Compared to the mitral valve, which can be imaged by transthoracic RT3DE with acceptable image quality, the aortic valve is more difficult to examine from a transthoracic approach because of its smaller size, the narrow LV outflow tract, the smaller surrounding blood pool, and the frequent thickening and sclerosis of the aortic valve apparatus [26]. With the introduction of RT3D TEE, examination of the aortic valve with satisfactory image quality became possible and is currently the recommended 3D approach for aortic valve assessment especially when a definite diagnosis cannot be made by 3D TTE [26]. As the aortic valve is smaller than the mitral valve and is oriented more orthogonal in the 3D volume and therefore is oriented more parallel to the ultrasound beam direction, a relatively narrow-angled 3D dataset with high spatial and temporal resolution, like in live 3D volume mode, can be acquired encompassing the entire aortic valve [26].

> RT3D TEE visualization of the aortic valve provides detailed morphologic information in aortic regurgitation.

Compared to 2D echocardiography, RT3DE has the advantage of being able to show the entire valve in an en face view from either the aortic root or the left ventricular outflow tract (LVOT). This 3D visualization provides detailed morphologic information on cusp tethering due to aortic root or annulus dilatation or on the extent of cusp degeneration with thickening, calcification, fusion, or prolapse which is critically relevant for planning aortic valve reconstruction [107]. In addition, RT3DE can provide information on the extent of cusp destruction from endocarditis (◘ Fig. 7.46) and is useful in evaluating the exact size and location of paravalvular leakage after surgical or interventional aortic valve replacement (◘ Fig. 7.47 and ◘ Fig. 7.48). This might also be of interest for evaluating the feasibility of RT3DE-guided interventional occluder device implantation into paravalvular leakage (see ▶ Chapter 12). The superiority of RT3DE in the description of the complex 3D anatomy in a rare case of a completely torn out and displaced prosthetic aortic valve and conduit within the ascending aorta is shown in ◘ Fig. 7.49.

Because quantitative measurements of aortic valve dimensions, e.g., annulus diameter and aortic valve area, are in principle more accurate in RT3DE datasets, an application like the mitral valve quantification (MVQ) tool is also desirable for the aortic valve. Echocardiographic quantification of AR severity is routinely based on vena contracta width and pressure half time by continuous wave Doppler [9], although accurate quantification of regurgitant flow volume or regurgitant fraction would be the ultimate goal. RT3DE, in principle, provides similar advantages for quantification of vena contracta area (VCA) and regurgitant volume like for MR (◘ Fig. 7.44). Several studies demonstrated

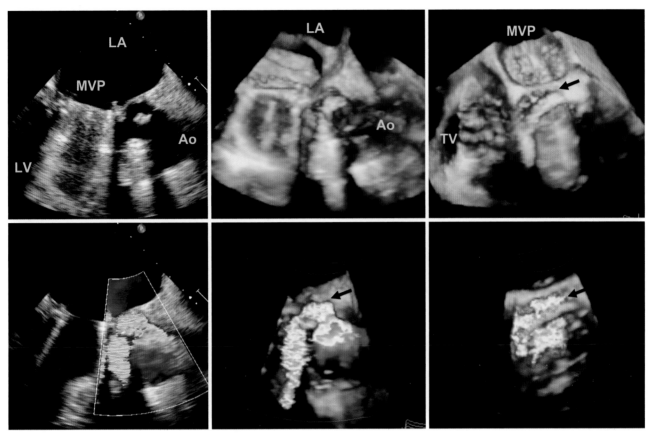

◘ Fig. 7.47 Example of a patient with a normal mechanical mitral valve prosthesis and a ruptured mechanical aortic valve prosthesis (*top left*) causing significant eccentric paravalvular regurgitation (*bottom left*). The 3D long-axis view to the outflow tract shows the dehiscence between the aortic valve prosthesis and the aortic ring (*top middle*). The 3D short-axis view to the aortic root clearly reveals the extent of the dehiscence even showing stretched sutures in the dehiscence space (*top right*). The 3D color Doppler long-axis (*bottom middle*) and short-axis views (*bottom right*) accurately represent extent and location of paravalvular aortic regurgitant flow (*arrows*). *Ao* aorta, *LA* left atrium, *LV* left ventricle, *MVP* mitral valve prosthesis, *TV* tricuspid valve. [→Videos 7.47A–F]

the advantage of using 3D TTE datasets to optimally identify a cross-sectional plane through the vena contracta perpendicular to the aortic regurgitant flow [108, 109]. Using angiographic grading for reference, Fang et al. [108] found good agreement for 3D vena contracta area measurements with aortic regurgitation severity grades and proposed a vena contracta area of <20 mm² and >60 mm² to define mild and severe aortic regurgitation, which has also been referenced in recent guidelines [11]. In a study with similar design, Chin et al. [109] also found good agreement of 3D vena contracta measurements with angiographic grading and derived a cutoff value for VCA of <30 mm² predicting mild aortic regurgitation and >50 mm² for predicting severe aortic regurgitation. Using 3Dl velocity-encoded MRI for reference, Ewe et al. [110] found aortic regurgitant volume

measurement by 3D transthoracic vena contracta area method to be significantly more accurate compared to the 2D transthoracic PISA method with a kappa value of 0.96 versus 0.53, the higher accuracy of 3D measurement being particularly evident in patients with eccentric jets.

Similar to 3D quantification of mitral regurgitation severity, the proximal isovelocity surface area method can be applied to determine the effective regurgitant orifice area which corresponds with the vena contracta area. Pirat et al. [111] performed an in vitro validation study of 3D reconstruction of the PISA surface based on manual tracing of the isovelocity surface contour in eight radial planes and found more accurate estimates of aortic regurgitant volume when compared to 2D methods which was most pronounced in noncircular orifices.

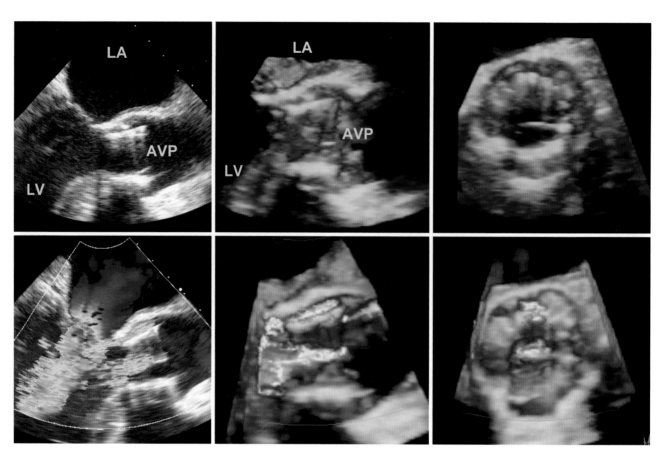

◻ Fig. 7.48 Comparison of 2D versus 3D image information in a patient during transfemoral implantation of an Edwards Sapien® aortic valve prosthesis. The 2D cross-sectional image shows the location of the prosthesis within the left ventricular outflow tract (*top left*) and moderate paravalvular and valvular regurgitation by 2D color Doppler (*bottom left*). Compared to this, the 3D image datasets provide long-axis (*top* and *bottom middle*) and short-axis views (*top* and *bottom right*) to the aortic valve within the same dataset allowing exact location and sizing of the regurgitant leaks (*bottom right*). *LA* left atrium, *LV* left ventricle, *AVP* aortic valve prosthesis. [→Videos 7.48A–F]

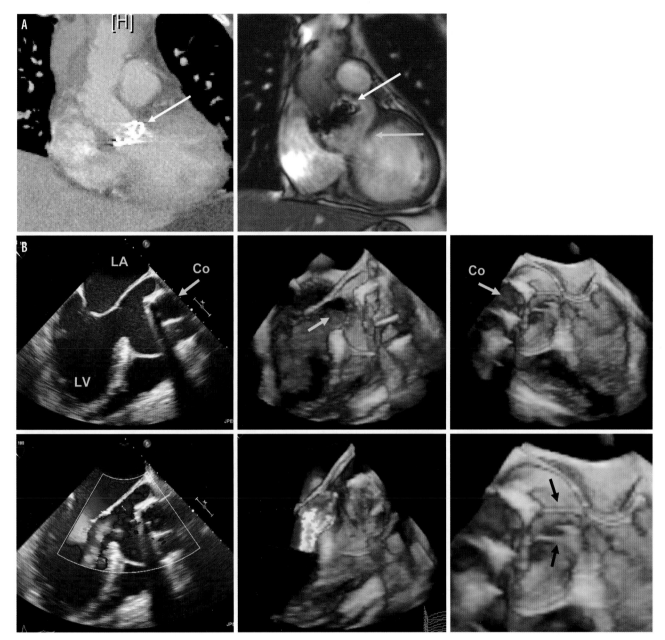

☐ **Fig. 7.49 A** Example of a 44-year-old man after surgical implantation of an aortic conduit with mechanical aortic valve prosthesis in the presence of aortic dissection type A 1 year previously. *Left* A cardio CT with detection of the valve prosthesis early after surgery (*white arrow*) is shown. *Right* A cardiac MRI 1 year later with an unclear finding, which was interpreted as formation of a new aneurysm proximal to the prosthesis (*white arrow*) in the aortic bulbus or LVOT with constriction between the aneurysm and LV (*yellow arrow*), is shown. **B** The 2D transesophageal echocardiography in the same patient provides a better image of the aneurysm formation proximal to the conduit (*Co; top left*). The 2D color Doppler reveals flow regurgitation through the narrow region between the LV and the aneurysm (*bottom left*). The RT3DE image in the same orientation as the 2D image with a view from postero-medial to the aneurysm shows a round opening between the aneurysm and the LV looking like an empty aortic ring (*arrow; top middle*). The RT3DE color Doppler image shows regurgitant flow filling the entire opening between the aneurysm and the LV (*bottom middle*). Cropping the RT3DE dataset from the other side providing a view from antero-lateral to the aneurysm reveals the true pathology by demonstrating two long sutures (*arrows*) stretched between the empty aortic ring and the torn out conduit (*top right* and *bottom right* with the view enhanced). This explains that the aneurysm is in fact the dilated aortic root; the regurgitant flow is caused by the blood volume filling and ballooning the aortic root aneurysm in systole and emptying back into the LV in diastole. *LA* left atrium, *LV* left ventricle. [→Videos 7.49B(a–e)]

7.3   Right-sided heart valves

Although insufficiencies of right-sided heart valves are similarly frequent as in their left-sided counterparts, they are commonly less clinically marked [8]. In principle, mechanisms of regurgitation in right-sided valves are the same as for left-sided valves, but degeneration is less marked. However, as a general limitation, right-sided heart valves are more difficult to examine by echocardiography.

Compared to left-sided heart valves, the tricuspid valve can only be assessed by RT3DE in a small percentage of patients, mainly because the leaflets are too thin for sufficient en face representation (◘ Fig. 7.50). The pulmonary valve is also too thin in most cases to be visualized successfully. From the transesophageal approach, image quality of the pulmonary valve is usually poor because it is located in the shadow of the aortic valve.

Grading of tricuspid valve regurgitation (TR) and pulmonary valve regurgitation (PR) severity, in principle, is based on similar parameters as for MR and AR with the same potential advantages of RT3DE over 2D echocardiography (◘ Fig. 7.51). However, clinical application of accurate TR grading is performed less frequently and little information is available in the current literature.

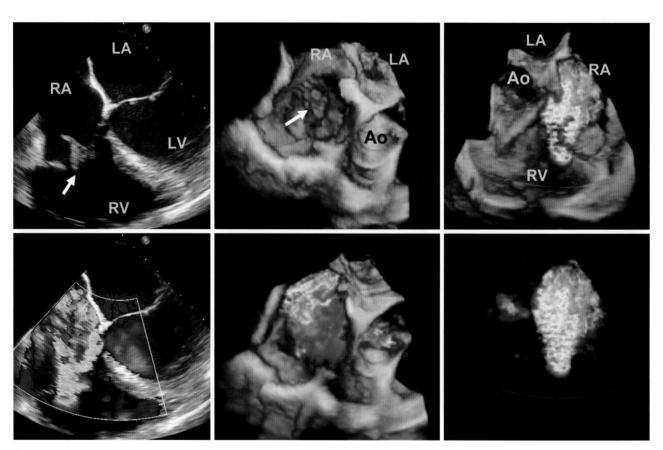

◘ **Fig. 7.50** Example of a patient with severe tricuspid regurgitation due to endocarditis. The 2D sector image shows a transesophageal 4-chamber view with detection of a huge vegetation on the tricuspid valve (*arrow; top left*) with severe tricuspid regurgitation detected by 2D color Doppler (*bottom left*). The RT3DE image shows a view from the RA to the tricuspid valve with the vegetation (*arrow; top middle*), while the RT3DE color Doppler image in the same orientation shows regurgitant flow back into the RA (*bottom middle*). The RT3DE color Doppler image (*top right*) with a perspective from the RV to the tricuspid valve shows the entire jet with PISA. *Bottom right* The same image as in the *top right* is shown but with tissue information suppressed. *LA* left atrium, *LV* left ventricle, *RA* right atrium, *RV* right ventricle, *Ao* aorta. [→Videos 7.50A–F]

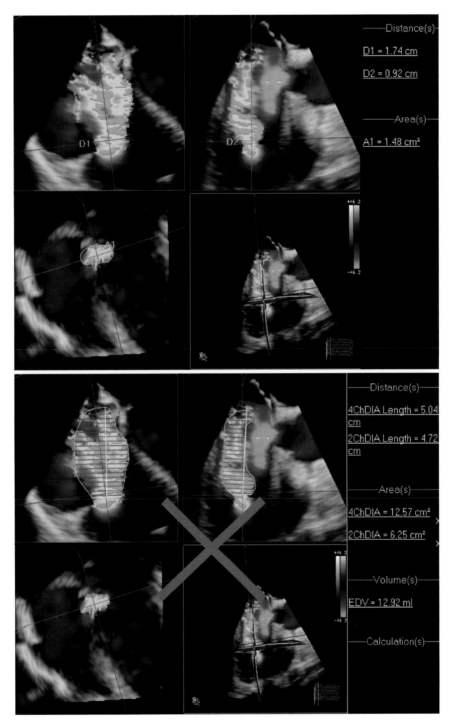

Fig. 7.51 The 3D color Doppler analysis of tricuspid regurgitation in the same case illustrated in **Fig. 7.50. *Left* Using multiplanar representation (MPR), the vena contracta width is measured in a 4-chamber (*top left*) and 2-chamber view (*top right*) and the vena contracta area measured in a cross-sectional plane through the vena contracta (*bottom left*). *Right* Measurement of the regurgitant jet volume in the views with a *red cross* is incorrect because the jet volume does not correlate with regurgitation severity, as the jet volume is mainly determined by the jet momentum which is determined by RV contractility [112]

References

1. Nkomo VT, Gardin JM, Skelton TN et al (2006) Burden of valvular heart diseases: a population-based study. Lancet 368:1005–1011
2. Iung B, Baron G, Butchart EG et al (2003) A prospective survey of patients with valvular heart disease in Europe: The Euro Heart Survey on Valvular Heart Disease. Eur Heart J 24:1231–1243
3. Avierinos JF, Gersh BJ, Melton LJ et al (2002) Natural history of asymptomatic mitral valve prolapse in the community. Circulation 106:1355–1361
4. Enriquez-Sarano M, Avierinos JF, Messika-Zeitoun D et al (2005) Quantitative determinants of the outcome of asymptomatic mitral regurgitation. New England Journal of Medicine 352:875–883
5. Zile MR (1991) Chronic aortic and mitral regurgitation. Clin Cardiol 9:239–253
6. Hetzer R, Dandel M (2011) Early detection of left ventricular dysfunction in patients with mitral regurgitation due to flail leaflet is still a challenge. Eur Heart J 32:665–667
7. Bonow RO, Carabello RA, Chatterjee K et al (2006) ACC/AHA 2006 guidelines for the management of patients with valvular heart disease. J Am Coll Cardiol 48:e1–e148
8. Vahanian A, Alfieri O, Andreotti F et al (2012) Guidelines on the management of valvular heart disease (version 2012). Eur Heart J 33:2451–2496
9. Grigioni F, Enriquez-Sarano M, Zehr KJ et al (2001) Ischemic mitral regurgitation: long-term outcome and prognostic implications with quantitative Doppler assessment. Circulation 103:1759–1764
10. Zoghbi WA, Enriquez-Sarano M, Foster E et al (2003) Recommendations for evaluation of the severity of native valvular regurgitation with two-dimensional and Doppler echocardiography. Journal of the American Society of Echocardiography 16:777–802
11. Lancellotti P, Moura L, Pierard LA et al (2010) European Association of Echocardiography recommendations for the assessment of valvular regurgitation. Part 2: mitral and tricuspid regurgitation (native valve disease). Eur J Echocardiogr 11:307–332
12. Grayburn PA, Weissman NJ, Zamorano JL (2012) Quantitation of mitral regurgitation. Circulation 126:2005–2017
13. Lang RM, Mor-Avi V, Sugeng L et al (2006) Three-dimensional echocardiography: the benefits of the additional dimension. J Am Coll Cardiol 48:2053-69
14. Kahlert P, Plicht B, Schenk IM et al (2008) Direct assessment of size and shape of noncircular vena contracta area in functional versus organic mitral regurgitation using real-time three-dimensional echocardiography. J Am Soc Echocardiogr 21:912–921
15. Pepi M, Tamborini G, Maltagliati A et al (2006) Head-to-head comparison of two- and three-dimensional transthoracic and transesophageal echocardiography in the localization of mitral valve prolapse. J Am Coll Cardiol 48:2524–2530
16. Grewal J, Mankad S, Freeman WK et al (2009) Real-time three-dimensional transesophageal echocardiography in the intraoperative assessment of mitral valve disease. J Am Soc Echocardiogr 22:34–41
17. Sugeng L, Shernan SK, Salgo IS et al (2008) Live 3-dimensional transesophageal echocardiography initial experience using the fully-sampled matrix array probe. J Am Coll Cardiol 52:446–449
18. Sugeng L, Coon P, Weinert L et al (2006) Use of real-time 3-dimensional transthoracic echocardiography in the evaluation of mitral valve disease. Journal of the American Society of Echocardiography 2006; 19:413–421
19. O'Gara P, Sugeng L, Lang R et al (2008) The role of imaging in chronic degenerative mitral regurgitation. JACC Cardiovasc Imaging 1:221–237
20. Carabello BA (2004) Indications for mitral valve surgery. J Cardiovasc Surg (Torino) 45:407–418
21. Walther T, Falk V, Mohr FW (2004) Minimally invasive mitral valve surgery. J Cardiovasc Surg (Torino) 45:487–495
22. Akins CW, Hilgenberg AD, Buckley MJ et al (1994) Mitral-valve reconstruction versus replacement for degenerative or ischemic mitral regurgitation. Annals of Thoracic Surgery 58:668–676
23. Seeburger J, Borger MA, Doll N et al (2009) Comparison of outcomes of minimally invasive mitral valve surgery for posterior, anterior and bileaflet prolapse. Eur J Cardiothorac Surg 36:532–548
24. Carpentier A (1983) Cardiac valve surgery – the »French correction«. J Thorac Cardiovasc Surg 86:323–337
25. Salcedo EE, Quaife RA et al (2009) A framework for systematic characterization of the mitral valve by real-time three-dimensional transesophageal echocardiography. J Am Soc Echocardiogr 22:1087–1099
26. Lang RM, Badano LP, Tsang W et al (2012) EAE/ASE recommendations for image acquisition and display using three-dimensional echocardiography. Eur Heart J Cardiovasc Imaging 13:1–46
27. Perloff JK, Roberts WC (1972) The mitral apparatus. Functional anatomy of mitral regurgitation. Circulation 46:227–239
28. Carpentier A, Lessana A, Relland JYM et al (1995) The »physio-ring«: an advanced concept in mitral valve annuloplasty. Ann Thorac Surg 60:1177–1186
29. Carpentier A, Chauvaud S, Fabiani JN et al (1980) Reconstructive surgery of mitral valve incompetence: ten-year appraisal. J Thorac Cardiovasc Surg 79:338–348
30. Al-Radi OO, Austin PC, Tu JV et al (2005) Mitral repair versus replacement for ischemic mitral regurgitation. Ann Thorac Surg 79:1260–1267
31. Barlow JB, Pocock WA (1988) Mitral valve billowing and prolapse: perspective at 25 years. Herz 13:227–234
32. Freed LA, Levy D, Levine RA et al (1999) Prevalence and clinical outcome of mitral-valve prolapse. New England Journal of Medicine 341:1–7
33. Anyanwu AC, Adams DH (2007) Etiologic classification of degenerative mitral valve disease: Barlow's disease and fibroelastic deficiency. Semin Thorac Cardiovasc Surg 19:90–96
34. Ling LH, Enriquez-Sarano M, Seward JB et al (1996) Clinical outcome of mitral regurgitation due to flail leaflet. N Engl J Med 335:1417–1423
35. La CG, Arendar I, Maisano F et al (2011) Real-time three-dimensional transesophageal echocardiography for assessment of mitral valve functional anatomy in patients with prolapse-related regurgitation. Am J Cardiol 107:1365–1374
36. Ring L, Rana BS, Ho SY, Wells FC (2013) The prevalence and impact of deep clefts in the mitral leaflets in mitral valve prolapse. Eur Heart J Cardiovasc Imaging 14:595–602
37. Foster GP, Isselbacher EM, Rose GA et al (1998) Accurate localization of mitral regurgitant defects using multiplane transesophageal echocardiography. Ann Thorac Surg 65:1025–1031
38. Mor-Avi V, Sugeng L, Lang RM (2009) Real-time 3-dimensional echocardiography: an integral component of the routine echocardiographic examination in adult patients? Circulation 119:314–329
39. Lang RM, Tsang W, Weinert L et al (2011) Valvular heart disease. The value of 3-dimensional echocardiography. J Am Coll Cardiol 58:1933–1944
40. Patel V, Hsiung MC, Nanda NC et al (2006) Usefulness of live/real time three-dimensional transthoracic echocardiography in the identification of individual segment/scallop prolapse of the mitral valve. Echocardiography 23:513–518
41. Sharma R, Mann J, Drummond L et al (2007) The evaluation of real-time 3-dimensional transthoracic echocardiography for the preoperative functional assessment of patients with mitral valve prolapse: a comparison with 2-dimensional transesophageal echocardiography. J Am Soc Echocardiogr 20:934–940
42. Barlow JB, Bosman CK (1966) Aneurysmal protrusion of the posterior leaflet of the mitral valve. An auscultatory-electrocardiographic syndrome. Am Heart J 71:166–178
43. Hayek E, Gring CN, Griffin BP (2005) Mitral valve prolapse. Lancet 365:507–518
44. Tanaka K, Takeda M (2004) Repair of Barlow's mitral valve: to do or not to do. Ann Thorac Surg 78:1879–1880
45. Chandra S, Salgo IS, Sugeng L et al (2011) Characterization of degenerative mitral valve disease using morphologic analysis of real-time three-dimensional echocardiographic images: objective insight into complexity and planning of mitral valve repair. Circ Cardiovasc Imaging 4:24–32
46. Fornes P, Heudes D, Fuzellier JF et al (1999) Correlation between clinical and histologic patterns of degenerative mitral valve insufficiency: a histomorphometric study of 130 excised segments. Cardiovasc Pathol 8:81–92

47. Sugeng L, Shernan SK, Weinert L et al (2008) Real-time three-dimensional transesophageal echocardiography in valve disease: comparison with surgical findings and evaluation of prosthetic valves. J Am Soc Echocardiogr 21:1347–1354

48. Chikwe J, Adams DH, Su KN et al (2012) Can three-dimensional echocardiography accurately predict complexity of mitral valve repair? Eur J Cardiothorac Surg 41:518–524.

49. Huang HL, Xie XJ, Fei HW et al (2013) Real-time three-dimensional transesophageal echocardiography to predict artificial chordae length for mitral valve repair. J Cardiothorac Surg 8:137

50. Chandra S, Salgo IS, Sugeng L et al (2011) A three-dimensional insight into the complexity of flow convergence in mitral regurgitation: adjunctive benefit of anatomic regurgitant orifice area. Am J Physiol Heart Circ Physiol 301:H1015–H1024

51. Vergnat M, Jassar AS, Jackson BM et al (2011) Ischemic mitral regurgitation: a quantitative three-dimensional echocardiographic analysis. Ann Thorac Surg 91:157–164

52. Nishimura RA, Schaff HV, Shub C et al (1983) Papillary muscle rupture complicating acute myocardial infarction: analysis of 17 patients. Am J Cardiol 51:373–7

53. Otsuji Y, Handschumacher MD, Schwammenthal E et al (1997) Insights from three-dimensional echocardiography into the mechanism of functional mitral regurgitation: direct in vivo demonstration of altered leaflet tethering geometry. Circulation 96:1999–2008

54. Hung J, Papakostas L, Tahta SA et al (2003) Mechanism of recurrent ischemic mitral regurgitation post-annuloplasty: Continued LV remodeling as a moving target. Circulation 108:476

55. Calafiore AM, Gallina S, Di MM et al (2001) Mitral valve procedure in dilated cardiomyopathy: repair or replacement? Ann Thorac Surg 71:1146–1152

56. Yamauchi T, Taniguchi K, Kuki S et al (2004) Evaluation of the mitral valve leaflet morphology after mitral valve reconstruction with a concept »coaptation length index«. J Card Surg 19:535–538

57. Watanabe N, Ogasawara Y, Yamaura Y et al (2006) Geometric differences of the mitral valve tenting between anterior and inferior myocardial infarction with significant ischemic mitral regurgitation: quantitation by novel software system with transthoracic real-time three-dimensional echocardiography. J Am Soc Echocardiogr 19:71–75

58. Watanabe N, Ogasawara Y, Yamaura Y et al (2005) Quantitation of mitral valve tenting in ischemic mitral regurgitation by transthoracic real-time three-dimensional echocardiography. J Am Coll Cardiol 45:763–769

59. Song JM, Fukuda S, Kihara T et al (2006) Value of mitral valve tenting volume determined by real-time three-dimensional echocardiography in patients with functional mitral regurgitation. Am J Cardiol 98:1088–1093

60. Yamaura Y, Watanabe N, Ogasawara Y et al (2005) Geometric change of mitral valve leaflets and annulus after reconstructive surgery for ischemic mitral regurgitation: real-time 3-dimensional echocardiographic study. J Thorac Cardiovasc Surg 130:1459–1461

61. Ryan LP, Jackson BM, Parish LM et al (2007) Mitral valve tenting index for assessment of subvalvular remodeling. Ann Thorac Surg 84:1243–1249

62. Yamada R, Watanabe N, Kume T et al (2009) Quantitative measurement of mitral valve coaptation in functional mitral regurgitation: In vivo experimental study by real-time three-dimensional echocardiography. J Cardiol 53:94–101

63. Daniel WG, Flachskampf FA (2006) Infective endocarditis. In: Camm AJ, Lüscher TF, Serruys PW (eds) The ESC textbook of cardiovascular medicine. Malden, MA, USA: Blackwell Publishing, pp 671–684

64. Click RL, Abel MD, Schaff HV (2000) Intraoperative transesophageal echocardiography: 5-year prospective review of impact on surgical management. Mayo Clin Proc 75:241–247

65. Freeman WK, Schaff HV, Khandheria BK et al (1992) Intraoperative evaluation of mitral valve regurgitation and repair by transesophageal echocardiography: incidence and significance of systolic anterior motion. J Am Coll Cardiol 20:599–609

66. Niwa Y, Yoshida K, Akasaka T et al (1996) [Intraoperative assessment of mitral valve plasty by transesophageal echocardiography]. J Cardiol 28:155–159

67. Kronzon I, Sugeng L, Perk G et al (2009) Real-time 3-dimensional transesophageal echocardiography in the evaluation of post-operative mitral annuloplasty ring and prosthetic valve dehiscence. J Am Coll Cardiol 2009; 53:1543–1547

68. Maffessanti F, Marsan NA, Tamborini G et al (2011) Quantitative analysis of mitral valve apparatus in mitral valve prolapse before and after annuloplasty: a three-dimensional intraoperative transesophageal study. J Am Soc Echocardiogr 24:405–413

69. Sinha A, Kasliwal RR, Nanda NC et al (2004) Live three-dimensional transthoracic echocardiographic assessment of isolated cleft mitral valve. Echocardiography 21:657–661

70. Kuperstein R, Feinberg MS, Carasso S et al (2006) The added value of real-time 3-dimensional echocardiography in the diagnosis of isolated cleft mitral valve in adults. J Am Soc Echocardiogr 19:811–814

71. Anwar AM, McGhie JS, Meijboom FJ, Ten Cate FJ (2008) Double orifice mitral valve by real-time three-dimensional echocardiography. Eur J Echocardiogr 9:731–732

72. Buck T, Plicht B, Erbel R (2006) [Current recommendations on echocardiographic evaluation of the severity of mitral regurgitation: standardization and practical application using a scoring system]. Herz 31:30–7

73. Yoganathan AP, Cape EG, Sung HW et al (1988) Review of hydrodynamic principles for the cardiologist: applications to the study of blood flow and jets by imaging techniques. J Am Coll Cardiol 12:1344–1353

74. Mascherbauer J, Rosenhek R, Bittner B et al (2005) Doppler echocardiographic assessment of valvular regurgitation severity by measurement of the vena contracta: an in vitro validation study. J Am Soc Echocardiogr 18:999–1006

75. Baumgartner H, Schima H, Kuhn P (1991) Value and limitations of proximal jet dimensions for the quantitation of valvular regurgitation: an in vitro study using Doppler flow imaging. J Am Soc Echocardiogr 4:57–66

76. Fehske W, Omran H, Manz M et al (1994) Color-coded Doppler imaging of the vena contracta as a basis for quantification of pure mitral regurgitation. Am J Cardiol 73:268–274

77. Mele D, Vandervoort PM, Palacios IF (1995) Proximal jet size by Doppler color flow mapping predicts severity of mitral regurgitation: clinical studies. Circulation 91:746–754

78. Hall SA, Brickner ME, Willett DL (1997) Assessment of mitral regurgitation severity by Doppler color flow mapping of the vena contracta. Circulation 95:636–642

79. Schwammenthal E, Chen C, Benning F (1994) Dynamics of mitral regurgitant flow and orifice area - physiologic application of the proximal flow convergence method: clinical data and experimental testing. Circulation 90:307–322

80. Khanna D, Vengala S, Miller AP et al (2004) Quantification of mitral regurgitation by live three-dimensional transthoracic echocardiographic measurements of vena contracta area. Echocardiography 21:737–743

81. Buck T, Plicht B, Kahlert P, Erbel R (2013) Understanding the asymmetrical vena contracta area: the difficult relationship between 2D and 3D measurements. JACC Cardiovasc Imaging 6:744

82. Little SH, Pirat B, Kumar R et al (2008) Three-dimensional color Doppler echocardiography for direct measurement of vena contracta area in mitral regurgitation: in vitro validation and clinical experience. JACC Cardiovasc Imaging 1:695–704

83. Yosefy C, Hung J, Chua S et al (2009) Direct measurement of vena contracta area by real-time 3-dimensional echocardiography for assessing severity of mitral regurgitation. Am J Cardiol 104:978–983

84. Hyodo E, Iwata S, Tugcu A et al (2012) Direct measurement of multiple vena contracta areas for assessing the severity of mitral regurgitation using 3D TEE. JACC Cardiovasc Imaging 5:669–676

85. Thavendiranathan P, Phelan D, Thomas JD et al (2012) Quantitative assessment of mitral regurgitation: validation of new methods. J Am Coll Cardiol 60:1470–1483

86. Iwakura K, Ito H, Kawano S et al (2006) Comparison of orifice area by transthoracic three-dimensional Doppler echocardiography versus proximal isovelocity surface area (PISA) method for assessment of mitral regurgitation. Am J Cardiol 97:1630–1637

87. Marsan NA, Westenberg JJ, Ypenburg C et al (2009) Quantification of functional mitral regurgitation by real-time 3D echocardiography: comparison with 3D velocity-encoded cardiac magnetic resonance. JACC Cardiovasc Imaging 2:1245–1252

88. Shanks M, Siebelink HM, Delgado V et al (2010) Quantitative assessment of mitral regurgitation: comparison between three-dimensional transesophageal echocardiography and magnetic resonance imaging. Circ Cardiovasc Imaging 2010; 3:694–700

89. Zeng X, Levine RA, Hua L et al (2011) Diagnostic value of vena contracta area in the quantification of mitral regurgitation severity by color Doppler 3D echocardiography. Circ Cardiovasc Imaging 4:506–513

90. Buck T, Plicht B, Kahlert P et al (2008) Effect of dynamic flow rate and orifice area on mitral regurgitant stroke volume quantification using the proximal isovelocity surface area method. J Am Coll Cardiol 52:767–778

91. Plicht B, Kahlert P, Goldwasser R et al (2008) Direct quantification of mitral regurgitant flow volume by real-time three-dimensional echocardiography using dealiasing of color Doppler flow at the vena contracta. J Am Soc Echocardiogr 2008; 21:1337–1346

92. Skaug TR, Hergum T, Amundsen BH et al (2010) Quantification of mitral regurgitation using high pulse repetition frequency three-dimensional color Doppler. J Am Soc Echocardiogr 23:1–8

93. Recusani F, Bargiggia GS, Yoganathan AP et al (1991) A new method for quantification of regurgitant flow rate using color flow imaging of the flow convergence region proximal to a discrete orifice: an vitro study. Circulation 83:594–604

94. Utsunomiya T, Ogawa T, Doshi R et al (1991) Doppler color flow »proximal isovelocity surface area« method for estimating volume flow rate: effects of orifice shape and machine factors. J Am Coll Cardiol 17:1103–1111

95. Buck T, Jansen CHP, Yoganathan AP et al (1998) Hemisphere Versus Hemiellipse: When Is Each Most Accurate for Proximal Isovelocity Calculation of Regurgitant Flows. (abstr). J Am Coll Cardiol 31:385

96. Yosefy C, Levine RA, Solis J et al (2007) Proximal flow convergence region as assessed by real-time 3-dimensional echocardiography: challenging the hemispheric assumption. J Am Soc Echocardiogr 20:389–396

97. Matsumura Y, Saracino G, Sugioka K et al (2008) Determination of regurgitant orifice area with the use of a new three-dimensional flow convergence geometric assumption in functional mitral regurgitation. J Am Soc Echocardiogr 21:1251–1256

98. Ziani AB, Latcu DG, Abadir S et al (2009) Assessment of proximal isovelocity surface area (PISA) shape using three-dimensional echocardiography in a paediatric population with mitral regurgitation or ventricular shunt. Arch Cardiovasc Dis 102:185–191

99. Matsumura Y, Fukuda S, Tran H et al (2008) Geometry of the proximal isovelocity surface area in mitral regurgitation by 3-dimensional color Doppler echocardiography: difference between functional mitral regurgitation and prolapse regurgitation. Am Heart J 155:231–238

100. Cobey FC, McInnis JA, Gelfand BJ et al (2012) A method for automating 3-dimensional proximal isovelocity surface area measurement. J Cardiothorac Vasc Anesth 26:507–511

101. Little SH, Igo SR, Pirat B et al (2007) In vitro validation of real-time three-dimensional color Doppler echocardiography for direct measurement of proximal isovelocity surface area in mitral regurgitation. Am J Cardiol 99:1440–1447

102. Li X, Shiota T, Delabays A et al (1999) Flow convergence flow rates from 3-dimensional reconstruction of color Doppler flow maps for computing transvalvular regurgitant flows without geometric assumptions: An in vitro quantitative flow study. J Am Soc Echocardiogr 12:1035–1044

103. Quaini A, Canic S, Guidoboni G et al (2011) A Three-Dimensional Computational Fluid Dynamics Model of Regurgitant Mitral Valve Flow: Validation Against in vitro Standards and 3D Color Doppler Methods. Cardiovasc Eng Technol 2:77–89

104. Grady L, Datta S, Kutter O et al (2011) Regurgitation quantification using 3D PISA in volume echocardiography. Med Image Comput Comput Assist Interv 14:512–519

105. de Agustin JA, Marcos-Alberca P, Fernandez-Golfin C et al (2012) Direct measurement of proximal isovelocity surface area by single-beat three-dimensional color Doppler echocardiography in mitral regurgitation: a validation study. J Am Soc Echocardiogr 25:815–823

106. Thavendiranathan P, Liu S, Datta S et al (2013) Quantification of chronic functional mitral regurgitation by automated 3-dimensional peak and integrated proximal isovelocity surface area and stroke volume techniques using real-time 3-dimensional volume color Doppler echocardiography: in vitro and clinical validation. Circ Cardiovasc Imaging 6:125–133

107. Khoury G, Glineur D, Rubay J et al (2005) Functional classification of aortic root/valve abnormalities and their correlation with etiologies and surgical procedures. Curr Opin Cardiol 20:115–121

108. Fang L, Hsiung MC, Miller AP et al (2005) Assessment of aortic regurgitation by live three-dimensional transthoracic echocardiographic measurements of vena contracta area: usefulness and validation. Echocardiography 22:775–781

109. Chin CH, Chen CH, Lo HS (2010) The correlation between three-dimensional vena contracta area and aortic regurgitation index in patients with aortic regurgitation. Echocardiography 27:161–166

110. Ewe SH, Delgado V, van der Geest R et al (2013) Accuracy of three-dimensional versus two-dimensional echocardiography for quantification of aortic regurgitation and validation by three-dimensional three-directional velocity-encoded magnetic resonance imaging. Am J Cardiol 112:560–566

111. Pirat B, Little SH, Igo SR et al (2009) Direct measurement of proximal isovelocity surface area by real-time three-dimensional color Doppler for quantitation of aortic regurgitant volume: an in vitro validation. J Am Soc Echocardiogr 22:306–313

112. Thomas JD, Liu CM, Flachskampf FA et al (1990) Quantification of jet flow by momentum analysis: an in vitro color Doppler flow study. Circulation 81:247–259

Valvular heart disease – stenoses

José Alberto de Agustin, José L. Zamorano

T. Buck et al. (Hrsg.), *Three-dimensional Echocardiography*,
DOI 10.1007/978-3-642-36799-1_8, © Springer-Verlag Berlin Heidelberg 2014

The benefits of three-dimensional (3D) echocardiography are particularly useful to evaluate valvular disease. Compared with two-dimensional (2D) echocardiography, 3D echocardiography improves the morphologic and quantitative assessment of valvular stenosis.

8.1   Evaluation of mitral valve stenosis

Mitral stenosis (MS) is mainly caused by two etiologies: a history of rheumatic carditis in the majority of patients or nonrheumatic calcific stenosis as a result of progressive atheromatous degeneration of the mitral annulus [1][2]. While surgical mitral valve replacement might be necessary in severe calcific MS in older patients, percutaneous mitral valvuloplasty [PMV, or commissurotomy (PMC)] remains a standard procedure in younger patients with rheumatic MS [3].

To define patients with mitral valve (MV) stenosis, clinical data, morphologic evaluation, and accurate measurements of the mitral valve orifice area (MVA) are necessary. Classic methods to determine MVA have important limitations. Real-time 3D echocardiography (RT3DE) provides not only different and superior morphologic evaluation of the MV apparatus, but also definition of the optimal plane of the smallest MV orifice and allows accurate measurement of the MVA.

> Real-time 3D echocardiography provides accurate definition of the optimal plane of the smallest MV orifice.

8.1.1   Morphological assessment of the mitral valve

Mitral valve stenosis (MS) is a disease associated with progressive morphologic changes of the MV apparatus. Selecting patients favorable for PMV requires precise evaluation of the MV apparatus and particularly commissural anatomy [3][4]. The morphologic assessment of the MV apparatus by transthoracic and transesophageal RT3DE is more accurate because it provides 3D views of the entire MV apparatus, particularly en face views from either the left atrium to the mitral valve (the surgeon's view) or from the left ventricle to the mitral valve (Fig. 8.1, Fig. 8.2, Fig. 8.3, Fig. 8.4, Fig. 8.5). Not only the location and degree of fusion, but also the thickening of the leaflets and chordae tendineae can be visualized clearly by RT3DE [5]. Earlier studies evaluated the interobserver variability of the Wilkins score using real-time 3D transthoracic echocardiography (RT3D TTE) compared to 2D echocardiography [6]. RT3DE assessment showed better inter- and intraobserver agreement for morphologic evaluation of rheumatic MS.

Recently, a new scoring system for the assessment of MS using transthoracic RT3DE has been proposed by Anwar et al. [7] [8]. They divided each leaflet into three scallops. Thickness, mobility, and calcification for each MV scallop were scored separately. The subvalvular apparatus was also divided into three cut sections, proximal (valve level), middle, and distal (papillary muscle level). The RT3DE score ranged from 0 to 31 points. The new proposed RT3DE score was feasible and reproducible and compared favorably with Wilkins's score. They also found that calcification by RT3DE score was the only predictor of the development of grade >2 mitral regurgitation after PMV, not only due to calcification extent but also due to the calcification site, because this complication was more common when the calcification was detected at the commissural segments of the MV leaflets by transthoracic RT3DE. However, morphologic assessment of a stenotic MV is much more rewarding through the application of transesophageal RT3DE (RT3D TEE) [9][10] [11][12].

8.1.2   Functional assessment of mitral stenosis

In the past, the gold standard method for determining MVA was invasive evaluation, using catheter-based data and Gorlin's equation. However, this invasive method was associated with complications and had important limitations. Most notably, it was inaccurate when significant valvular regurgitation was present. Today, 2D echocardiography is the standard method to determine MVA in routine clinical practice [3][11]. MVA can be assessed indirectly by the pressure half-time (PHT) method or by direct planimetry. These methods have several limitations. PHT-derived MVA can be obtained easily, but may be influenced by hemodynamic factors (e.g., heart rate, cardiac rhythm, cardiac index, left ventricular systolic and diastolic dysfunction, left ventricular and atrial compliance, left ventricular hypertrophy, and concomitant valvular disease) [13][14]. The main advantage of planimetry is that it provides a relatively hemodynamic-independent assessment of the MVA. Until now, direct measurements of the MVA could be only performed using planimetry in 2D short-axis views, but this method has several limitations: the most important is that there is no controlled sectioning of the mitral funnel orifice. Thus, 2D measurements of the MVA are made in the short-axis view with no simultaneous, independent imaging to verify that the imaging plane corresponds to the smallest and most perpendicular view of the MV orifice. Therefore, this method requires significant experience and operator skill to obtain the correct imaging plane that displays the true MV orifice. In addition, 2D planimetry is limited to patients with favorable image quality from a parasternal window.

> Planimetry of MVA using 2D short-axis views is mainly limited by the lack of controlled sectioning of the funnel-shaped mitral orifice.

The assessment of patients with MV stenosis is one of the most rewarding clinical applications of RT3DE. Not only does RT3DE show the anatomic structure of the MV, but also shows the optimal plane of the smallest MV orifice at the leaflet tips at the smaller end of the funnel-shaped valve (Fig. 8.6, Fig. 8.7) as already demonstrated in early studies using reconstructive 3D echocardiography [15][16]. Thereby, overestimation of mitral valve opening area due to malpositioning of the short-axis cut plane can be obviated. In contrast, RT3DE provides unique orientations of the image planes not obtainable by routine 2D echocardiography [17].

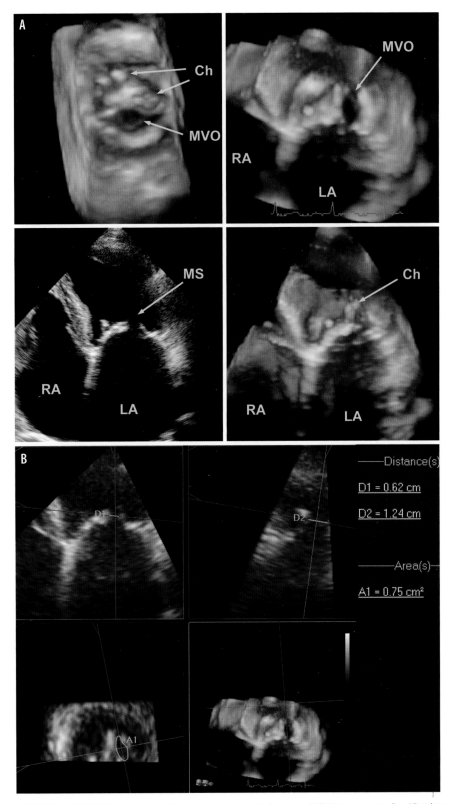

■ **Fig. 8.1** **A** Comparison of 2D TTE and RT3D TTE visualization of severe rheumatic mitral stenosis (*MS*). Using a narrow live 3D volume, the en face view from the left ventricle to the mitral valve clearly shows the shape and size of the mitral valve orifice (*MVO*) as well as the thickened chordae (*Ch*). It also shows typical commissural fusion but without signs of heavy calcification along the commissure (*top left*). Tilting and cropping the 3D dataset provides a cross-sectional view to the mitral valve and the MVO as well as the left atrium (*LA; top right*). The RT3DE 4-chamber view (*bottom right*) provides additional information about the mitral apparatus compared to 2D 4-chamber view (*bottom left*), such as thickening of the chordae. **B** RT3D TTE measurement of the mitral valve orifice area. The multiplane representation (*MPR*) allows exact definition of the smallest orifice area at the leaflet tips in a 4-chamber view (*green plane; top left*), the 2-chamber view (*red plane; top right*), and short-axis view (*blue plane; bottom left*). *RA* right atrium. [→Videos 8.1A (a–d)]

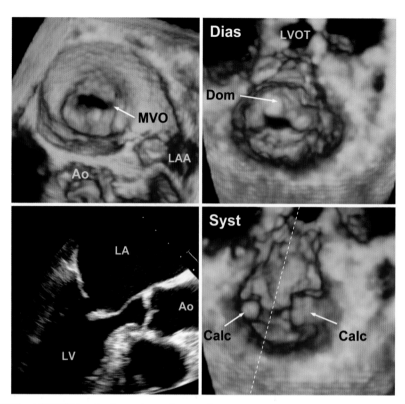

⬛ **Fig. 8.2** Comparison of 2D TEE and RT3D TEE imaging in a patient with severe rheumatic mitral stenosis. Using a live 3D zoom volume, en face view from the left atrium (*LA*) shows the narrow, elliptic mitral valve orifice (*MVO; top left*). The en face view from the left ventricle (*LV*) to the mitral valve shows typical doming (*Dom*) of the anterior leaflet in diastole (*top right*). In systole, the en face view reveals solid sclerotic-calcific (*Calc*) thickening in the region of the antero-lateral (*right* (larger)) and postero-medial (*left* (smaller)) commissure as an important finding, thus, making percutaneous commissurotomy less suitable (*bottom right*). The 2D long-axis view (*bottom left*) with its orientation through the middle of the mitral valve and LVOT (*white dashed line* in *bottom right image*) fails to detect the calcification. *Ao* aorta, *LAA* left atrial appendage, *LVOT* left ventricular outflow tract, *Dias* diastolic, *Syst* systolic. [→Videos 8.2A–C]

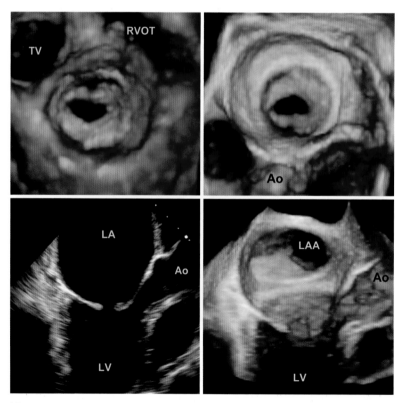

⬛ **Fig. 8.3** A typical example of rheumatic mitral stenosis with comparison of image information by 2D TEE versus RT3D TEE. Using a RT3DE full volume, en face view from the left ventricle (*LV*) to the mitral valve shows commissural fusion of the two leaflets resulting in a restricted, narrow valve opening with smooth and only mildly thickened leaflet edges (*top left*). The en face view from the left atrium (*LA*) to the mitral valve shows the smooth funnel-shaped leaflets (*top right*). Comparison of the 2D and the RT3DE long-axis views reveals the superior spatial information of RT3DE (*bottom left* and *right*). *TV* tricuspid valve, *RVOT* right ventricular outflow tract, *Ao* aorta, *LAA* left atrial appendage. [→Videos 8.3A–D]

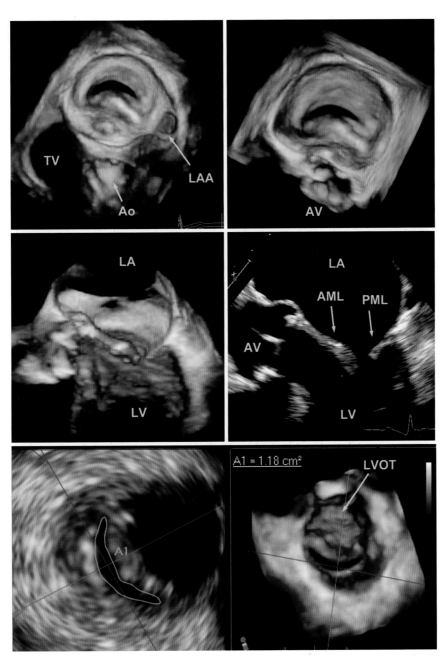

■ **Fig. 8.4** Unusual case of mitral stenosis shown by RT3D TEE with severely thickened and restricted leaflets but no commissural fusion resulting in a smile-shaped mitral valve orifice. The patient reported a history of repeated mitral valve endocarditis but no rheumatic fever. The two en face views from the left atrium to the mitral valve show a comparison of a full volume dataset (*top left*) and a live 3D zoom dataset (*top right*). Both en face views reveal smooth leaflets and leaflet edges. The RT3DE and 2D long-axis views show severely thickened and retracted leaflet tips (*middle left* and *right*). Measurement in the 3D dataset provided a mitral valve opening area of 1.18 cm², indicating moderate MS (*bottom*). *TV* tricuspid valve, *Ao* aorta, *LAA* left atrial appendage, *AV* aortic valve, *LA* left atrium, *LV* left ventricle, *AML* anterior mitral leaflet, *PML* posterior mitral leaflet, *LVOT* left ventricular outflow tract. [→Videos 8.4A–D]

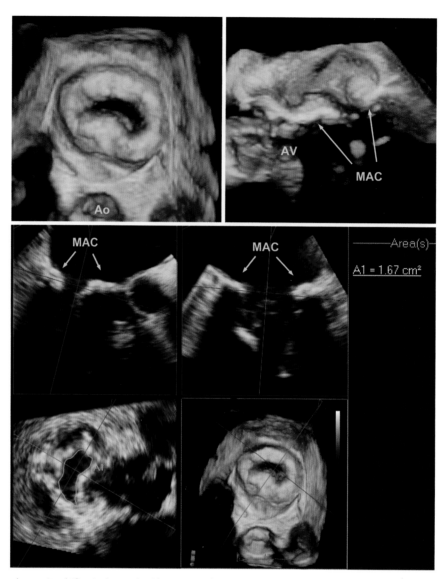

◘ **Fig. 8.5** Example of nonrheumatic calcific mitral stenosis with severe circular mitral annular calcification (*MAC*). The RT3D TEE en face surgeon's view from a full volume dataset clearly shows circular annular thickening with calcified plaques (*top left*). The RT3DE angulated long-axis view provides a perspective to the circular calcified annulus as well as a cross-sectional view to the calcified thickening of the annulus and basal anterior and posterior leaflet (*top right*). The multiplane representation shows 2D cross-sectional views of the annular calcification and allows direct planimetry of the MVA at the annular level. *AV* aortic valve, *Ao* aorta. [→Videos 8.5A,B]

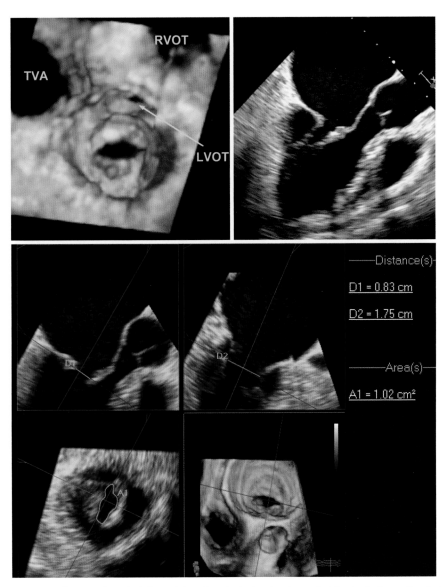

◘ **Fig. 8.6** Transesophageal RT3DE en face view from the left ventricle to the mitral valve showing typical doming in rheumatic mitral valve stenosis (*top left*). The en face view clearly shows the absence of significant sclerotic leaflet thickening or calcification indicating suitability of this valve for percutaneous commissurotomy. The multiplane representation (*below*) of the funnel-shaped mitral valve within the 3D dataset allows the smallest orifice at the smaller end of the funnel for measurement of mitral valve orifice to be defined (see ◘ Fig. 8.7). *TVA* tricuspid valve annulus, *RVOT* right ventricular outflow tract, *LVOT* left ventricular outflow tract. [→Videos 8.6A,B]

◻ Fig. 8.7 Demonstration of the importance of an optimal measurement plane position at the leaflet tips for the measurement of mitral valve orifice area within a funnel-shaped mitral valve in the same patient shown in ◻ Fig. 8.6. The *lower images* represent the image plane with mitral valve orifice areas at the respective cross-section levels indicated in the upper images

Planimetry using transthoracic 3D echocardiography is not limited to the parasternal window but also allows MVA measurement from an apical window (◻ Fig. 8.1). An initial study compared RT3D TEE with current 2D echocardiographic methods for the assessment of MVA [2D planimetry, PHT method, and proximal isovelocity surface area (PISA) method] in patients with rheumatic MS [6]. Invasive determination of MVA using Gorlin's equation was used for reference. RT3DE planimetry was performed at the ideal cross-section of the MV during its greatest diastolic opening. The ideal cross-section was defined as the most perpendicular view on the plane with the smallest MV orifice. Analysis showed better agreement when comparing the invasively determined MVA with RT3DE-determined MVA than when comparing it with conventional 2D echocardiographic methods. Similar results have been reported by others [18][19] [20][21]. Kasliwal et al. [22] compared the MVA obtained by 3D echocardiography with the true mitral orifice measured directly during operation and found a high degree of agreement versus the anatomic finding.

> **RT3DE might replace the invasive Gorlin method as the gold standard for the quantification of the MVA.**

There is sufficient evidence that RT3DE is superior to 2D echocardiography and can be routinely used for the quantification of MVA in MS [6]. The exceptional quality of the images of the MV suggests that this modality will become the new gold standard for MVA quantification. In addition, a recent study found RT3DE planimetry to be more accurate than the Gorlin method for estimation of MVA [23]. Thus, in the future, RT3DE might replace

the Gorlin method as the gold standard for the quantification of the MVA and may eventually make routine preoperative cardiac catheterization unnecessary [24].

Beside planimetry of the MVA, unconventional 3D echocardiographic indices like the geometry of the mitral stenosis and mitral valve volume (i.e., the volume of the leaflet funnel) assessed by 3D transesophageal echocardiography (TEE) have been evaluated [25]. In two recent studies, the mitral valve volume before PMV was found to be inversely correlated to a successful PMV procedure [26][27].

In recent years, RT3D TEE has become a valuable complementary tool guiding PMV [28][29]30] and accurately managing and diagnosing possible complications. Real-time 3DTEE supplies superior imaging quality and is capable of facilitating interventions with unprecedented detail and ease (see ▶ Fig. 12.25). Real-time 3D TEE provides wide fields of view with superior depth resolution allowing safe navigation by monitoring the spatial relationships between cardiac structures and interventional devices simultaneously. Positioning of the interatrial transseptal puncture is essential for minimizing the risk of ardiac tamponade and successfully navigating the balloon catheter toward the mitral orifice. Fine corrections in position and alignment are more easily performed with 3D TEE, as seen in navigating the balloon catheter just beyond the plane of MV coaptation. The distal half of the balloon must be placed just beyond the MV plane of coaptation, inflated, and then retracted against the MV prior to full inflation (see ▶ Fig. 12.25). Appreciation of incorrect positioning in the left ventricle may be helpful in avoiding potential complications. After inflating

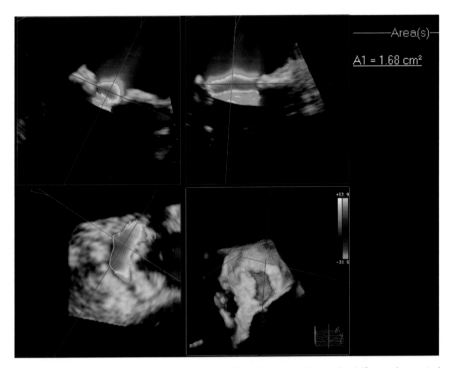

Fig. 8.8 Example of the 3D measurement of the MVA using RT3DE color Doppler in the same patient with calcific mitral stenosis shown in ▪ Fig. 8.5. The color Doppler flow cross-sectional area is measured where flow is narrowest, which is at the annular level in patients with calcific MS

the balloon, success can be assessed using 3D TEE to confirm commissural fissuring and search for possible leaflet tears.

RT3DE color Doppler has also shown to be of clinical usefulness in patients with mitral stenosis. In patients with nonrheumatic calcific mitral stenosis, where circular calcification and thickening of the annulus and basal portion of the mitral leaflets is the main cause of restricted mitral valve opening compared to funnel-shaped rheumatic MS, the RT3DE color Doppler en face view to the flow cross-section at the limiting anatomic orifice area at the annular level has been demonstrated to be more accurate compared to PHT (▪ Fig. 8.8) [31]. Moreover, because the effective and anatomic orifice areas are essentially equal in calcific MS with a tubular valve geometry, the RT3D color Doppler measurement of the flow cross-sectional area (representing effective orifice area) should provide results similar to those obtained using Gorlin's equation and, therefore, might supplant invasive evaluation.

The RT3DE color Doppler representation using the multiplane mode also allows accurate analysis of the flow field proximal to the stenotic orifice by using the PISA method [6]. Visualization of the PISA in two perpendicular planes as well as an en face cross-section provides important information on the PISA shape. In principle, the same requirements for PISA application should be valid for MS as they are for mitral regurgitation (MR; ▶ Chapter 7). To apply the conventional PISA method, PISA needs to be nearly hemispheric. An example where PISA is asymmetric requiring a hemielliptic PISA method is shown in ▪ Fig. 8.9.

8.2 Evaluation of aortic valve stenosis

8.2.1 Morphological assessment of aortic stenosis

By its unique 3D visualization and the surgeon's en face perspective of the aortic valve, RT3DE adds important information for the understanding of aortic valve pathologies in aortic stenosis. Due to the limited spatial resolution of currently available transthoracic RT3DE transducers, visualization of the aortic valve has been unsatisfactory, because aortic valve leaflets are thinner than the mitral valve, but on the other hand in a diseased stage often highly calcified and are usually orientated more parallel to the ultrasound beam, rather than perpendicular to it. Morphologic and functional assessment of the aortic valve using RT3DE technology only became satisfactory once the RT3D TEE probe became available (▶ Chapter 2), which provides a direct en face view from the aorta to the aortic valve, giving detailed morphologic information on leaflet anatomy, atheromatous degeneration and thickening, calcific lesions, cusp mobility, commissural fusion (▪ Fig. 8.10), and the location of the LCA ostium in relation to the left coronary cusp (▪ Fig. 8.11) [17]. As a consequence, detailed morphologic assessment of the aortic valve morphology by RT3D TEE has been demonstrated clinically feasible and useful for example before and during transcatheter aortic valve implantation (▶ Chapter 12) [32].

> Transesophageal RT3DE provides a direct en face view of the aortic valve, thus, giving detailed morphologic information.

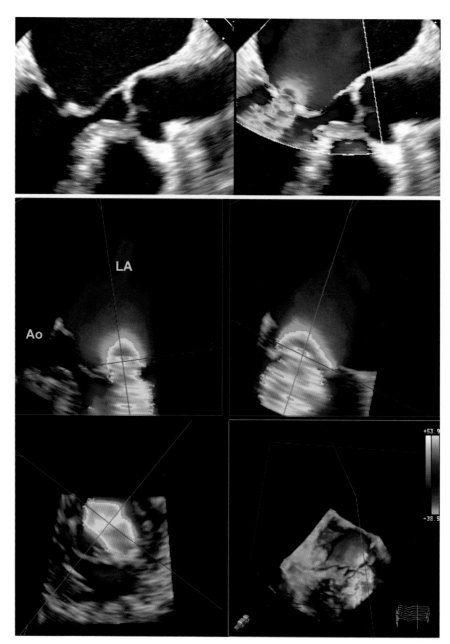

☐ Fig. 8.9 The RT3DE color Doppler dataset in the same patient shown in ☐ Fig. 8.2 demonstrates the hemielliptic shape of the PISA in the flow field proximal to the elliptic valve orifice shown in ☐ Fig. 8.2. *Ao* aorta, *LA* left atrium. [→Videos 8.9A,B]

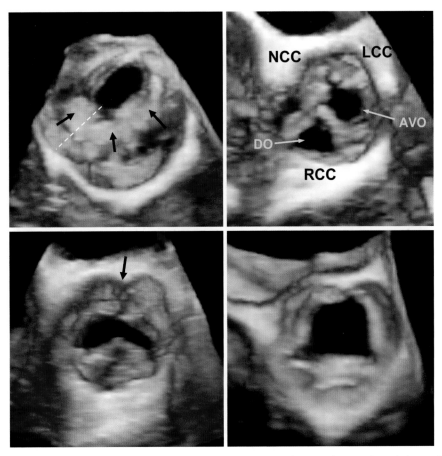

☐ **Fig. 8.10** RT3D TEE en face views from the aortic root to the aortic valve (surgeon's view) in different etiologies and morphologies of aortic valve stenosis. *Top left* Bicuspid valve with severe atheromatous thickening (*arrows*) (*white dashed line* indicating commissural line). *Top right* Rheumatic valve stenosis with commissural fusion between the right coronary cusp (*RCC*) and noncoronary cusp (*NCC*) as well as partly between the NCC and left coronary cusp (*LCC*) resulting in opening (*AVO*) of the LCC only. Dropout artifact (*DO*) indicates thin leaflets. *Bottom left* Degenerative thickened valve with restricted valve opening and commissural fusion between the NCC and LCC (*arrow*). *Bottom right* As a nearly normal aortic valve, this valve shows only moderately thickened leaflets with no signs of atheromatous degeneration and normal leaflet separation. [→Videos 8.10A–D]

◘ Fig. 8.11 Example of RT3D TEE visualization of combined mitral and aortic stenosis in an 82-year-old woman. RT3DE provides a modified en face view to a severely atheromatous thickened aortic valve with minimal opening in systole (*Syst; top left*) and a degenerated mitral valve (*MV*) with restricted opening in diastole (*Dias; top right*). The RT3DE en face view (*top left*) and long-axis view (*bottom left*) reveal the proximity of the solid thickened left coronary cusp (*LCC*) to the ostium of the left coronary artery (*LCA*) as a potential risk for LCA occlusion during transcatheter aortic valve implantation. This relationship cannot be represented by 2D echocardiography (*bottom right*) because neither the 2D short-axis nor 2D long-axis planes provide a cross-section through both the LCA ostium and aortic valve. *TV* tricuspid valve. [→Videos 8.11A–C]

8.2.2   Functional assessment of aortic stenosis

The accurate assessment of aortic valve area (AVA) is crucial in making decisions in patients with aortic valve stenosis (AS). While cardiac catheterization using the Gorlin formula was historically the gold standard to assess AVA, today 2D echocardiography is the standard diagnostic technique for assessing the severity of AS through the measurement of transvalvular gradients and calculation of the effective AVA using the continuity equation [3][11]. However, Doppler-derived methods are limited in patients with subvalvular obstruction, a small aorta, eccentric jet in bicuspid aortic valves, significant aortic regurgitation, or depressed left ventricular function [33][34][35]. Another potential limitation of 2D Doppler-derived methods is the assumption of the left ventricular outflow tract (LVOT) being circular, while in many cases it is more elliptical [35].

Direct planimetry of the anatomic AVA, in principle, is more accurate but is highly dependent on image quality. Compared to the transthoracic 2D approach, which frequently offers only limited visualization of the AV, multiplane 2D TEE provides proper representation of the aortic valve cusps in a short-axis cross-sectional view through the aortic root. However, the major limitation of 2D TEE for direct planimetry of the AVA is the dif-

ficulty in obtaining the cross-sectional view at the level of the tips of the aortic valve cusps where AVA is smallest. Two prior studies found clinically important overestimation of anatomic valve area by 2D TEE planimetry compared with flow-derived methods [36][37].

> The major limitation of 2D TEE for direct planimetry of the AVA is the difficulty in obtaining the cross-sectional view at the tips of the aortic valve cusps where AVA is smallest.

Recently, RT3DE has been found to provide superior accuracy in detecting the smallest AVA by controlled orientation of the measurement plane in either two simultaneous image planes (xPlane mode, ◘ Fig. 8.12) or three cut planes through the 3D dataset (◘ Fig. 8.13). Early studies using RT3D TTE demonstrated good correlation with intraoperative 3D TEE measurements [38] and good agreement with 2D TEE planimetry and 2D TTE using the continuity equation [39][40]. In addition, the 3D method showed lower interobserver variability. However, as mentioned above, visualization of the aortic valve using currently available transthoracic matrix array transducer technology is limited, thus, preventing AVA determination in most patients.

Therefore, most studies that examined the role of 3D echocardiography in aortic stenosis have been performed using the

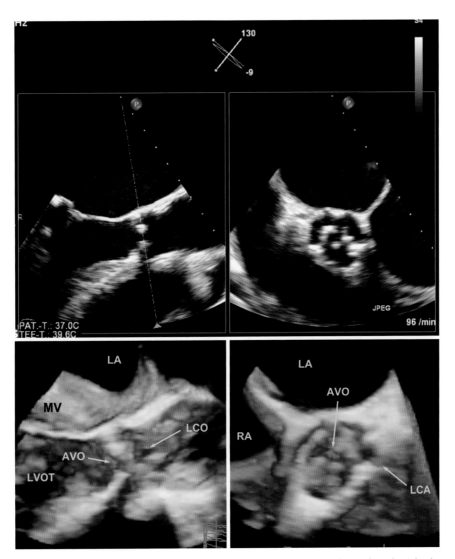

Fig. 8.12 Example showing two simultaneous image planes (xPlane mode) using the matrix array transducer, where the right plane can be electronically rotated and swept to provide optimal representation of the smallest aortic valve orifice (*AVO*) at the leaflet tips (*dashed white line* in *upper left image plane*). Compared to this, RT3D TEE provides superior anatomic information of the aortic valve morphology and neighboring structures. The RT3DE long-axis view (*bottom left*) depicts the severely sclerotic thickened aortic valve (*AV*) cusps, the proximity of the left coronary cusp to the left coronary ostium (*LCO*), and provides an en face view to the severe atheromatous aortic wall. The RT3DE en face view (*bottom right*) shows severely thickened aortic valve cusps with fusion of all three commissures. *LA* left atrium, *RA* right atrium, *MV* mitral valve, *LVOT* left ventricular outflow tract, *LCA* left coronary artery. [→Videos 8.12A–C]

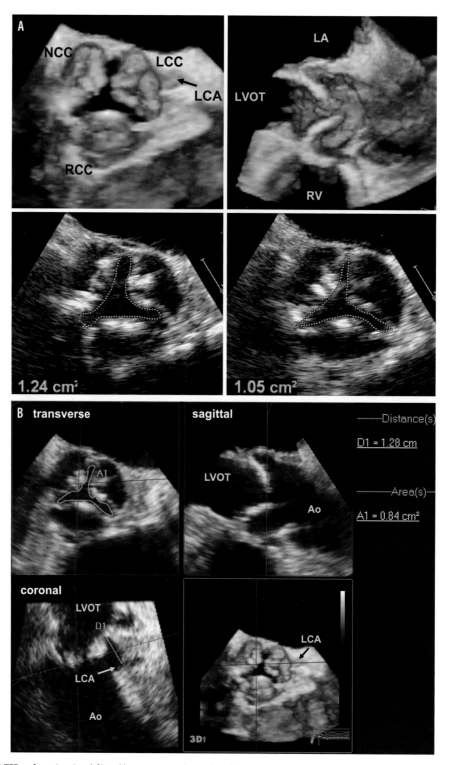

☐ **Fig. 8.13 A** The RT3D TEE en face view (*top left*) and long-axis view (*top right*) of an atheromatous thickened and restricted aortic valve. The 2D planimetry resulted in varying dimensions of 1.24 cm² and 1.05 cm² for the aortic valve opening area. **B** Measurement of aortic valve area (*AVA*) within the 3D data set in the same patient shown in **A**. Optimal positioning of the green plane at the leaflet tips resulted in a significantly smaller AVA of 0.84 cm² compared to 2D measurements in **A**. Note the detection of the aortic annulus and the ostium of the left coronary artery (*LCA*) in one view only in the coronal plane (*lower left panel*) which can be reconstructed from the RT3D dataset, but cannot be acquired by 2D imaging. In the coronal plane, the annulus-to-left main distance can be accurately measured (1.2 cm)

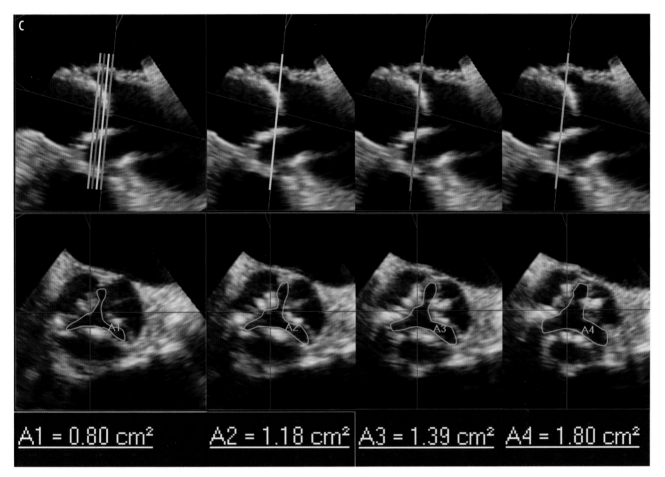

⬛ Fig. 8.13 (continued) **C** Demonstration of the importance of optimal positioning of the cross-sectional measurement plane at the narrowest part of the funnel-shaped aortic valve at the leaflet tips for obtaining the smallest AVA (same patient as shown in **A** and **B**). *NCC* noncoronary cusp, *LCC* left coronary cusp, *LCA* left coronary artery, *RCC* right coronary cusp, *LA* left atrium, *LVOT* left ventricular outflow tract, *RV* right ventricle, *Ao* aorta. [→Videos 8.13A(a, b), B]

3D TEE approach. Several early studies [41][42][43][44][45] confirmed that planimetry of the 3D aortic valve opening area is feasible and accurate using reconstructive 3D TEE, compared with 2D TEE-based data and invasive measurements. More recently, feasibility of RT3D TEE in the direct assessment of AVA in patients with aortic stenosis was validated in several studies [46][47]. Utility of 3D echocardiography in children with congenital aortic stenosis before and after balloon valvuloplasty has also been demonstrated by Bharucha et al. [48].

As a result of anatomically correct visualization of the 3D structure of the aortic valve, RT3D TEE can accurately measure AVA even with unusual 3D valve geometry, like in degenerated bicuspid valves (⬛ Fig. 8.14) [49] or unicuspid aortic valve stenosis [50]. Recognizing bicuspid aortic stenosis in patients referred for transcatheter aortic valve implantation is another important utility of RT3D TEE, because it is still a contraindication for the procedure [51]. The utility of 3D TEE in characterizing morphology and diagnosis of unicuspid aortic valve stenosis has also been reported [52].

Beside a more accurate planimetry of AVA, RT3DE provides accurate assessment of the noncircular LVOT area (⬛ Fig. 8.15) for AVA assessment using the continuity equation. While the elliptic shape of the LVOT has already been described as a potential cause of AVA underestimation by 2D methods in early studies [53], RT3DE is ideally suited to demonstrate the true shape of the LVOT [17]. Several investigators demonstrated significant underestimation of the true LVOT area by 2D echocardiography compared to transthoracic and transesophageal RT3DE measurements [54][55][56][57].

To eliminate the inaccuracy of the AVA calculation caused by invalid geometric assumption of LVOT area when using the continuity equation, RT3DE has been used to measure LVOT stroke volume independent from the LVOT area measurement. Gutierrez-Chico et al. [58] validated a new method substituting the Doppler-derived systolic stroke volume by directly obtained systolic SV from semiautomated RT3DE LV volumetry (▶ Chapter 3). Poh et al. [59] used RT3DE color Doppler to measure LVOT systolic stroke volume directly by the integral of color Doppler velocities times the flow cross-sectional area within the LVOT sampled over systole. They found that measuring LVOT systolic volume by RT3DE improves accuracy of the AVA calculation by the continuity equation, including situations such as upper septal hypertrophy, common in the elderly, which modifies LVOT geometry [59].

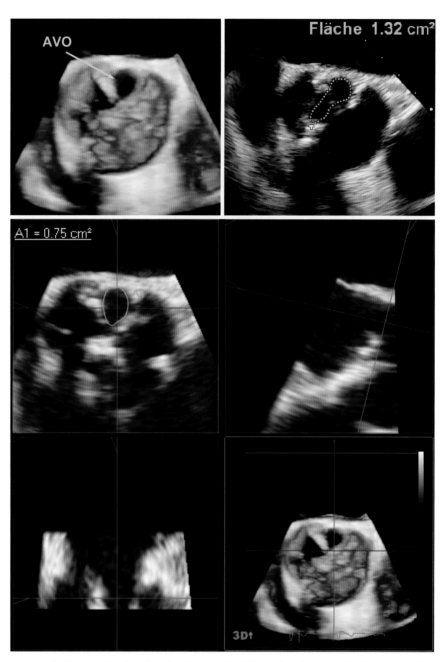

◻ **Fig. 8.14** *Top right* Unusual case of a »buttonhole«-shaped aortic valve stenosis which could not be appropriately represented in a standard 2D cross-sectional plane. *Top left* The RT3D TEE en face view revealed the true shape and size of the aortic valve orifice (*AVO*) in a bicuspid aortic valve with subtotal commissural fusion and marked atheromatous thickening. Three-dimensional navigation of the measurement plane to the leaflet tips using multiplane representation (*MPR*) of the 3D dataset provided an AVO area of 0.75 cm^2 compared to 1.32 cm^2 by 2D echocardiography. [→Video 8.14]

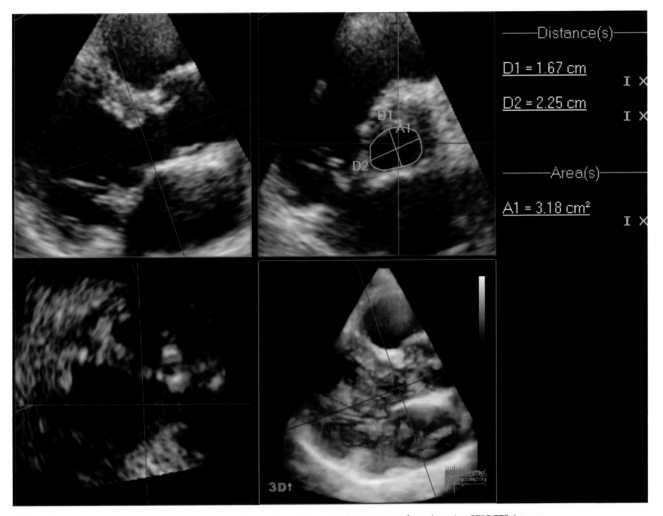

Distance(s)

D1 = 1.67 cm   I ×

D2 = 2.25 cm   I ×

Area(s)

A1 = 3.18 cm²   I ×

Fig. 8.15 Representation of noncircular cross-sectional area of the LVOT using 3D orientation of cut planes in a RT3D TTE dataset

Exact measurement of the aortic annulus is critical before transcatheter aortic valve implantation. Ng et al. [60] and other investigators [61][62]63] demonstrated direct planimetry of the aortic annular area by 3D TEE has better agreement with multislice computed tomography (gold standard method) than 2D measurements of the aortic annulus. A more detailed consideration of this aspect is provided in ► Chapter 12.

In addition, RT3DE has been demonstrated to provide superior estimation of AVA in patients with combined stenotic lesions in tandem, like supravalvular stenosis (SVAS) or subaortic stenosis (SAS) [64]. Moreover, RT3DE can provide unique 3D visualization of a subvalvular membrane in patients with subaortic stenosis permitting accurate measurement of the subvalvular stenotic area (◘ Fig. 8.16). RT3DE was also used to define congenitally severe aortic stenosis, and the results from RT3DE were compared with the valve morphology observed during surgery. The sites of fusion of the leaflets were correctly identified by RT3DE in all cases [65].

> RT3DE can provide unique 3D visualization of a subvalvular membrane permitting accurate measurement of subvalvular stenotic area.

8.3 Evaluation of tricuspid and pulmonary valve stenosis

Compared with the mitral and aortic valves, fewer studies have been published about the clinical application of 3D echocardiography in tricuspid or pulmonary valve disease. The 3D shape of the tricuspid annulus is complex and does not conform to a flat ring. It has been described as pear-shaped in the postmortem human heart [66]. The asymmetric shape of the right ventricle and the position in relation to the usual acoustic windows limit accurate assessment of tricuspid valve disease for conventional 2D echocardiographic assessments, especially the posterior leaflet. Unlike evaluation of mitral stenosis, short-axis 2D imaging of the tricuspid valve orifice is rarely feasible. Thus, it is not possible to visualize all three cusps simultaneously in one cross-sectional view. Nor is it possible to obtain detailed anatomical information of the tricuspid valve annulus, leaflets, and commissures in tricuspid valve disease leading to stenosis, like rheumatic carditis or carcinoid disease. However, in patients with good image quality 3D echocardiography overcomes this limitation of 2D echocardiography and provides a 3D en face view from the atrial and ventricular side to the tricuspid valve annulus and all three tri-

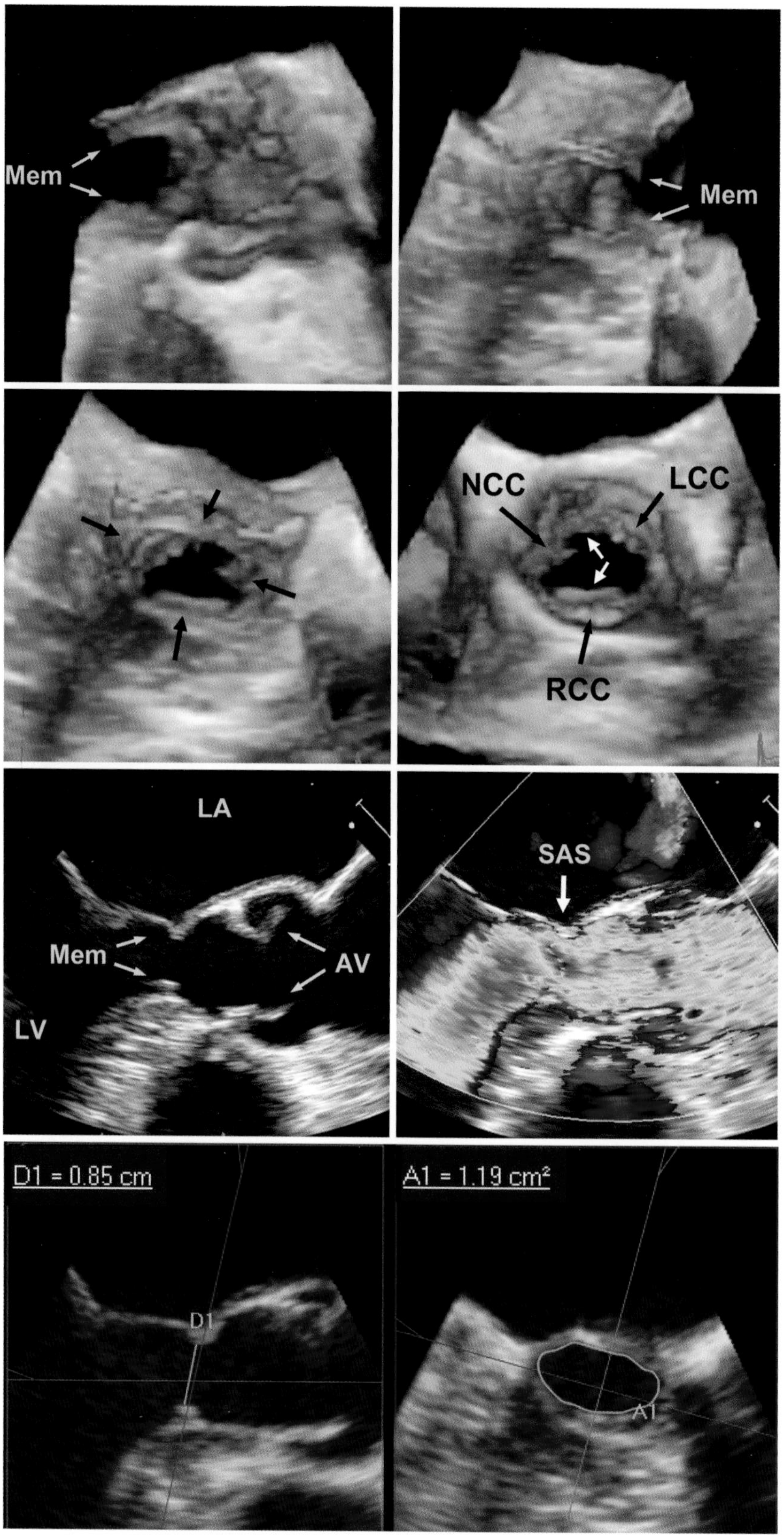

■ **Fig. 8.16** The RT3D TEE representation of membranous subaortic stenosis (*SAS*). The RT3DE tilted views from the aortic root to the SAS (*top left*) and from the left ventricular outflow tract (*LVOT*) to the SAS (*top right*) show a cross-section of the membrane (*Mem*), the SAS orifice, and its relation to the aortic valve. The RT3DE en face view from the LVOT to the SAS shows the circular membrane (*arrows; second row left*) and the en face surgeon's perspective reveals a view through the opened aortic valve cusps to the SAS membrane behind (*white arrows; second row right*). The 2D long-axis view depicts the SAS within the LVOT (*third row left*) and the beginning of flow turbulence due to the stenosis using color Doppler (*third row right*). Measurement within the 3D dataset yielded a SAS area of 1.19 cm² indicating moderate stenosis (*bottom*). *AV* aortic valve, *LV* left ventricle, *LA* left atrium, *RCC* right coronary cusp, *LCC* left coronary cusp, *NCC* noncoronary cusp. [→Videos 8.16A–D]

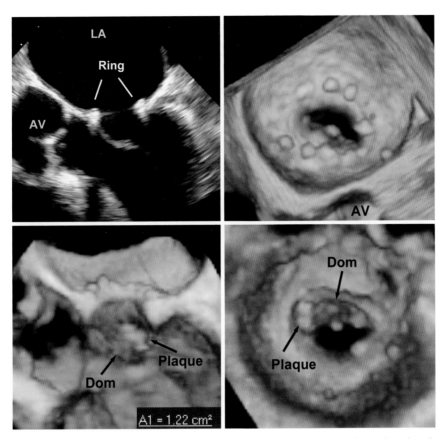

◻ **Fig. 8.17** Mitral stenosis after mitral valve reconstruction with ring implantation. The 2D TEE cross-section only reveals a relatively narrow ring diameter and restricted motion of the anterior mitral leaflet (*AML; top left*). The RT3DE en face surgeon's view shows a significantly smaller orifice compared to the ring size indicated by the knots, most likely due to degenerative thickening of tissue growth within the implanted ring (*top right*). In addition, the RT3DE long-axis view (*bottom left*) and the en face view from the left ventricle (*bottom right*) reveal a solid plaque with fusion of the AML to the postero-medial ring as a likely cause of AML doming (*Dom*). The 3D measurement provided a mitral valve opening area of 1.22 cm². *LA* left atrium, *AV* aortic valve. [→Videos 8.17A–D]

cuspid valve leaflets, which enables direct planimetry of tricuspid valve area [67][68][69]70].

Henein et al. [71] characterized the tricuspid apparatus in patients with rheumatic heart disease with mitral stenosis and severe tricuspid regurgitation using gated 3D TEE. They found thickened leaflets with restricted motion, together with annular dilatation. In addition, 3D echocardiography is particularly valuable in assessing patients with carcinoid disease, due to its ability to visualize simultaneously all three tricuspid valve leaflets and their chordal attachments from unique perspectives [72]. The valvular involvement consists of leaflet thickening with excessive fibrosis and markedly restricted motion. The fibrotic leaflets move in a stiff board-like fashion rather than the normal undulating motion, and their restricted opening leads to RV inflow obstruction. The tricuspid valve leaflets are usually retracted and held partially open during both systole and diastole, thus, resulting in a combined tricuspid stenosis and regurgitation, the latter being predominant [72]. However, RT3DE requires further validation studies before being used for clinical decision-making in tricuspid disease. The utility of RT3DE in the evaluation of pulmonary valve disease has been less explored. The visualization of pulmonary valve details with 3D echocardiography is limited, except when it is thickened or calcified. Kelly et al. [73] recently demonstrated the feasibility of live 3D echocardiography in the morphologic assessment of the pulmonary valve in para-

sternal short-axis view, providing incremental value in the RT3D TTE examination.

❯ RT3DE requires further validation studies before being used for clinical decision-making in tricuspid disease.

8.4 Evaluation of prosthetic and reconstructed valves

Entire views and the motions of prosthetic heart valves can also be well displayed by 3D echocardiography for anatomic detail and function (see ▶ Fig. 7.22, Fig. 7.23, Fig. 7.24 in ▶ Chapter 7). In addition, 3D echocardiography can be used to obtain accurate valve planimetry in bioprostheses. Mannaerts et al. [74] studied the feasibility of bioprosthetic orifice area measurement by reconstructive 3D TEE in patients with normally functioning valve prostheses in the mitral and aortic positions compared with Doppler methods. The orifice area obtained by 3D TEE correlated better than the orifice area obtained by Doppler compared with the orifice area indicated by the manufacturer. The orifice area by 3D echocardiography may also provide better insight into the extent and mechanisms of valvular obstruction in prosthetic and reconstructed valves (◻ Fig. 8.17 and ▶ Fig. 11.9 in ▶ Chapter 11) and may be useful to better differentiate pathologic obstruction from patient-

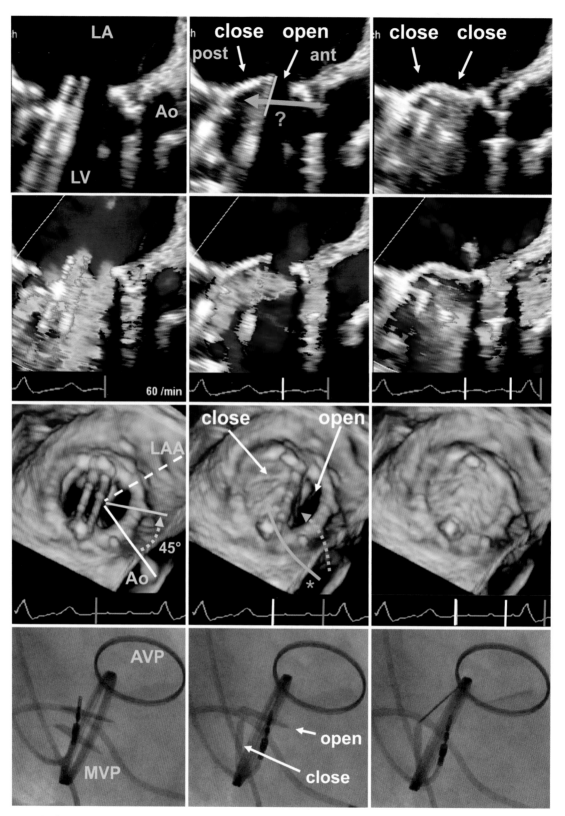

Fig. 8.18 Example of transesophageal RT3DE imaging in a case of asynchronous mitral valve prosthesis (*MVP*) leaflet closure with consequent prosthesis stenosis caused by eccentric paraprosthetic aortic regurgitation. *Top row* Transesophageal echocardiographic visualization of the asynchronous leaflet closure pattern of the MVP. After synchronous opening of both MVP leaflets in early diastole (*left*), the posterior leaflet (*post*) closes prematurely (*middle*), while the anterior leaflet (*ant*) stays open until end-diastole (*right*). *Second row* Color-Doppler imaging shows the eccentric paraprosthetic aortic regurgitation jet striking the posterior MVP leaflet (*middle*). RT3D TEE (*third row*) and fluoroscopic (*bottom row*) illustration of the asynchronous closing pattern of MVP leaflets. RT3DE images show the MVP in an en face perspective from the left atrium with a 45° rotation from an anatomic orientation (*left*) and the assumed streamlines of paraprosthetic aortic regurgitation flow striking the anterior and posterior leaflets (*middle*). *Ao* aorta, *LV* left ventricle, *LA* left atrium, *LAA* left atrial appendage, *AVP* aortic valve prosthesis

prosthesis mismatch. In a recent report, RT3D TEE imaging was demonstrated to be crucial for understanding in a case of stenosis of a mechanical mitral valve prosthesis caused by an eccentric paraprosthetic aortic regurgitation (◻ Fig. 8.18) [75].

Furthermore, 3D-TEE provides a unique anatomical imaging diagnostic capability for prosthetic valve thrombosis [76][77] and pannus overgrowth [78]. In addition, RT3D TEE has been shown to provide additional information in the evaluation of prosthetic valve endocarditis [79]. Sugeng et al. [10] studied the ability of RT3D TEE to preoperatively assess prosthetic valve pathology, including stenosis, comparing 3D image information with surgical findings. They found 96% agreement of RT3D TEE with surgical findings.

References

1. Iung B, Baron G, Butchart EG et al (2003) A prospective survey of patients with valvular heart disease in Europe: The Euro Heart Survey on Valvular Heart Disease. European Heart Journal 24:1231–1243

2. Akram MR, Chan T, McAuliffe S, Chenzbraun A (2009) Non-rheumatic annular mitral stenosis: prevalence and characteristics. Eur J Echocardiogr 10:103–105

3. Bonow RO, Carabello RA, Chatterjee K, et al (2006) ACC/AHA 2006 guidelines for the management of patients with valvular heart disease. J Am Coll Cardiol 48:e1–e148

4. Wilkins GT, Weyman EA, Abascal VM et al (1988) Percutaneous balloon dilatation of the mitral valve: an analysis of echocardiographic variables related to outcome and the mechanism of dilatation. Br Heart J 60:299–308

5. Messika-Zeitoun D, Brochet E, Holmin C et al (2007) Three-dimensional evaluation of the mitral valve area and commissural opening before and after percutaneous mitral commissurotomy in patients with mitral stenosis. Eur Heart J 28:72–79

6. Zamorano J, Cordeiro P, Sugeng L et al (2004) Real-time three-dimensional echocardiography for rheumatic mitral valve stenosis evaluation: an accurate and novel approach. J Am Coll Cardiol 2004; 43:2091–2096

7. Anwar AM, Attia WM, Nosir YF et al (2010) Validation of a new score for the assessment of mitral stenosis using real-time three-dimensional echocardiography. J Am Soc Echocardiogr 2010; 23:13–22

8. Soliman OI, Anwar AM, Metawei AK et al (2011) New scores for the assessment of mitral stenosis using real-time three-dimensional echocardiography. Curr Cardiovasc Imaging Rep 4:370–377

9. Salcedo EE, Quaife RA, Seres T, Carroll JD (2009) A framework for systematic characterization of the mitral valve by real-time three-dimensional transesophageal echocardiography. J Am Soc Echocardiogr 2009; 22:1087–1099

10. Sugeng L, Shernan SK, Weinert L et al (2008) Real-time three-dimensional transesophageal echocardiography in valve disease: comparison with surgical findings and evaluation of prosthetic valves. J Am Soc Echocardiogr 21:1347–1354

11. Vahanian A, Alfieri O, Andreotti F et al (2012) Guidelines on the management of valvular heart disease (version 2012). Eur Heart J 33:2451–2496

12. Krapf L, Dreyfus J, Cueff C et al (2013) Anatomical features of rheumatic and non-rheumatic mitral stenosis: Potential additional value of three-dimensional echocardiography. Arch Cardiovasc Dis 106:111–115

13. Hatle L, Angelsen B, Tromsdal A (1979) Noninvasive assessment of atrio-ventricular pressure half-time by Doppler ultrasound. Circulation 60:-1096–1104

14. Rodriguez L, Thomas JD, Monterroso V et al (1993) Validation of the proximal flow convergence method - calculation of orifice area in patients with mitral-stenosis. Circulation 88:1157–1165

15. Chen Q, Nosir YF, Vletter WB et al (1997) Accurate assessment of mitral valve area in patients with mitral stenosis by three-dimensional echocardiography. J Am Soc Echocardiogr 10:133–140

16. Kupferwasser I, Mohr-Kahaly S, Menzel T et al (1996) Quantification of mitral valve stenosis by three-dimensional transesophageal echocardiography. Int J Card Imaging 12:241–247

17. Lang RM, Badano LP, Tsang W et al (2012) EAE/ASE recommendations for image acquisition and display using three-dimensional echocardiography. Eur Heart J Cardiovasc Imaging 13:1–46

18. Zamorano J, Perez d, I, Sugeng L et al (2004) Non-invasive assessment of mitral valve area during percutaneous balloon mitral valvuloplasty: role of real-time 3D echocardiography. Eur Heart J 25:2086–2091

19. Binder TM, Rosenhek R, Porenta G et al (2000) Improved assessment of mitral valve stenosis by volumetric real-time three-dimensional echocardiography. J Am Coll Cardiol 36:1355–1261

20. Xie MX, Wang XF, Cheng TO et al (2005) Comparison of accuracy of mitral valve area in mitral stenosis by real-time, three-dimensional echocardiography versus two-dimensional echocardiography versus Doppler pressure half-time. Am J Cardiol 95:1496–1499

21. Sebag IA, Morgan JG, Handschumacher MD et al (2005) Usefulness of three-dimensionally guided assessment of mitral stenosis using matrix-array ultrasound. Am J Cardiol 96:1151–1156

22. Kasliwal RR, Trehan N, Mittal S (1996) A new '«gold standard» for the measurement of mitral valve area: Surgical Validation of Volume Rendered Three-Dimensional Echocardiography (abstr). Circulation 94:355

23. Perez d, I, Casanova C, Almeria C et al (2007) Which method should be the reference method to evaluate the severity of rheumatic mitral stenosis? Gorlin's method versus 3D-echo. Eur J Echocardiogr 8:470–473

24. Mannaerts HF, Kamp O, Visser CA (2004) Should mitral valve area assessment in patients with mitral stenosis be based on anatomical or on functional evaluation? A plea for 3D echocardiography as the new clinical standard. Eur Heart J 25:2073–2074

25. Limbu YR, Shen X, Pan C et al (1998) Assessment of mitral valve volume by quantitative three-dimensional echocardiography in patients with rheumatic mitral valve stenosis. Clin Cardiol 21:415–418

26. Langerveld J, Valocik G, Plokker HW et al (2003) Additional value of three-dimensional transesophageal echocardiography for patients with mitral valve stenosis undergoing balloon valvuloplasty. J Am Soc Echocardiogr 16:841–849

27. Valocik G, Kamp O, Mannaerts HF, Visser CA (2007) New quantitative three-dimensional echocardiographic indices of mitral valve stenosis: new 3D indices of mitral stenosis. Int J Cardiovasc Imaging 2007; 23:707–716

28. Dobarro D, Gomez-Rubin MC, Lopez-Fernandez T et al (2009) Real time three-dimensional transesophageal echocardiography for guiding percutaneous mitral valvuloplasty. Echocardiography 26:746–748

29. Shin JJ, Alfirevic A, Navia JL (2013) Complications of percutaneous mitral balloon valvotomy: usefulness of real-time 3-dimensional technology. J Cardiothorac Vasc Anesth 27:546–548

30. Eng MH, Salcedo EE, Quaife RA, Carroll JD (2009) Implementation of real time three-dimensional transesophageal echocardiography in percutaneous mitral balloon valvuloplasty and structural heart disease interventions. Echocardiography 26:958–966

31. Chu JW, Levine RA, Chua S et al (2008) Assessing mitral valve area and orifice geometry in calcific mitral stenosis: a new solution by real-time three-dimensional echocardiography. J Am Soc Echocardiogr 21:1006–1009

32. Janosi RA, Kahlert P, Plicht B et al (2009) Guidance of percutaneous transcatheter aortic valve implantation by real-time three-dimensional transesophageal echocardiography – A single-center experience. Minim Invasive Ther Allied Technol142–148

33. Danielsen R, Nordrehaug JE, Vik-Mo H (1989) Factors affecting Doppler echocardiographic valve area assessment in aortic stenosis. Am J Cardiol 63:1107–11

34. Rahimtoola SH (2000) Severe aortic stenosis with low systolic gradient:the good and bad news. Circulation 101:1892–4

35. Baumgartner H, Hung J, Bermejo J et al (2009) Echocardiographic assessment of valve stenosis: EAE/ASE recommendations for clinical practice. Eur J Echocardiogr 10:1–25

36. Bernard Y, Meneveau N, Vuillemenot A et al (1997) Planimetry of aortic valve area using multiplane transoesophageal echocardiography is not a reliable method for assessing severity of aortic stenosis. Heart 1997; 78:68–73

37. Gilon D, Cape EG, Handschumacher MD et al (2002) Effect of three-dimensional valve shape on the hemodynamics of aortic stenosis: Three-dimensional echocardiographic stereolithography and patient studies. Journal of the American College of Cardiology 40:1479–1486

38. Vengala S, Nanda NC, Dod HS et al (2004) Images in geriatric cardiology. Usefulness of live three-dimensional transthoracic echocardiography in aortic valve stenosis evaluation. Am J Geriatr Cardiol 13:279–284

39. Blot-Souletie N, Hebrard A, Acar P et al (2007) Comparison of accuracy of aortic valve area assessment in aortic stenosis by real time three-dimensional echocardiography in biplane mode versus two-dimensional transthoracic and transesophageal echocardiography. Echocardiography 24:1065–1072

40. Goland S, Trento A, Iida K et al (2007) Assessment of aortic stenosis by three-dimensional echocardiography: an accurate and novel approach. Heart 93:801–807

41. Nanda NC, Roychoudhury D, Chung SM et al (1994) Quantitative assessment of normal and stenotic aortic valve using transesophageal three-dimensional echocardiography. Echocardiography 11:617–625

42. Kasprzak JD, Salustri A, Roelandt JR et al (1998) Three-Dimensional Echocardiography of the Aortic Valve: Feasibility, Clinical Potential, and Limitations. Echocardiography 15:127–138

43. Ge S, Warner JG, Jr., Abraham TP et al (1998) Three-dimensional surface area of the aortic valve orifice by three-dimensional echocardiography: clinical validation of a novel index for assessment of aortic stenosis. Am Heart J 136:1042–50

44. Menzel T, Mohr-Kahaly S, Kolsch B et al (1997) Quantitative assessment of aortic stenosis by three-dimensional echocardiography. J Am Soc Echocardiogr 10:215–223

45. Handke M, Schafer DM, Heinrichs G et al (2002) Quantitative assessment of aortic stenosis by three-dimensional anyplane and three-dimensional volume-rendered echocardiography. Echocardiography 19:45–53

46. de la MG, Saura D, Oliva MJ et al (2010) Real-time three-dimensional transoesophageal echocardiography in the assessment of aortic valve stenosis. Eur J Echocardiogr 11:9–13

47. Nakai H, Takeuchi M, Yoshitani H et al (2010) Pitfalls of anatomical aortic valve area measurements using two-dimensional transoesophageal echocardiography and the potential of three-dimensional transoesophageal echocardiography. Eur J Echocardiogr 11:369–376

48. Bharucha T, Fernandes F, Slorach C et al (2012) Measurement of effective aortic valve area using three–dimensional echocardiography in children undergoing aortic balloon valvuloplasty for aortic stenosis. Echocardiography 29:484–491

49. Plicht B, Janosi RA, Kahlert P et al (2008)[Aortic valve with »calcified valvular stenosis«: precise clarification of morphology and severity using transesophageal three dimensional echocardiography]. Herz 33:315–316

50. Brantley HP, Nekkanti R, Anderson CA, Kypson AP (2012) Three-dimensional echocardiographic features of unicuspid aortic valve stenosis correlate with surgical findings. Echocardiography 29:E204–E207

51. Unsworth B, Malik I, Mikhail GW (2010) Recognising bicuspid aortic stenosis in patients referred for transcatheter aortic valve implantation: routine screening with three-dimensional transoesophageal echocardiography. Heart 96:645

52. Matsumoto K, Tanaka H, Hiraishi M et al (2011) A case of unicommissural unicuspid aortic valve stenosis diagnosed by real time three-dimensional transesophageal echocardiography. Echocardiography 28:E172–E173

53. Baumgartner H, Kratzer H, Helmreich G, Kuehn P (1990) Determination of aortic valve area by Doppler echocardiography using the continuity equation: a critical evaluation. Cardiology 77:101–111

54. Doddamani S, Bello R, Friedman MA et al (2007) Demonstration of left ventricular outflow tract eccentricity by real time 3D echocardiography: implications for the determination of aortic valve area. Echocardiography 24:860–866

55. Khaw AV, von Bardeleben RS, Strasser C et al (2009) Direct measurement of left ventricular outflow tract by transthoracic real-time 3D-echocardiography increases accuracy in assessment of aortic valve stenosis. Int J Cardiol 136:64–71

56. Perez d, I, Zamorano J, Perez de la YR et al (2008) [Quantification of aortic valve area using three-dimensional echocardiography]. Rev Esp Cardiol 61:494–500

57. Saitoh T, Shiota M, Izumo M et al (2012) Comparison of left ventricular outflow geometry and aortic valve area in patients with aortic stenosis by 2–dimensional versus 3-dimensional echocardiography. Am J Cardiol 109:1626–1631

58. Gutierrez-Chico JL, Zamorano JL, Prieto-Moriche E et al (2008) Real-time three-dimensional echocardiography in aortic stenosis: a novel, simple, and reliable method to improve accuracy in area calculation. Eur Heart J 9:1296–1306

59. Poh KK, Levine RA, Solis J et al (2008) Assessing aortic valve area in aortic stenosis by continuity equation: a novel approach using real-time three-dimensional echocardiography. Eur Heart J 29:2526–35

60. Ng AC, Delgado V, van der KF et al (2010) Comparison of aortic root dimensions and geometries before and after transcatheter aortic valve implantation by 2- and 3-dimensional transesophageal echocardiography and multislice computed tomography. Circ Cardiovasc Imaging 3:94–102

61. Messika-Zeitoun D, Serfaty JM, Brochet E et al (2012) Multimodal assessment of the aortic annulus diameter: implications for transcatheter aortic valve implantation. J Am Coll Cardiol 55:186–194

62. Shahgaldi K, da Silva C, Back M et al (2013) Transesophageal echocardiography measurements of aortic annulus diameter using biplane mode in patients undergoing transcatheter aortic valve implantation. Cardiovasc Ultrasound 11:5

63. Calleja A, Thavendiranathan P, Ionasec RI, et al (2013) Automated quantitative 3-dimensional modeling of the aortic valve and root by 3-dimensional transesophageal echocardiography in normals, aortic regurgitation, and aortic stenosis: comparison to computed tomography in normals and clinical implications. Circ Cardiovasc Imaging 6:99–108

64. Rajdev S, Nanda NC, Patel V et al (2006) Live/real-time three-dimensional transthoracic echocardiographic assessment of combined valvar and supravalvar aortic stenosis. Am J Geriatr Cardiol 15:188–190

65. Sadagopan SN, Veldtman GR, Sivaprakasam MC et al (2006) Correlations with operative anatomy of real time three-dimensional echocardiographic imaging of congenital aortic valvar stenosis. Cardiol Young 16:490–494

66. Deloche A, Guerinon J, Fabiani JN et al (1973) [Anatomical study of rheumatic tricuspid valve diseases: Application to the study of various valvuloplasties]. Ann Chir Thorac Cardiovasc 12:343–349

67. Faletra F, La MU, Bragato R, De Chiara F (2005) Three dimensional transthoracic echocardiography images of tricuspid stenosis. Heart 2005; 91:499

68. Pothineni KR, Duncan K, Yelamanchili P et al (2007) Live/real time three-dimensional transthoracic echocardiographic assessment of tricuspid valve pathology: incremental value over the two-dimensional technique. Echocardiography 24:541–552

69. Anwar AM, Geleijnse ML, Soliman OI et al (2007) Evaluation of rheumatic tricuspid valve stenosis by real-time three-dimensional echocardiography. Heart 93:363–364

70. Badano LP, Agricola E, Perez d et al (2009) Evaluation of the tricuspid valve morphology and function by transthoracic real-time three-dimensional echocardiography. Eur J Echocardiogr 10:477–484

71. Henein MY, O'Sullivan CA, Li W et al (2003) Evidence for rheumatic valve disease in patients with severe tricuspid regurgitation long after mitral valve surgery: the role of 3D echo reconstruction. J Heart Valve Dis 12:566–572

72. Bhattacharyya S, Toumpanakis C, Burke M et al (2010) Features of carcinoid heart disease identified by 2- and 3-dimensional echocardiography and cardiac MRI. Circ Cardiovasc Imaging 3:103–11

73. Kelly NF, Platts DG, Burstow DJ (2010) Feasibility of pulmonary valve imaging using three-dimensional transthoracic echocardiography. J Am Soc Echocardiogr 23:1076–1080

References

74. Mannaerts H, Li Y, Kamp O et al (2001) Quantitative assessment of mechanical prosthetic valve area by 3-dimensional transesophageal echocardiography. J Am Soc Echocardiogr 14:723–731

75. Buck T, Plicht B, Kahlert P et al (2013) Stenosis of a mechanical mitral valve prosthesis by eccentric paraprosthetic aortic regurgitation. JACC Cardiovasc Imaging 6:278–280

76. Faletra FF, Moschovitis G, Auricchio A (2009) Visualisation of thrombus formation on prosthetic valve by real-time three-dimensional trans-oesophageal echocardiography. Heart 95:482

77. Paul B, Minocha A (2010) Thrombosis of a bileaflet prosthetic mitral valve: a real-time three-dimensional transesophageal echocardiography perspective. Int J Cardiovasc Imaging 26:367–368

78. Ozkan M, Gunduz S, Yildiz M, Duran NE (2010) Diagnosis of the prosthetic heart valve pannus formation with real-time three-dimensional trans-oesophageal echocardiography. Eur J Echocardiogr 11:E17

79. Kort S (2006) Real-time 3-dimensional echocardiography for prosthetic valve endocarditis: initial experience. J Am Soc Echocardiogr 19:130–139

Congenital heart disease in adults

Folkert J. Meijboom, Heleen van der Zwaan, Jackie McGhie

T. Buck et al. (Hrsg.), *Three-dimensional Echocardiography*,
DOI 10.1007/978-3-642-36799-1_9, © Springer-Verlag Berlin Heidelberg 2014

Due to the success of cardiac surgery in infancy and childhood, starting some 40 years ago and improving ever since, the survival for patients with congenital heart disease has improved dramatically. Over 85% of all patients born with a congenital cardiac defect now survive beyond childhood, often well into adult life. Many of these patients have residual abnormalities, which may be morphological, functional or (most often) both, and these residua tend to change with time. As an example, the patient with repaired tetralogy of Fallot will require long-term monitoring of problems such as pulmonary regurgitation with consequent volume loading of the right ventricle, ventricular dysfunction, and associated arrhythmias. Patients with repaired coarctation will require monitoring of associated lesions, such as bicuspid aortic valve, aortic valve stenosis/regurgitation, recurrent aortic arch obstruction, and systemic arterial blood pressure. The result is that the vast majority of patients, who had their congenital cardiac malformation »repaired« or »corrected« at a young age, require follow-up throughout childhood and adult life. Imaging plays a major role in this follow-up. In current clinical practice, more than 90% of the imaging involves echocardiography.

> ❯ **Even experienced echocardiographers are often challenged by the spatial interpretation of complex congenital cardiac malformations.**

Echocardiography of congenital heart disease is often considered to be one of the most difficult aspects of the technique. The examination should be performed by cardiologists, pediatric cardiologists, or sonographers with great expertise and skill in this specific domain. Most of these professionals are content with two-dimensional (2D) echocardiography and are confident that they can image and evaluate even the most complex congenital cardiac malformation. However, even experienced operators are often challenged by the spatial interpretation of complex congenital cardiac malformations.

This is where three-dimensional (3D) imaging comes in as a very helpful technique: it can show the anatomy of the heart as it is, in its real 3D nature. Even if 3D imaging is broadly accessible and its understanding is more intuitive to a wider audience, ranging from medical students to electrophysiologists and cardiac surgeons, RT3DE scanning of congenital malformations is demanding and should remain in the hands of the more experienced subspecialized echocardiographers. Current 3D platforms have lower spatial and temporal resolution compared with 2D echocardiography, but the added dimension enhances the understanding of congenital heart defects. Unique projections, such as en face views of intracardiac structures, including not only the semilunar and atrioventricular valves but also the interatrial and interventricular septums, can be created using 3D echocardiograms.

> ❯ **Even if the understanding of 3D images is more intuitive to a wider audience, RT3DE scanning of congenital malformations is demanding and should remain in the hands of the more experienced echocardiographers.**

Another very useful feature of 3D echocardiography is the possibility to image the entire heart in one full volume dataset (► Chapter 2) [1]. Off-line analysis allows cross-sections through the heart in any desired plane. For beginners in 3D analysis, it is very useful to start with the preprogrammed orthogonal cross-sections, giving rise to 2D planes that are perpendicular to each other: sagittal (left–right), coronal (superior–inferior), and transverse (anterior–posterior) orientation (see ► Fig. 2.23). In most current 3D analysis systems, like Philips Qlab and in the Tomtec Cardio View, these three planes can be shown in the multiplane representation (MPR) view (► Chapter 2), together with a fourth image, in which these planes are shown in a 3D rendered view (◻ Fig. 9.1).

Apart from these three cross-sectional planes which can be moved and rotated in any direction, the anyplane mode allows cropping of the 3D image in any orientation or direction (◻ Fig. 9.2). It is no longer necessary to memorize or to mentally reconstruct the transducer position that was necessary to create the cross-section: this can be displayed visually.

Beside the advantage that multiple 2D cross-sections can be shown (and understood!) simultaneously in the 3D anatomy, the 3D hologram that can be produced (on the flat screen of the computer) allows visualization of the actual anatomy in its true 3D sense. For complex anatomy in particular, both the multiple 2D cross-sections visible in the 3D anatomy and the rendered 3D images have proven to be very useful to both expert users of 2D echocardiography as well as those having less experience.

In current practice, real-time 3D echocardiography (RT3DE) has become an integral part of the analysis of congenital heart disease in many labs. If, in the future, 3D could match 2D echocardiography in terms of spatial and temporal resolution (which is a matter of increased computing performance and intelligent signal processing (► Chapter 1), then the role of 3D echocardiography is likely to increase further and the complementary nature of the techniques would be enhanced.

> ❯ **In current practice, real-time 3D echocardiography has become an integral part of the analysis of congenital heart disease in many labs.**

Dedicated high-frequency pediatric probes (► Chapter 2) are mandatory for transthoracic 3D echocardiographic studies in pediatric patients, providing excellent results with image resolution good enough to visualize even very thin and delicate intracardiac structures. High-frequency 3D transducers (2–7 MHz) lack acoustic power and are not suitable for larger adult patients with a congenital cardiac malformation. The image resolution of the transthoracic adult 3D transducer, with a lower frequency of 1–5 MHz (X5-1 Philips), is certainly adequate for left ventricular (LV) volume calculations. In congenital heart disease practice, reliable assessment of LV function by RT3DE is important. The 2D analysis of LV function depends on assumptions about LV geometry, which are not reliable in the often deformed LV in patients with congenital heart disease. Some have reported excellent correlation between RT3DE-derived LV volumes, ejection fraction, and stroke volume with magnetic resonance imaging (MRI)-derived volumes [2][3][4][5].

Reliable measurement of right ventricular (RV) volumes and function would be of great help, since the RV plays a more important role in congenital heart disease than in general cardiology. The last section of this chapter will elaborate on RV

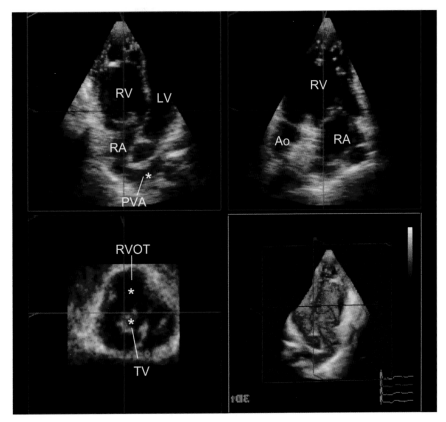

■ **Fig. 9.1** Example of multiplane representation (*MPR*) of three orthogonal cross-sectional planes from a full volume 3D dataset in a patient with transposition of the great arteries after a Mustard-type atrial switch. *RV* right ventricle, *LV* left ventricle, *RA* right atrium, *PVA* pulmonary venous atrium, *RVOT* right ventricular outflow tract, *Ao* aorta, *TV* tricuspid valve [→Video 9.1]

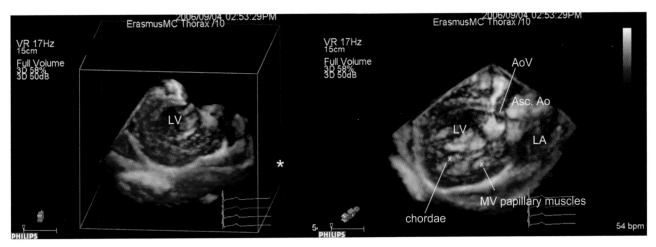

■ **Fig. 9.2** Example of cropping. *Left* The anyplane – *purple* and marked with an asterisk (*) – as seen in the crop box. *Right* The cross section that is made with this anyplane and the view into the heart from this anyplane is shown. *LV* left ventricle, *LA* left atrium, *Asc Ao* ascending aorta, *AoV* aortic valve, *MV* mitral valve

analysis with 3D echocardiography. Application of transthoracic RT3DE for analysis of intracardiac morphology produces less spectacular images in adults than in the pediatric population due to the limited spatial resolution of the low-frequency transducers. Despite this limitation, it provides important additional information that cannot be obtained with 2D imaging, justifying its use to supplement 2D echocardiographic analysis [6][7]. However, in all cases where a more detailed morphologic assessment is required a transesophageal RT3DE examination can be performed providing high quality 3D imaging.

Because of the enormous diversity of congenital heart disease (e.g., both unrepaired and repaired, with many different surgical techniques, creating different sequelae and residua) in adult patients, it is impossible to give a complete overview of the possibilities and added value of 3D echocardiography for all diagnostic categories. Moreover, many of the common congenital anomalies will be dealt with in the pediatric cardiology chapter (► Chapter 10). Instead, illustrative examples of congenital abnormalities that are common in adults are described in the following section with emphasis on the added value of 3D echocardiography in these cases.

9.1   Patent foramen ovale

A patent foramen ovale (PFO) is present in approximately one third of the population and, therefore, is not considered as a congenital cardiac anomaly. Increasingly, it has become the focus of medical attention since transient ischemic attacks (TIAs), cerebral vascular accidents (CVAs), and migraine have been attributed to paradoxical embolization through a foramen ovale. The role of RT3DE is limited, since functional assessment, demonstration of right-to-left shunting through the foramen using echo contrast, is the essence of the diagnosis. However, as described in ► Chapter 11, the RT3D TEE en face view from the left atrium (LA) to the interatrial septum can be useful to detect the exact location of the shunt orifice. In selected cases (e.g., if an atrial septal aneurysm is present), RT3DE may contribute to assessing the exact anatomy of the interatrial septum and the extent of the fossa ovalis membranous aneurysm.

9.2   Atrial septal defect

The nomenclature of atrial septal defects (ASD) has gradually changed over the past few decades. It used to be customary to differentiate between a primum and secundum type ASD, which is no longer done. The term primum ASD is considered obsolete and is classified as a partial atrioventricular septal defect (pAVSD) and is discussed always as such, because of the abnormality of the atrioventricular valves inherent to a partial AVSD. This section deals with secundum type ASD and sinus venosus defects.

The exact size and shape of ASDs and their exact position within the interatrial septum have become more important since transcatheter closure of ASDs has developed into a serious alternative to surgical closure [8]. Not all defects are amenable for transcatheter closure: they should not be too large, the rims

should be sufficient to provide good anchoring of the device, and the defects should not be too close to important intracardiac structures (e.g., the mitral and tricuspid valves or orifices of veins that drain into the left or right atrium). In children, transthoracic 2D echocardiography is often diagnostic because, in contrast to adult patients, the subcostal view can virtually always be used and it is this view that provides the most information. Without this view, 2D transesophageal echocardiography (TEE) is often indicated to identify all rims and the relation of the defect to relevant structures. The optimal 3D dataset is acquired from the subcostal position, but this is rarely feasible in adults. A foreshortened 4-chamber position or a parasternal long-axis view angulated to the right, with the ASD between the dotted lines and not further than 15 cm away from the transducer is next best option (◘ Fig. 9.3).

The added value that RT3DE has for analysis of an ASD is the possibility to create an en face view of the interatrial septum [9][10][11]. The entire interatrial septum can be seen with the defect within it. It can be viewed and measured both from the left and right atrial side (◘ Fig. 9.4, ◘ Fig. 9.5, ◘ Fig. 9.6).

The rims around the defect can be seen in one view. From the right-sided view, distances to important anatomical landmarks (e.g., the tricuspid valve, the ostium of the coronary sinus, and the ostia of the caval veins) can be measured. Mathewson et al. [12] proposed a standardized orientation and nomenclature for the rims (◘ Fig. 9.5).

Something that is difficult to appreciate with 2D echocardiography – the change of the size of the ASD during the cardiac cycle – is easy to see in the en face view using RT3DE [13]. The area of the defect is largest during atrial relaxation and is smallest during atrial contraction. During atrial contraction, the area was reported to be >50% smaller than during atrial relaxation [9][14]. This implies that the choice for the size of a closure device should be based on the measurement during atrial relaxation, when the ASD is at its largest.

In patients who have sufficient transthoracic echocardiographic (TTE) image quality, a RT3DE study might provide all the answers to the questions about feasibility of transcatheter closure and a TEE might be omitted [8][15]. However, besides RT3D TTE with all its additive information, RT3D TEE provides far more detailed information about spatial relationships of atrial septal defects and surrounding structures (◘ Fig. 9.5, ◘ Fig. 9.6, ◘ Fig. 9.7, ◘ Fig. 9.8) as well as much higher spatial resolution for more accurate quantification of ASD size (◘ Fig. 9.7, ◘ Fig. 9.9).

> ◗ RT3DE provides detailed information about spatial relationships of atrial septal defects and surrounding structures as well as high spatial resolution for accurate quantification of ASD size.

Because of the above stated additional information that 3D echocardiography provides, we believe that RT3DE should be included in all echocardiographic work-ups of ASDs, in addition to the standard modalities, especially when transcatheter closure is considered. RT3D TEE, apart from offering additional diagnostic accuracy because of its superior image resolution when compared to RT3D TTE, can be used as guidance for device closure of the defect [16][17] as covered in detail in ► Chapter 12.

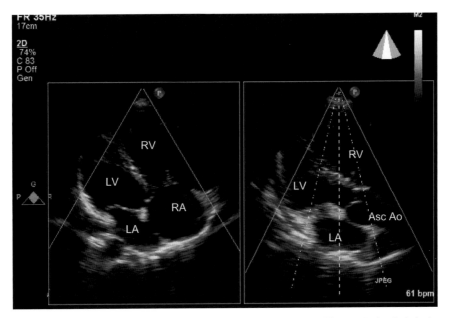

■ **Fig. 9.3** *Left* Foreshortened 4-chamber view. *Right* The dotted lines represent the subvolumes that will be acquired and stitched together to construct a full volume 3D dataset. *RV* right ventricle, *LV* left ventricle, *RA* right atrium, *LA* left atrium, *RVOT* right ventricular outflow tract, *Asc Ao* ascending aorta. [→Video 9.3]

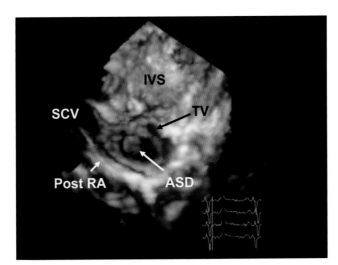

■ **Fig. 9.4** The right lateral view onto the interatrial septum reveals a large, centrally located ASD II with adequate rims around the defect. The patient is probably a good candidate for transcatheter closure. *SCV* superior vena cava, *IVS* interventricular septum, *TV* tricuspid valve, *ASD* atrial septal defect, *Post RA* posterior right atrial wall. [→Video 9.4]

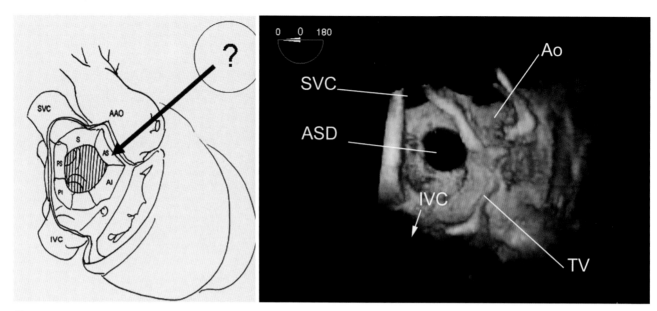

◘ Fig. 9.5 Right atrial view as proposed by Mathewson et al. [5]. *Left* In the schematic drawing, all rims can be identified, except the anterior–superior rim, indicated by the question mark. It is not possible to differentiate between the real anterior–superior rim and the wall of the aortic sinus. Source [5]; Copyright Elsevier. *Right* For comparison, the RT3DE image of the right atrial view is shown. *SVC* superior vena cava, *AAO* ascending aorta, *IVC* inferior vena cava, *ASD* atrial septal defect, *Ao* aorta, *TV* tricuspid valve. [→Video 9.5]

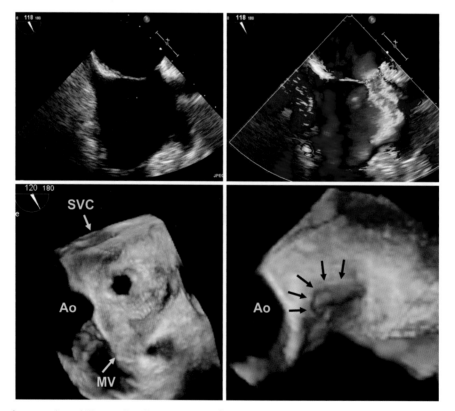

◘ Fig. 9.6 Comparison of transesophageal 2D versus live 3D representation of an ostium secundum ASD with a small rim towards the aortic wall (anterior-superior). The 3D en face view from the left atrium towards the interatrial septum (*IAS*) shows the exact shape and size of the defect and its anterior-superior location in the IAS (*bottom left*). The zoomed 3D representation allows exact detection of the extent and width of the anterior–superior rim and its relation to the aortic wall (*bottom right*). *SVC* superior vena cava, *Ao* aortic root, *MV* mitral valve. [→Videos 9.6A–D]

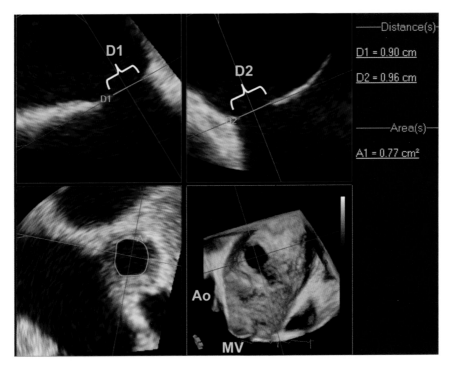

Fig. 9.7 The 3D measurement of atrial septal defect (*ASD*) diameters and area in the same case as shown in ◘ Fig. 9.6. *Ao* aortic root, *MV* mitral valve

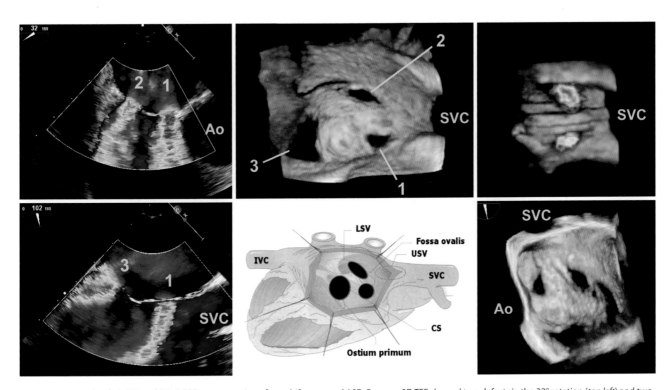

Fig. 9.8 Example of 2D TEE and RT3D TEE representation of a multifenestrated ASD. Because 2D TEE showed two defects in the 32° rotation (*top left*) and two defects in the 102° rotation (*bottom left*), there had to be at least three defects that could not be visualized in one 2D image plane. The RT3DE en face view from the right atrium (*top middle*) and from the left atrium to the interatrial septum (*IAS*) (*bottom right*) clearly visualized the orientation of the three defects to each other as well as the location within the IAS and the spatial relation to surrounding cardiac structures. RT3D color Doppler en face view from the right atrium clearly identifies the flow passing through the three defects (top right). Defect 1 (*1*) is located anterior–superior, defect 2 (*2*) posterior–superior, and defect 3 (*3*) anterior–inferior. The RT3DE en face view from the right atrium to the IAS shows the location of the three defects on a nonplanar, domed IAS which makes 2D representation and planimetry of each defect very difficult (*top middle*). *Ao* aortic root, *SVC* superior vena cava, *IVC* inferior vena cava, *LSV* lower sinus venosus, *UVS* upper sinus venosus, *CS* coronary sinus. [→Videos 9.8A–E]

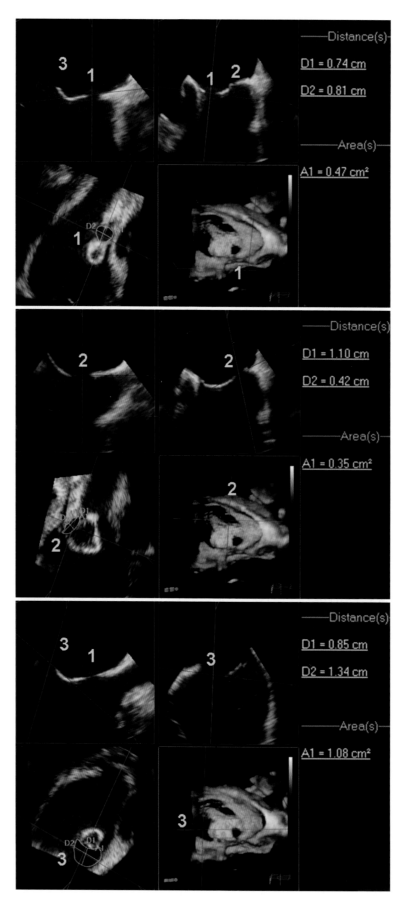

Fig. 9.9 The 3D measurement of each of the three ASDs demonstrated in ◘ Fig. 9.8 is shown. Note that the spatial orientation of the three cross-sectional planes must be individually adjusted for each defect

9.3   Ventricular septal defect

The interventricular septum (IVS) has a complex, curved shape which cannot be visualized in its entirety in a single 2D plane. It is again the en face view of the IVS that brings added value by showing its curved structure, the ventricular septal defect (VSD) within it, and the relation to other intracardiac structures. The spatial relationship of the VSD to other parts of the intracardiac anatomy can directly be assessed during data acquisition or offline in one 3D dataset [18][19][20][21].

Transthoracic datasets are acquired from the apical 4-chamber position and from the parasternal long-axis view. The subcostal view is very rewarding, but can be challenging to obtain in adult patients. In the chapter about 3D echocardiography in congenital heart disease in the pediatric population (▶ Chapter 10), more can be read about 3D analysis of VSDs.

During cropping of the 3D dataset, the images from the left ventricle onto the IVS and the VSD are easier to obtain than the images from the right side of the IVS. From the left side, the defect is directly visible, showing its exact location, size, and relation to landmark structures like the mitral and aortic valves (◘ Fig. 9.10, ◘ Fig. 9.11). The problem with the view from the right side of the heart for the most common form of the VSD, the perimembranous VSD, is the fact that the right side of the VSD is partially (if not entirely) covered by the septal leaflet of the tricuspid valve, its chordae, and papillary muscles. Only by digitally »cutting away« these structures that obscure the view can the VSD be visualized in a 3D fashion from the right side. In addition, muscular VSDs are usually better seen from the left side of the heart where the IVS has a rather smooth wall, than from the right side of the heart. The many, coarse trabeculation on the right side of the IVS can obscure the defect (◘ Fig. 9.12 and ◘ Fig. 9.13). If the 3D en face view from the right side of the IVS does not provide the desired information, scrolling of a 2D cutting plane from right to left (and vice versa) through the IVS might be helpful to find the delineation of the borders of the VSD.

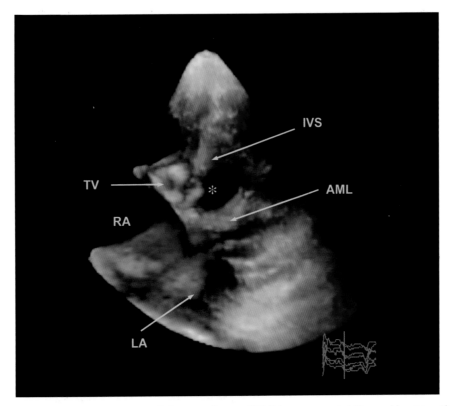

◘ **Fig. 9.10** Example of transthoracic RT3DE representation of a large membranous VSD (*) in a non-operated 61-year-old woman with Eisenmenger's syndrome and severe right heart dilatation. *TV* tricuspid valve, *RA* right atrium, *IVS* interventricular septum, *AML* anterior mitral leaflet, *LA* left atrium. [→Video 9.10]

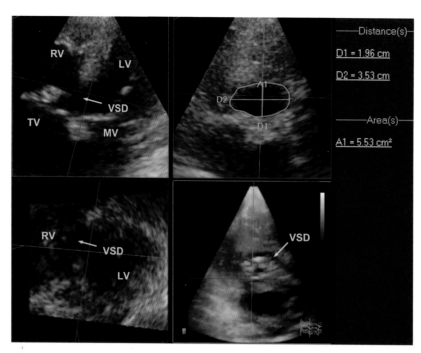

▣ Fig. 9.11 Representation of the same ventricular septal defect (*VSD*) shown in ▣ Fig. 9.10 in three cross-sectional planes, allowing exact detection of the VSD and measurement of diameters and area. The RT3DE en face view from the left ventricle (*LV*) to the interventricular septum (*IVS*) shows the exact size, shape, and location of the VSD as well as a view through the VSD to the tricuspid valve (*TV*) behind it. *RV* right ventricle, *MV* mitral valve

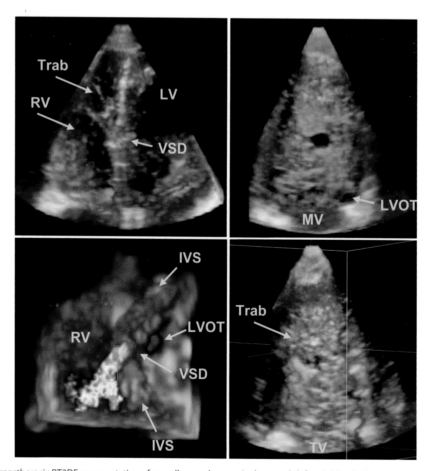

▣ Fig. 9.12 Example of transthoracic RT3DE representation of a small muscular ventricular septal defect (*VSD*) which is covered by marked trabeculation (*Trab*) on the right ventricular side of the interventricular septum (*IVS; top left*). The 3D en face view from the left ventricle (*LV*) to the IVS provides clear visualization of size, shape, and location of the VSD (*top right*), whereas the en face view from the right ventricle (*RV*) to the VSD is obscured by the trabeculation (*bottom right*). The 3D color Doppler short-axis view from the apex to the IVS shows the eccentric direction of shunt flow through the VSD (*bottom left*). *LVOT* left ventricular outflow tract, *MV* mitral valve, *TV* tricuspid valve. [→Videos 9.12A–D]

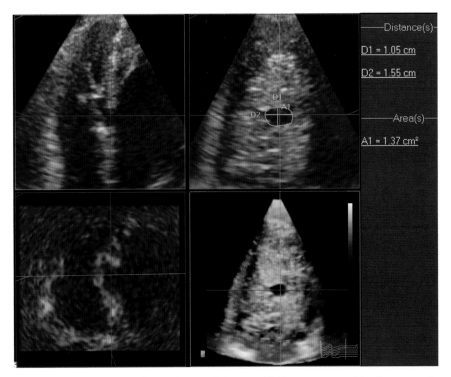

Fig. 9.13 Multiplane representation of the same muscular VSD shown in ◻ Fig. 9.12 with 3D measurement of the diameters and area

9.4 Atrioventricular septal defects

RT3DE analysis of an atrioventricular septal defect (AVSD) is extremely rewarding [22][23][24][25]. In the pediatric cardiology chapter (► Chapter 10), some illustrative examples are shown. Adult patients with an AVSD can have a defect repaired in childhood or an unrepaired form of AVSD. Patients with an AVSD, repaired or unrepaired, either complete or incomplete, invariably have abnormalities at the level of the atrioventricular valves: the essence of an AVSD is that it has a common atrioventricular junction, guarded by five leaflets [right mural leaflet, anterior–superior leaflet, superior (or anterior) bridging leaflet, left mural leaflet, and inferior (or posterior) bridging leaflet]. In the complete form, there is only one orifice between atria and ventricles (◻ Fig. 9.14, ◻ Fig. 9.15, ◻ Fig. 9.17). The septal defect of an AVSD is one large defect, extending both into the interatrial and into the interventricular septum, and should not be confused with separate atrial and ventricular septal defects that happen to be adjacent. This can occur in the presence of normal atrioventricular valves, but the anatomy is completely different from an AVSD. In partial or incomplete AVSD, there is fusion of the anterior and posterior bridging leaflet in the midline, where these two leaflets are also attached to the intact interventricular septum (◻ Fig. 9.17). This creates a separate left and right valve opening, in what is anatomically still one common atrioventricular junction. An incomplete AVSD or a surgically repaired complete AVSD has two atrioventricular orifices, but these should not be confused with the mitral and tricuspid valves. The entirely different anatomy is difficult to appreciate with 2D echocardiography, but is unmistakable with the en face view of the valves that is only possible with 3D echocardiography. The en face view from the ventricular side is usually of a better quality than the view from the atrial side. This is unfortunate, since a good surgical view can rarely be produced with adequate image quality. RT3D TEE is able to provide these images (◻ Fig. 9.14, ◻ Fig. 9.17). As described in the pediatric cardiology chapter (► Chapter 10), the size and shape of the septal defects can be depicted in an excellent manner with transthoracic 3D echocardiography.

> ❯ The entirely different anatomy of atrioventricular orifices in AVSD is difficult to appreciate with 2D echocardiography, but is unmistakable with a 3D en face view.

In patients with AVSD, a septal commissure can be erroneously described as a »cleft« (◻ Fig. 9.15). However, several characteristic differences between the two exist. In AVSD, the clues are
- characteristic interatrial communication,
- a common atrioventricular junction,
- no differential insertion of AV valves,
- the line of apposition between the superior and inferior bridging leaflets points to the ventricular septum, and
- the mural leaflet of the left AV valve is typically small and relatively triangular in shape.

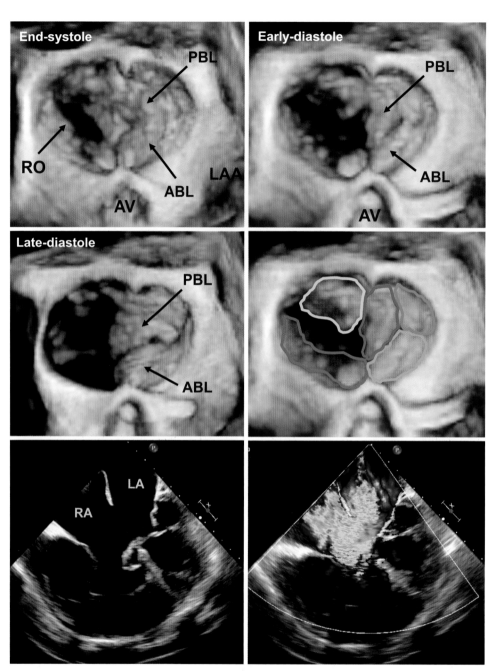

◘ Fig. 9.14 Example of a complete AVSD shown by a transesophageal live 3D acquisition. The 3D en face view clearly depicts a single valve. The 3D dataset is cropped to the valve level so no parts of the atrial septum are visible. *Upper left* A mid-systolic frame with the valve closed is presented but shows a large regurgitant orifice (*RO*). *Upper right* The valve in an early diastolic frame with the leaflets starting to open is shown. *Middle right* Clearly, different leaflets can be identified, with right mural leaflet (*yellow*), anterior–superior leaflet (*purple*), anterior bridging leaflet (*turquoise*), left mural leaflet (*green*), and posterior bridging leaflet (*red*). The posterior (*PBL*) and anterior bridging leaflet (*ABL*) are presented most prominent in a late-diastolic frame (*middle left*). *Bottom* Shown is the complex anatomy in the standard 2D view with color Doppler representation of severe regurgitation on the *right*. A large atrial septal defect is presented in the videos. *AV* aortic valve, *LAA* left atrial appendage, *RA* right atrium, *LA* left atrium. [→Videos 9.14A(a-d),B,C]

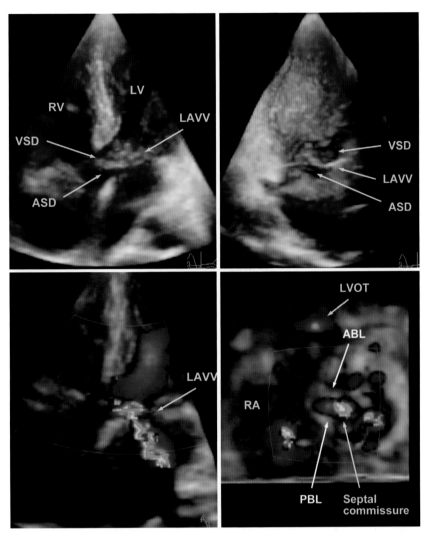

◘ **Fig. 9.15** Example of a complete AVSD in a 46-year-old woman. The septal commissure, often (but actually erroneously) referred to as »cleft« in the left atrioventricular valve (*LAVV*) is indicated with an arrow. *Top right* The 3D en face view from left ventricle (*LV*) to the interventricular septum (*IVS*) clearly shows the atrial side of the AVSD below the LAVV and the ventricular side of the AVSD above the LAVV. *Bottom left* The 3D color Doppler 4-chamber view illustrating the regurgitant jet through the septal commissure in a typical location. *Bottom right* The 3D color Doppler short-axis en face view from the apex to the base shows the LAVV with a posterior bridging leaflet (*PBL*), an anterior bridging leaflet (*ABL*) and a septal commissure pointing to the ventricular septum. *RV* right ventricle, *RA* right atrium, *ASD* atrial septal defect, *VSD* ventricular septal defect, *LVOT* left ventricular outflow tract. [→Videos 9.15A–D]

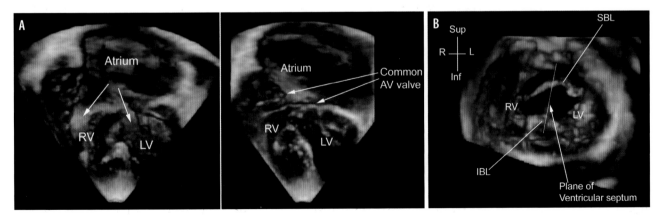

◘ **Fig. 9.16** **A** Complete atrioventricular septal defect with a common atrium in an 11-year-old patient. *Left* The common atrioventricular valve is shown in an open position with the left and right ventricular components (*arrows*). *Right* The 4-chamber view demonstrates the common atrioventricular (*AV*) valve in the closed position. There is no differential insertion of left and right ventricular components. **B** The en face view of the common atrioventricular junction from the ventricular aspect of the common atrioventricular valve is shown. The superior bridging leaflet (*SBL*) and inferior bridging leaflet (*IBL*) are indicated. These leaflets »bridge« across the plane of the ventricular septum (marked by the line). *LV* left ventricle, *RV* right ventricle, *L* left, *R* right, *Sup* superior, *Inf* inferior. [→Videos 9.16A,B]

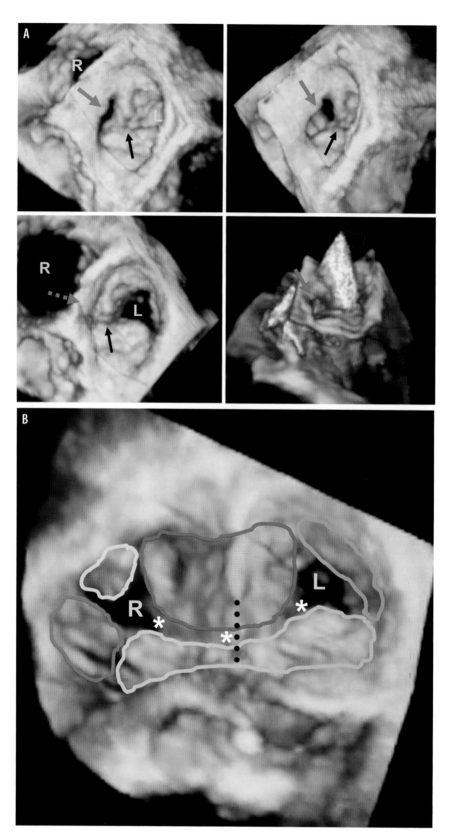

⬚ **Fig. 9.17 A** Example of transesophageal RT3DE full volume representation of an incomplete AVSD in a 70-year-old man. The upper left RT3DE perspective shows an en face view to a cleft-like connection (*black arrow*) from the left valve opening (*L*) to the atrial septal defect (*red arrow*). Tilted to the right, the *upper right* perspective shows a direct view to the atrial septal defect (*red arrow*) and tilted to the left, the *lower left* perspective shows an en face view to the left atrioventricular valve. *Lower right* Shown is severe regurgitation through the insufficient left atrioventricular valve. **B** The transesophageal RT3DE dataset cropped to the level of the atrial septal defect (*black dotted line*) provides an en face view to the entire atrioventricular valve with an anterior bridging leaflet (*turquoise*), a posterior bridging leaflet (*red*), with a septal commissure in between (*three white asterisks*), and on further left leaflet (*green*) and two further right leaflets (*yellow, purple*)

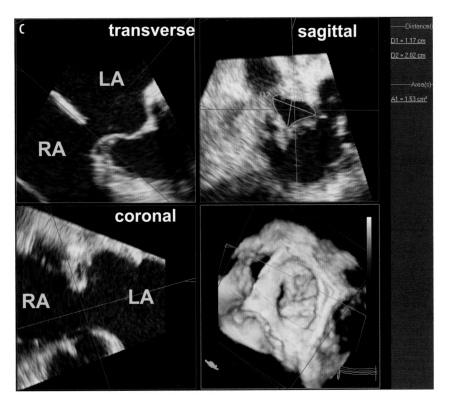

Fig. 9.17 (continued) **C** Multiplanar representation of the transesophageal RT3DE dataset with a transverse plane showing the atrial septal defect between left (*LA*) and right atrium (*RA*) (*upper left*), a sagittal plane showing the size and planimetry of the atrial septal defect (*upper right*), and a coronal plane through the atrial septal defect (*lower left*). *R* right valve opening. [→Videos 9.17A(a-d),B]

Whereas in a real cleft mitral valve (Fig. 9.18), characteristic clues include the following:

- the cleft typically runs toward the aortic valve,
- there are separate AV valves and a normal morphology of the right (tricuspid) valve,
- no »primum« atrial communication exists,
- the cleft never crosses the ventricular septum, and
- differential insertion of the AV valves is usually maintained.

9.5 Ebstein's anomaly

Echocardiographic analysis of the tricuspid valve (TV) is notoriously difficult (see ▶ Chapter 10). In the standard 2D echocardiographic views, only two leaflets are visible and it can be difficult to differentiate between the septal and the postero-inferior leaflet [26]. TEE is sometimes very helpful in the evaluation of the tricuspid valve, but since the TV is positioned anteriorly, away from the transducer located in the esophagus, the results can be disappointing. In adults, the transgastric view is helpful for the evaluation of the TV with TEE. If the tricuspid valve is abnormal, as in the case of Ebstein's anomaly, the most common congenital malformation of the tricuspid valve, it becomes even more difficult.

The transthoracic acquisition of 3D data with the TV as the region of interest is best achieved from the apical or foreshortened 4-chamber position. It will encompass the entire tricuspid valve. A high parasternal view with the transducer angulated to the right towards the right hip can also provide a useable 3D dataset. In a 3D dataset acquired from these positions, Ebstein's malformation of the TV can be analyzed. The leaflets, their attachment to the septum and to the anterior wall, and the degree displacement of the functional TV orifice towards the pulmonary valve or the apex can be seen (Fig. 9.19 and Fig. 9.20).

In order to assess the size and (sometimes very irregular) shape of the actual TV orifice – often remote from the anatomic TV annulus – an en face view is very helpful (Fig. 9.19). However, creating this en face view can be very challenging; there is no standardized approach due to the wide variety of the degree and direction of displacement of the TV opening. Once a good en face view is obtained, not only the orifice can be seen but also the sail-like anterior–superior leaflet is visualized. In the same view, the right ventricular anterior wall and the presence (or absence) of attachment of the anterior–superior leaflet to the RV free wall can be judged. The en face view can be used for planimetry of the orifice, which is relevant in case of TV stenosis.

Both the en face and the right lateral views will provide extra anatomical information in addition to that from the 2D analysis. Combination of RT3DE with color Doppler provides more insight into the mechanism of tricuspid regurgitation [27]. In our experience, the TV and Ebstein's disease are more difficult to assess (even with 3D echocardiography) than abnormalities situated on the left side of the heart. However, actually seeing, in one image, that a tricuspid valve has three leaflets is already an improvement over 2D imaging.

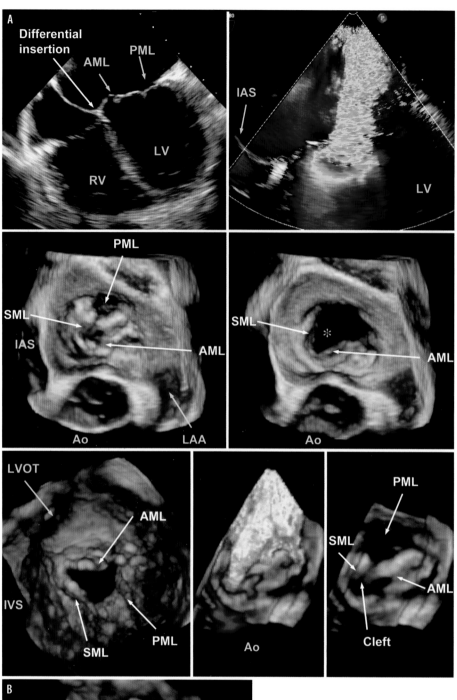

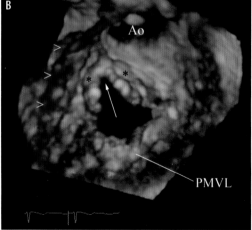

Fig. 9.18 **A** Transesophageal 2D and RT3DE representation of a true cleft mitral valve with severe regurgitation in a 26-year-old woman. *Top left* The 2D image clearly depicts differential insertion of atrioventricular valves suggesting a real cleft. The RT3DE en face view from the left atrium to the mitral valve (*middle row*) shows the prolapsing mitral valve with the cleft (*), a septal (*SML*), anterior (*AML*) and posterior mitral leaflet (*PML*) in systole (*middle left*) and diastolic opening (*middle right*). The 3D en face view from the apex to the mitral valve clearly shows the cleft and the chordae attachment to the SML and AML (*bottom left*). The 3D en face view from the left atrium towards the cleft MV with color Doppler (*bottom middle*) and without color Doppler (*bottom right*) clearly depicts the anatomy of the regurgitant lesion. **B** Magnified view of the true cleft in the anterior leaflet of the mitral valve (*arrow*). Note that the cleft is orientated toward the aorta and does not extend to the ventricular septum (>). The posterior mitral valve leaflet (*PMVL*) is indicated. The asterisks (*) mark the two parts of the cleft anterior mitral valve leaflet. *RV* right ventricle, *LV* left ventricle, *IAS* interatrial septum, *Ao* aortic root, *LAA* left atrial appendage, *LVOT* left ventricular outflow tract.
[→Videos 9.18A(a–e), B(a)]

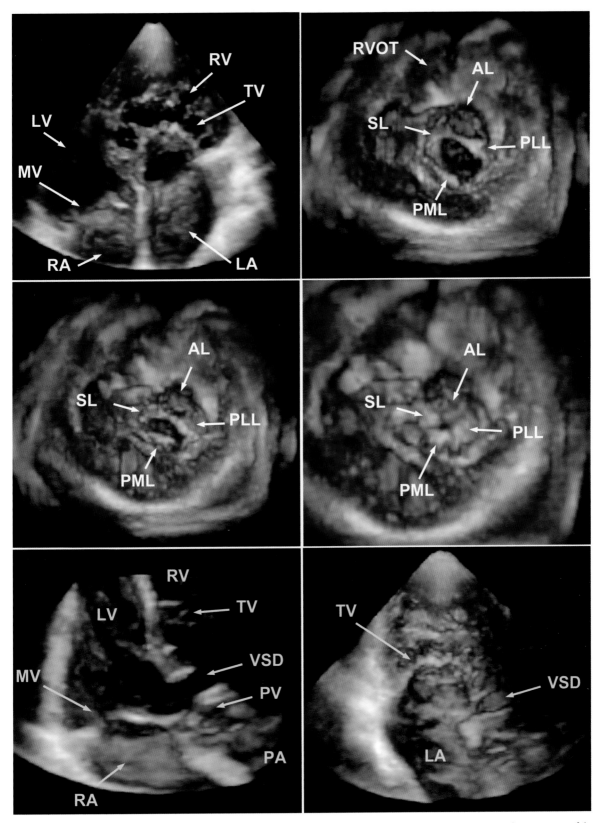

■ **Fig. 9.19** Example of transthoracic RT3DE representation of Ebstein's disease in a 22-year-old woman with congenitally corrected transposition of the great arteries (*ccTGA*) in combination with a perimembranous ventricular septal defect (*VSD*) and pulmonary valve (*PV*) stenosis. The 3D en face view from the apex to the tricuspid valve (*TV*) reveals detailed information about TV leaflet anatomy during valve opening (*top right*), valve mid closure (*middle left*), and complete closure (*middle right*) showing four leaflets: a septal (*SL*), anterior (*AL*), postero-medial (*PML*) and postero-lateral (*PLL*) with the SL and the PLL connected by a bridge like a natural Alfieri stitch. A modified 3D 5-chamber view clearly shows the spatial relation between the VSD, the LVOT, and the stenotic PV (*bottom left*). The 3D en face view from the right ventricle (*RV*) to the interventricular septum shows the exact size, shape, and location of the VSD (*bottom right*). *LV* left ventricle, *MV* mitral valve, *RA* right atrium, *LA* left atrium, *RVOT* right ventricular outflow track, *PA* pulmonary artery. [→Videos 9.19A–D]

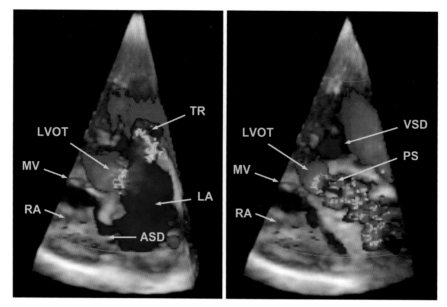

☐ **Fig. 9.20** The RT3DE color Doppler information in the same patient with Ebstein's disease shown in ☐ Fig. 9.19. The 3D color Doppler reveals not only mild tricuspid regurgitation (*TR*) but also a secundum type ASD in the same view (*left*). The flow propagation zone entering through the left ventricular outflow tract (*LVOT*) into the LA is an illusion (*left*), with the flow propagation belonging to the pulmonary valve stenosis (*PS*) as shown in the 3D view cropped more anteriorly (*right*) with depiction of flow through the VSD. *MV* mitral valve, *RA* right atrium, *LA* left atrium, *ASD* atrial septal defect, *VSD* ventricular septal defect. [→Videos 9.20A,B]

9.6   Transposition of the great arteries

In adult congenital heart disease, almost all patients with a simple transposition of the great arteries (TGA) have had either a Mustard or a Senning atrial switch procedure. The LV sustains the (low-resistance) pulmonary circulation and has, as a consequence, low systolic pressure. The RV sustains the systemic circulation and has systemic ventricular pressures. Due to these pressure differences, the ventricular septum bulges to the left and the LV is squashed behind the high-pressured RV. Assessment of LV ejection fraction by 2D echocardiography is not very reliable in these patients, because the assumptions underlying Simpson's biplane planimetry method (round shape and concentric contractions) are not valid in abnormally shaped, squashed LVs. It is reported that RT3DE can measure LV function more reliably than 2D echocardiography in these circumstances [3]. Assessment of RV function remains difficult. The systemic RV lies anteriorly in the chest and is, in adults, very often dilated. From an apical 4-chamber position, it is a challenge to encompass the entire RV in a 3D dataset. Analysis of RV function with dedicated software is difficult, but sometimes feasible (it is addressed separately at the end of this chapter).

The anatomy of atrioventricular and semilunar valves are usually normal and the interventricular septum is most often intact; RT3DE has nothing extra to offer in this respect. »Piece de resistance« in the echocardiographic analysis of a patient with a Mustard or Senning repair is the analysis of the systemic venous pathways that are created to connect the superior and inferior vena cava with the left atrium. These intraatrial tunnels are usually referred to as atrial baffles (☐ Fig. 9.21).

Many (sometimes even very experienced sonographers and cardiologists) have difficulties in understanding how the atrial

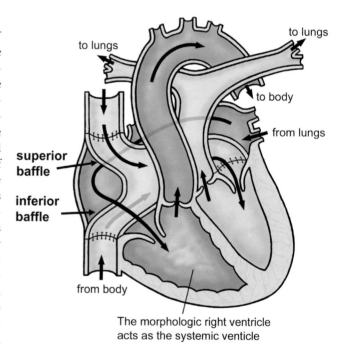

☐ **Fig. 9.21** A schematic drawing of an atrial switch according to Mustard. The baffles are the intratunnels created by the surgeon to transport the systemic venous return from the superior and inferior vena cava towards the left atrium and the mitral valve in such a way that the pulmonary veins, which enter the posterior wall of the left atrium, have unobstructed communication with the right atrium. Crown Copyright 2002–2008

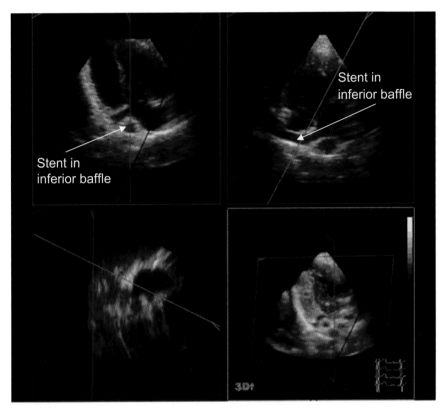

◘ Fig. 9.22 TGA after Mustard type atrial repair and stent in inferior baffle as treatment of baffle stenosis. The multiplane view is shown. The angles of the cutting planes are seen in the 3D image (*right bottom*). The relation between the *green plane* and *red plane* is better visualized in the upper images. [→Video 9.22]

baffles actually run inside the right atrium, how they are related to each other, how they drain into the remains of the left atrium, and how they relate to the pulmonary veins. These pulmonary veins drain, unaltered and untouched by the surgical procedure, into the posterior wall of the left atrium. The pulmonary venous blood is directed toward the right atrium and should not be obstructed by the atrial baffles. RT3DE of an atrial switch repair is a good example how 3D echocardiography can be used in the analysis of complex anatomy. Analysis using the MPR mode in which the three orthogonal cross sections are shown together with the 3D dataset (▶ Chapter 2) is the first very helpful step in the analysis of a transposition after atrial switch (◘ Fig. 9.22).

> ❯ RT3DE of an atrial switch repair in TGA is a good example how 3D echocardiography can be used in the analysis of complex anatomy.

By scrolling through the sagittal plane from posterior to anterior, the inferior baffle is seen first, with its course almost purely from right to left (◘ Fig. 9.22). At this level, the pulmonary venous atrium is seen, posterior from this inferior baffle, with the left pulmonary veins draining from the left lateral side into this compartment. If one scrolls slightly more towards the anterior, the inferior baffle disappears from this plane and the right pulmonary veins can now be seen entering the pulmonary venous atrium as well as the connection between the pulmonary venous atrium and the right atrium (◘ Fig. 9.23).

Most of these 2D cross-sections, now derived from the 3D dataset, can be acquired during the standard 2D echocardiographic workup, implicating that there would be no real added value of RT3DE. However, in our experience, the added value consists of the possibility to establish and appreciate, off-line, the exact level and orientation of these cross-sections in the intracardiac anatomy. Both superior and inferior baffles can be followed over their course, from the caval veins to their entrance in the remnants of the original left atrium. If a baffle stenosis is present, the area and length of a narrowed segment in the baffle can be seen and measured with planimetry. If a patient with TGA after a Mustard or Senning type repair has an endocardial pacemaker, the superior vena cava and the superior baffle are identified easily because they contain a pacemaker wire. If a patient has a stent in the superior or inferior baffle, identification of the anatomic structure that contains the stent is easier (◘ Fig. 9.22).

For patients with a complex transposition and a Rastelli-type repair, the intracardiac conduit from the left ventricle towards the anteriorly positioned aortic valve can be visualized and shown in relation to the adjacent structures. It is difficult, just as in 2D echocardiography, to assess the conduit from the right ventricle to the pulmonary artery, because of its anterior–superior position in the chest, just behind the sternum.

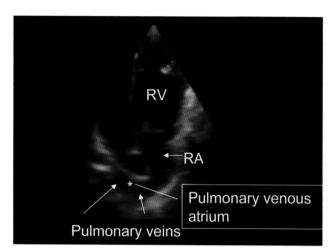

Fig. 9.23 A cross section through the 3D dataset mimicking an apical 4-chamber view in a patient with a TGA after Mustard repair. The pulmonary veins are shown along with the connection to the right atrium. Atrial baffles are not seen in this view, because they are in other levels. If one scrolls through the dataset more towards the posterior, the inferior baffle would be seen, while scrolling more anteriorly would show the superior baffle. *RV* right ventricle, *RA* right atrium. [→Video 9.23]

9.7 Congenitally corrected transposition of the great arteries

The now preferred name for this rare anomaly is atrioventricular and ventriculoarterial discordance, but in clinical practice it is still often referred to as congenitally corrected transposition of the great arteries (ccTGA). A more modern term is double-disco heart.

It is a challenge to analyze these patients with 2D echocardiography. A former echocardiographic definition was »if you lose your way in a heart, it is a ccTGA.« The most difficult part was the identification of the connections between the ventricles and the great arteries: in one plane it might look like the aorta was connected to the right ventricle (RV) and in another view it looked as if the pulmonary artery was connected to the RV. The advantage of 3D echocardiography is that the entire anatomy is in a full volume 3D dataset and the anatomic relations and connections of the great arteries can be unequivocally shown. In ▪ Fig. 9.24, ▪ Fig. 9.25, and ▪ Fig. 9.26, illustrations are shown that demonstrate the added value of 3D echocardiography in the case of complex anatomy.

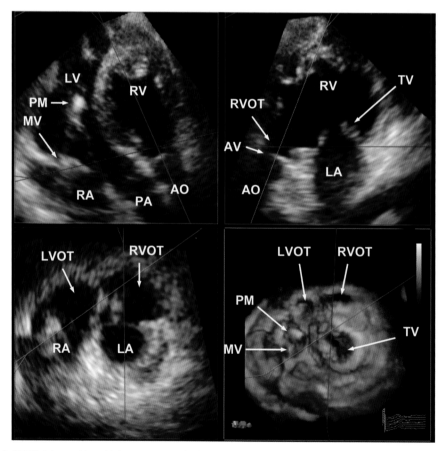

Fig. 9.24 Transthoracic RT3DE dataset with multiplane representation in a 42-year-old woman with ccTGA with the aortic valve (connected to RVOT) left and anterior (*bottom right*). Individual orientation of the three image planes (*red, green, blue*) allows for the most comprehensive cross-sectional representation of the abnormal anatomic relationships. *LV* left ventricle, *RV* right ventricle, *RA* right atrium, *LA* left atrium, *MV* mitral valve, *TV* tricuspid valve, *LVOT* left ventricular outflow tract, *RVOT* right ventricular outflow tract, *AO* aorta, *PA* pulmonary artery, *PM* pacemaker lead. [→Video 9.24]

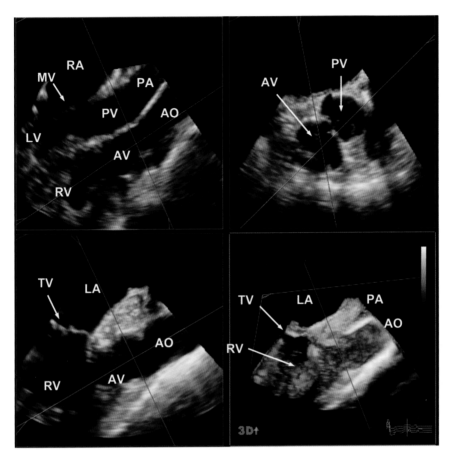

Fig. 9.25 Transesophageal RT3DE dataset with multiplane representation in the same patient with congenitally corrected TGA shown in ▢ Fig. 9.24 with clear demonstration of the abnormal, parallel orientation of the aorta (*AO*) and aortic valve (*AV*) to the pulmonary artery (*PA*) and pulmonary valve (*PV*) (*top left*). *LV* left ventricle, *RV* right ventricle, *RA* right atrium, *LA* left atrium, *MV* mitral valve, *TV* tricuspid valve. [→Video 9.25]

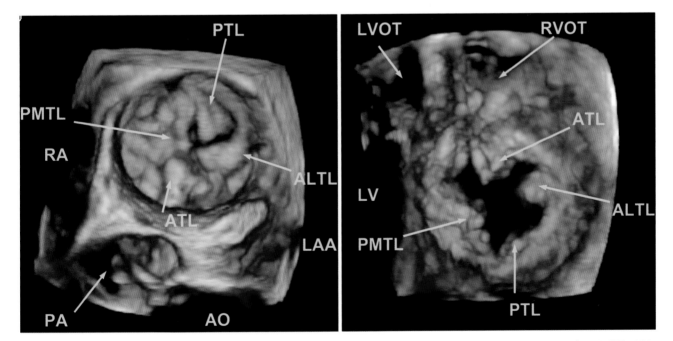

Fig. 9.26 The RT3DE en face view from the left atrium to the tricuspid valve (*TV; left*) and from the apex to the TV (*right*) in the same case shown in ▢ Fig. 9.24 and ▢ Fig. 9.25. The TV appears to have four leaflets. Note the abnormal left and anterior position of the aorta (*AO*) in relation to the pulmonary artery (*PA*). Naming of abnormal anatomic structures, as in this case the abnormal TV, according to its position in the patient's heart (anterior–posterior, superior–inferior, and left–right) is the best way to describe these very rare anomalies. Orientation in the heart is made much easier with 3D echocardiography when compared with 2D echocardiography. *LAA* left atrial appendage, *PTL* posterior tricuspid leaflet, *PMTL* posterior–medial tricuspid leaflet, *RA* right atrium, *ALTL* antero-lateral tricuspid leaflet, *ATL* anterior tricuspid leaflet, *LVOT* left ventricular outflow tract, *RVOT* right ventricular outflow tract, *LV* left ventricle. [→Videos 9.26A,B]

9.8   Tetralogy of Fallot

In a complex congenital malformation like tetralogy of Fallot, RT3DE can be of great value for understanding the exact morphology and spatial relationships as demonstrated in ◘ Fig. 9.27. However, in adults, the pulmonary valve might be difficult to assess with RT3DE. In normal hearts, LV ejection fraction can be assessed more reliably with RT3DE than with 2D echocardiography. This is also probably true for the LV assessment in tetralogy of Fallot, in which the shape of the LV is almost always compromised by a substantially dilated RV. Assessment of RV volumes and ejection fraction is extremely relevant in this population [28], which is addressed separately at the end of this chapter.

9.9   RT3DE in other congenital cardiac malformations

There is very little experience published in the literature about the added value of RT3DE in other malformations than the ones described above. Case reports about subaortic stenosis (◘ Fig. 9.28, see ▶ Fig. 8.16 in Chapter 8) [29], double orifice mitral valve (see ▶ Fig. 7.30 in Chapter 7) [30], cleft mitral valve (◘ Fig. 9.18, see also ▶ Fig. 7.31 in Chapter 7) [31], double aortic arch [32], right atrial aneurysm [33], infective endocarditis of a patent foramen ovale [34], and cor triatriatum sinister [35] have been reported. These are examples of the growing awareness of the potential for RT3DE in congenital heart disease, but more experience is needed and the exact role of RT3DE in the analysis of these complex congenital cardiac lesions remains to be established.

9.10   Role of RT3DE in the analysis of right ventricular function

No geometric assumptions have been proven accurate for the measurement of right ventricular (RV) volumes and function by 2D echocardiography. However, RT3DE is free of geometric assumptions and foreshortened views and would, in principle, be an ideal tool for RV functional analysis (▶ Chapter 6). Some studies have shown that RV function using RT3DE is feasible: with cardiac MRI as a reference, this technique proved to be accurate in experimental settings. However, both acquisition and analysis of a 3D dataset are challenging. Some »tips and tricks« are summarized below.

> ❯ RT3DE is free of geometric assumptions and foreshortened views and is, in principle, an ideal tool for RV function analysis in congenital heart disease.

9.10.1 Acquisition

A 3D dataset containing a RV can be acquired as follows. The patient is positioned in the left lateral decubitus position. In most cases, the patient needs to be turned slightly back towards a supine position. The aim is to optimize the quality of the initially displayed 2D image and to have the RV centrally positioned within the ultrasound sector. Attention needs to be paid to use the minimum angle mode (large, medium, or small) and depth possible to assure optimal frame rates. Dilated or hypertrophic RVs (e.g., after an atrial switch procedure for transposition of the great arteries) may be difficult to visualize completely in combination with acceptable frame rates. Frame rates generally vary between 25 and 55 frames per cardiac cycle. Although the 3D transducer has a footprint that is not larger than a normal 2D transducer, the transducer itself is somewhat larger (▶ Chapter 2). Movement of the transducer in the intercostal spaces may thereby be limited.

After optimization of the 2D view, a switch to the real-time display is made where two orthogonal views are shown (◘ Fig. 9.29). Attention is needed for the inclusion of the RV apex and lateral wall, while checking the orthogonal view for visualization of the RV outflow tract. In patients with tetralogy of Fallot, the RV outflow tract may be dilated due to an operatively placed patch to relieve RV outflow tract obstruction. In order to visualize this, a more superior angulation of the probe is needed. In most healthy persons, the long axis of the heart is almost purely superior–inferior (vertical), with the RV positioned just behind the sternum. This position implies that imaging of the RV outflow tract, anterior, just behind the sternum and superior, can be quite challenging. In patients with moderately dilated or hypertrophic ventricles, the long axis of the RV is often more horizontal. The sternum compromises the image quality to a lesser extent and imaging of the entire RV is more often possible. During one single end-expiratory breath hold, four or seven wedge-shaped subvolumes gated to the R wave are acquired to form a full volume dataset containing the whole RV (◘ Fig. 9.30).

With increasing survival of patients with congenital heart disease, rhythm disturbances with consequently an irregular heart rhythm become more frequent, thereby limiting the use of RT3DE, where steering of subvolumes is needed. However, in newer 3D systems that provide one-beat full volume acquisition this problem is largely solved (▶ Chapter 2).

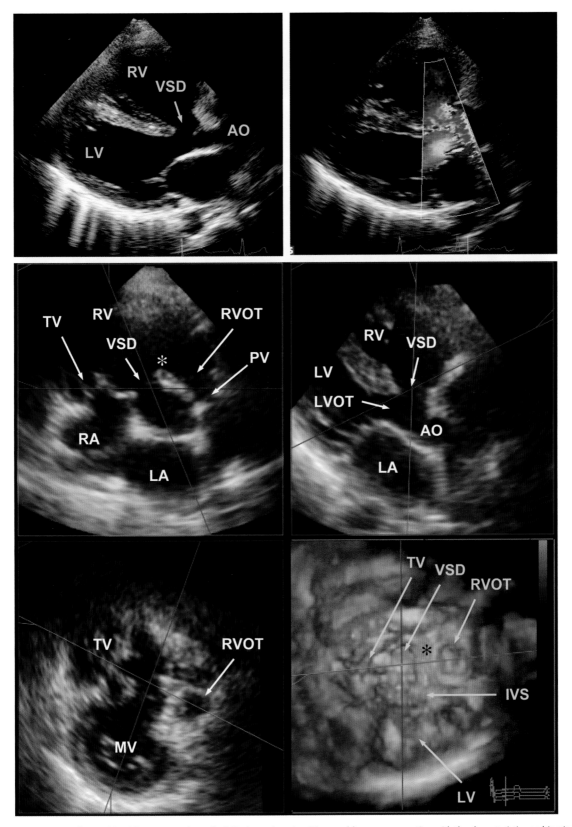

Fig. 9.27 Comparison of 2D and RT3DE representations of a Fallot's tetralogy in a 25-year-old woman presenting with the characteristic combination of overriding aorta, perimembranous (subaortic) ventricular septal defect (*VSD*), pulmonary valve (*PV*) stenosis, and right ventricular hypertrophy. The 2D color Doppler image clearly shows direct right ventricular outflow (*blue*) towards the overriding aorta (*AO; top right*). The 3D en face view from the apex to base (*bottom right*) shows the location of the VSD – connecting the RV to the aorta – located on a (green) line between the tricuspid valve (TV) and right ventricular outflow tract (*RVOT*). The RVOT is quite wide for a tetralogy of Fallot. The *green* plane (*middle left*) also depicts the relation between the TV, VSD, and RVOT with the typical ventricular infundibulum deviated anteriorly (∗) between the LVOT and RVOT, the hallmark of Fallot's tetralogy. *LV* left ventricle, *RV* right ventricle, *RA* right atrium, *LA* left atrium, *MV* mitral valve, *LVOT* left ventricular outflow tract, *IVS* interventricular septum. [→Videos 9.27A–C]

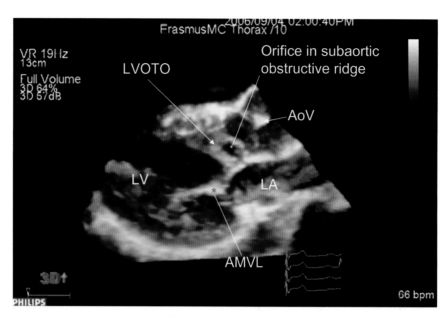

■ **Fig. 9.28** Left lateral view onto the interventricular septum and cutting through the left ventricular outflow tract (LVOT). A complex left ventricular outflow tract obstruction (*LVOTO*) is indicated (*arrow*) with only one small orifice. The attachment not only to the ventricular septum but also the mitral valve is nicely shown here. A discrete subaortic stenosis is always a circular structure; in order to visualize this, the en face view of the LVOTO would provide this additional information. *AoV* aortic valve, *LV* left ventricle, *LA* left atrium, *AMVL* anterior mitral valve leaflet. [→Video 9.28]

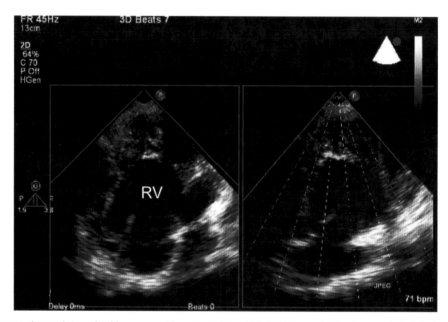

■ **Fig. 9.29** Optimally, two orthogonal views should encompass the entire right ventricle (*RV*). The most difficult part to include is the right ventricular outflow tract. [→Video 9.29]

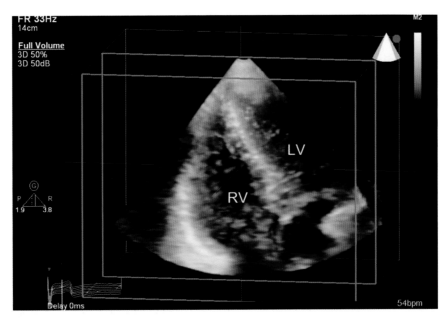

◘ **Fig. 9.30** Full volume 3D data set of the right ventricle (*RV*). *LV* left ventricle

9.10.2 Analysis

Analysis of the right ventricular datasets is best performed with dedicated software (4D RV-Function©, TomTec Imaging Systems, Unterschleissheim, Germany), which offers semiautomatic contour detection of the endocardial borders (► Chapter 6). Hereafter, the program calculates RV volumes and ejection fraction (EF) with the possibility of manual contour revision (◘ Fig. 9.31).

Analysis of patients who have a RV that functions as asystemic ventricle (e.g., in congenitally corrected transposition of the great arteries or transposition of the great arteries after a Mustard or Senning repair) is difficult. At present, the role of 3D echocardiography for RV assessment in clinical practice is limited. Extensive validation of 3D echocardiographic measurements is needed before it will be applicable in clinical practice.

In summary, both acquisition and analysis of the right ventricle by RT3DE is feasible in most congenital heart diseases and forms a practical approach, but its value for clinical purposes remains to be established [36][37][38][39].

9.11 Conclusion

RT3DE is a very useful tool for the analysis of adult congenital heart disease; however, it still has substantial shortcomings in terms of spatial and temporal resolution particularly when obtaining one-beat full volume 3D datasets. It provides additional information that cannot be obtained without a 3D technique. Analysis of ventricular function, which is as important as in »regular« cardiology, is performed better with 3D imaging than with 2D imaging. Understanding of the intracardiac morphology is enhanced by the en face view, which is a unique feature of 3D echocardiography. At present, it has not replaced other echocardiographic modalities because of its apparent weaknesses in resolution, but the strengths of RT3DE justify its use in all regular echocardiographic work-ups of patients with congenital heart disease.

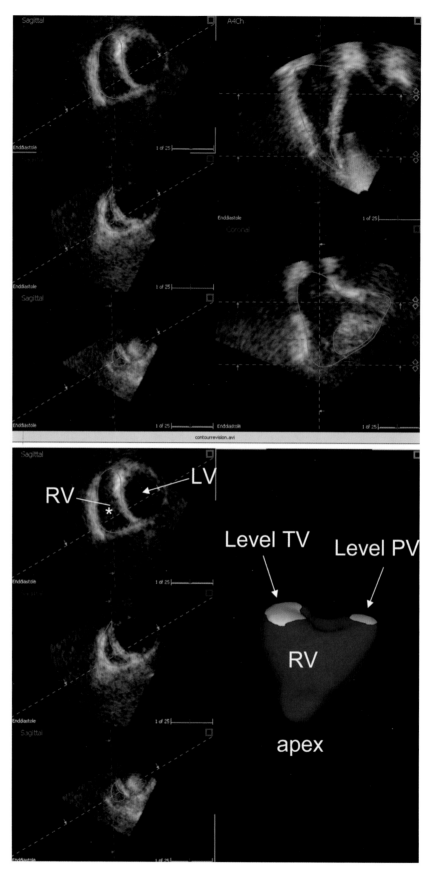

◻ Fig. 9.31 RV volume analysis. *Top* The endocardial borders are traced manually in three orthogonal planes. Through automated contour detection the endocardial wall is analyzed automatically, based on algorithms. After automatic contour detection, it is possible to go through the entire dataset to see how the lines are drawn. If necessary, the borders can be corrected manually. *Bottom* Finally, a RV »beutel« is reconstructed, shown (in *green*). *RV* right ventricle, *PV* pulmonary vein, *TV* tricuspid valve, *LV* left ventricle. [→Video 9.31]

References

1. Balestrini L, Fleishman C, Lanzoni L et al (2000) Real-time 3-dimensional echocardiography evaluation of congenital heart disease. J Am Soc Echocardiogr 13:171–176
2. Altmann K, Shen Z, Boxt LM et al (1997) Comparison of three-dimensional echocardiographic assessment of volume, mass, and function in children with functionally single left ventricles with two-dimensional echocardiography and magnetic resonance imaging. Am J Cardiol 80:1060–1065
3. van den Bosch AE, Robbers-Visser D, Krenning BJ et al (2006) Real-time transthoracic three-dimensional echocardiographic assessment of left ventricular volume and ejection fraction in congenital heart disease. J Am Soc Echocardiogr 19:1–6
4. Riehle TJ, Mahle WT, Parks WJ et al (2008) Real-time three-dimensional echocardiographic acquisition and quantification of left ventricular indices in children and young adults with congenital heart disease: comparison with magnetic resonance imaging. J Am Soc Echocardiogr 21:78–83
5. Raedle-Hurst TM, Mueller M, Rentzsch A et al (2009) Assessment of left ventricular dyssynchrony and function using real-time 3-dimensional echocardiography in patients with congenital right heart disease. Am Heart J 157:791–798
6. Simpson JM, Miller O (2011) Three-dimensional echocardiography in congenital heart disease. Arch Cardiovasc Dis. 104:45–56
7. Broberg C, Meadows AK (2011) Advances in imaging: the impact on the care of the adult with congenital heart disease. Prog Cardiovasc Dis 53:293–304
8. Seo JS, Song JM, Kim YH et al (2012) Effect of atrial septal defect shape evaluated using three-dimensional transesophageal echocardiography on size measurements for percutaneous closure. J Am Soc Echocardiogr 25:1031–1040
9. Saric M, Perk G, PurgessJR, Kronzon I (2010) Imaging atrial septal defects by real-time three-dimensional transesophageal echocardiography: step-by-step approach. J Am Soc Echocardiogr 23:1128–1135
10. Marx GR, Fulton DR, Pandian NG et al (1995) Delineation of site, relative size and dynamic geometry of atrial septal defects by real-time three-dimensional echocardiography. J Am Coll Cardiol 25:482–490
11. Roberson DA, Cui W, Patel D et al (2011) Three-dimensional transesophageal echocardiography of atrial septal defect: a qualitative and quantitative anatomic study. J Am Soc Echocardiogr 24:600–610
12. Mathewson JW, Bichell D, Rothman A, Ing FF (2004) Absent postero-inferior and anterosuperior atrial septal defect rims: Factors affecting nonsurgical closure of large secundum defects using the Amplatzer occluder. J Am Soc Echocardiogr 17:62–69
13. van den Bosch AE, Ten Harkel DJ, McGhie JS et al (2006) Characterization of atrial septal defect assessed by real-time 3-dimensional echocardiography. J Am Soc Echocardiogr 19:815–821
14. Franke A, Kuhl HP, Rulands D et al (1997) Quantitative analysis of the morphology of secundum-type atrial septal defects and their dynamic change using transesophageal three-dimensional echocardiography. Circulation 96:II-7
15. Mehmood F, Vengala S, Nanda NC et al (2004) Usefulness of live three-dimensional transthoracic echocardiography in the characterization of atrial septal defects in adults. Echocardiography 21:707–713
16. Acar P Massabuau P, Elbaz M (2008) Real-time 3D transoesophageal echocardiography for guiding Amplatzer septal occluder device deployment in an adult patient with atrial septal defect. Eur J Echocardiogr 9:822–823
17. Lodato JA, Cao QL, Weinert L et al (2009) Feasibility of real-time three-dimensional transoesophageal echocardiography for guidance of percutaneous atrial septal defect closure. Eur J Echocardiogr 10:543–548
18. Chen FL, Hsiung MC, Nanda N et al (2006) Real time three-dimensional echocardiography in assessing ventricular septal defects: an echocardiographic-surgical correlative study. Echocardiography 23:562–568
19. Mehmood F, Miller AP, Nanda et al (2006) Usefulness of live/real time three-dimensional transthoracic echocardiography in the characterization of ventricular septal defects in adults. Echocardiography 23:421–427
20. Hsu JH, Wu JR, Dai ZK, Lee MH (2007) Real-time three-dimensional echocardiography provides novel and useful anatomic insights of perimembranous ventricular septal aneurysm. Int J Cardiol 118:326–331
21. van den Bosch AE, Ten Harkel DJ, McGhie JS et al (2006) Feasibility and accuracy of real-time 3-dimensional echocardiographic assessment of ventricular septal defects. J Am Soc Echocardiogr 19:7–13
22. Seliem MA, Fedec A, Szwast A et al (2007) Atrioventricular valve morphology and dynamics in congenital heart disease as imaged with real-time 3-dimensional matrix-array echocardiography: comparison with 2-dimensional imaging and surgical findings. J Am Soc Echocardiogr 20:869–876.
23. van den Bosch AE, Ten Harkel DJ, McGhie JS et al (2006) Surgical validation of real-time transthoracic 3D echocardiographic assessment of atrioventricular septal defects. Int J Cardiol 112:213–218
24. Takahashi K, Mackie AS, Thompson R et al (2012) Quantitative real-time three-dimensional echocardiography provides new insight into the mechanisms of mitral valve regurgitation post-repair of atrioventricular septal defect. J Am Soc Echocardiogr 25:1231–1244
25. Kutty S, Smallhorn JF (2012) Evaluation of atrioventricular septal defects by threedimensional echocardiography: benefits of navigating the third dimension. J Am Soc Echocardiogr 25:932–944
26. Anwar AM, Geleijnse ML, Ten Cate FJ, Meijboom FJ (2006) Assessment of tricuspid valve annulus size, shape and function using real-time three-dimensional echocardiography. Interact Cardiovasc Thorac Surg 5:683–687
27. Paranon S, Acar P. Ebstein's anomaly of the tricuspid valve: from fetus to adult: congenital heart disease. Heart. 2008 Feb;94(2):237-43
28. van der Hulst AE et al. Real-time three-dimensional echocardiography: segmental analysis of the right ventricle in patients with repaired tetralogy of fallot. J Am Soc Echocardiogr. 2011 Nov;24(11):1183-90
29. Miyamoto, K., et al., Detection of discrete subaortic stenosis by 3-dimensional transesophageal echocardiography. Echocardiography, 2005. 22(9): p. 783-4
30. Anwar AM, McGhie JS, Meijboom FJ, ten Cate FJ (2008) Double orifice mitral valve by real-time three-dimensional echocardiography. Eur J Echocardiogr 9:731–732
31. Nomoto K, Hollinger I, DiLuozzo G, Fischer GW (2009) Recognition of a cleft mitral valve utilizing real-time three-dimensional transoesophageal echocardiography. Eur J Echocardiogr 10:367–369
32. Sivaprakasam MC, Vettukattil JJ (2006) 3-D echocardiographic imaging of double aortic arch. Eur J Echocardiogr 7:476–477
33. Guerra VC, Coles J, Smallhorn JF (2005) Aneurysm of right atrium diagnosed by 3-dimensional real-time echocardiogram. J Am Soc Echocardiogr 18:1221
34. Acar P, Abadir S, Bassil R (2007) Images in congenital heart disease. Infective endocarditis of the patent oval fossa assessed by three-dimensional echocardiography. Cardiol Young 17:113
35. Patel V, Nanda NC, Arellano I et al (2006) Cor triatriatum sinister: assessment by live/real time three-dimensional transthoracic echocardiography. Echocardiography 23:801–802
36. van der Zwaan HB Geleijnse ML, Soliman OI et al (2011) Test-retest variability of volumetric right ventricular measurements using real-time three-dimensional echocardiography. J Am Soc Echocardiogr 24:671–679
37. van der Zwaan HB, Helbing WA, Boersma E et al (2010) Usefulness of real-time three-dimensional echocardiography to identify right ventricular dysfunction in patients with congenital heart disease. Am J Cardiol 106:843–850
38. van der Zwaan HB, Helbing WA, McGhie JS et al (2010) Clinical value of real-time three-dimensional echocardiography for right ventricular quantification in congenital heart disease: validation with cardiac magnetic resonance imaging. J Am Soc Echocardiogr 23:134–140
39. Khoo NS, Young A, Occleshaw C et al (2009) Assessments of right ventricular volume and function using threedimensional echocardiography in older children and adults with congenital heart disease: comparison with cardiac magnetic resonance imaging. J Am Soc Echocardiogr 22:1279–1288

Congenital heart disease in children

John M. Simpson, Owen I. Miller

T. Buck et al. (Hrsg.), *Three-dimensional Echocardiography*,
DOI 10.1007/978-3-642-36799-1_10, © Springer-Verlag Berlin Heidelberg 2014

An understanding of the morphology of congenital heart defects is essential for the practice of pediatric cardiology. The anatomy of cardiac lesions is, by its nature, three-dimensional and the introduction of imaging techniques, including echocardiography, which can represent cardiac lesions three-dimensionally have the potential to refine diagnosis and understanding of spatial relationships which is essential to plan surgical or catheter intervention [1]. In children with congenital heart disease (CHD) three-dimensional (3D) echocardiography is particularly attractive because of favorable acoustic windows permitting high quality echocardiographic images. The painless, portable and noninvasive nature of the technique means that it can be repeated easily compared to other imaging techniques.

10.1 Technical and patient-specific factors

Technical aspects of the acquisition and interrogation of 3D datasets are discussed elsewhere in this book but there are several factors relevant to the pediatric age range which merit emphasis. Heart rates in early infancy are often between 120 and 150 beats per minute, roughly double the typical adult heart rate. The average newborn infant weighs 3.0–3.5 kg compared to an adult weight of more than twenty times this size. Thus, for 3D techniques to be feasible in this age range there needs to be high temporal and spatial resolution. The initial real-time 3D ultrasound systems did not lend themselves to pediatric practice because of the low frequency of the ultrasound and sparse array of the matrix probe [2][3] which led to images of insufficient quality for widespread clinical application. Additional factors included the physical size of the ultrasound probes which were initially so large that they were incompatible with the small acoustic windows, generally between rib spaces, in small children. Alternatives included rotational transthoracic or transesophageal echocardiography probes which reconstructed serial cross-sectional images into a 3D dataset [4][5][6][7]. Recent advances in probe technology now mean that 3D probes are available for pediatric use which are of high frequency (up to 7 MHz currently) and with a footprint which is no larger than conventional ultrasound probes used in the pediatric age range (▶ Chapter 2.2) [8]. Depending on the 3D modality employed, frame rates in excess of 60 frames/s are now achievable.

> For 3D echocardiographic techniques to be feasible
> in small children, high temporal and spatial resolution
> are needed.

Movement artifact is another important consideration in the pediatric age range where most echocardiographic studies are performed in children who are awake and unsedated. In this regard, the choice of 3D imaging modality is relevant. Live 3D imaging provides truly real-time 3D images albeit at the expense of the size of the sector which can be interrogated and acquired. Recent advances in image processing give the operator greater flexibility in terms of the area of interest and optimization of frame rates than was previously possible. Live 3D color is a further enhancement which is particularly useful to assess (e.g., valvular regurgitation without the problem of stitch artifacts). A full volume acquisition has a much larger field of view but with the potential for artifacts caused by stitching of sequential segments during the acquisition process (▶ Chapter 2). An alternative is the acquisition of a manually defined volume of interest in the live 3D zoom acquisition mode. This technique avoids the problem of stitch artifacts but does have the disadvantage that if a very large portion of the image is included in the acquired volume, frame rates will drop significantly which can be a problem in smaller, younger children with rapid heart rates (▶ Chapter 2). In practice, many infants and children who merit 3D echocardiography are studied on the intensive care unit, and some may require general anesthesia for other reasons. In such situations, simple measures such as brief suspension of ventilation permit acquisition of high quality 3D datasets without movement or respiration leading to suboptimal imaging.

10.2 Selection of imaging probes in children

At present the choices of 3D imaging probes in children include a high frequency transthoracic imaging probe (currently up to 7 MHz) which is typically used in children up to the age of 4–5 years depending on the region of interest. In children older than this, the »adult« 3D probes with a larger footprint and lower frequency are normally used with excellent results. The latest generation of 3D ultrasound probes have a sonographic footprint similar to standard imaging probes. Three-dimensional imaging during surgery or catheter intervention is being increasingly used and demanded by surgeons and interventionists. There are 3D transesophageal probes available which are of a similar size to a conventional adult probe (▶ Chapter 2.2). This has been used widely in adult patients, particularly to guide interventions such as closure of atrial septal defects (▶ Chapter 12) [9][10][11]. Such a probe can be used in children down to a body weight of around 25 kg. At present, there is no pediatric 3D transesophageal echocardiography probe small enough to permit imaging in infants and smaller children. At these authors' institution the approach we have taken for smaller surgical patients has been to use a 3D epicardial approach with a 3D matrix probe [12]. This has permitted the acquisition of excellent quality 3D images without intervening structures between the probe and the heart coupled with absence of patient movement or respiration. Acquisition of images prior to surgical opening of the pericardial sac or using alternative sonographic windows such as placement of the probe on the atrial rather than ventricular wall help to reduce problems of epicardial contact related to cardiac motion. In the absence of a pediatric 3D transesophageal probe, adoption of an epicardial approach has removed the obstacle presented by the large size of current »adult« 3D transesophageal echocardiography probes allowing intraoperative 3D imaging in smaller patients.

> For transesophageal 3D imaging the adult probe can be
> used in children down to a weight of around 25 kg.

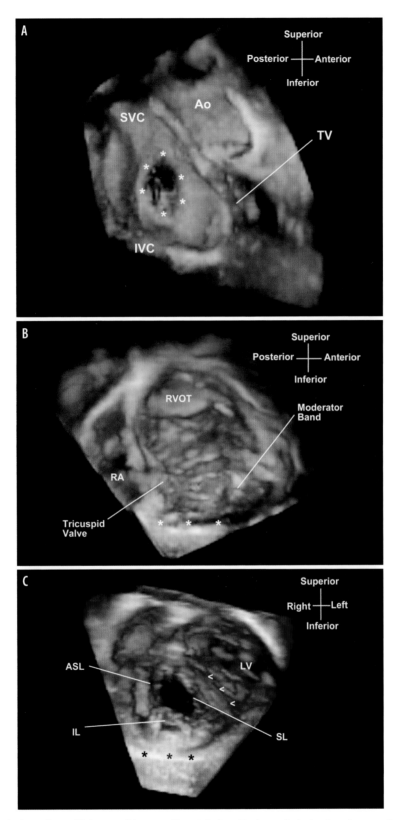

Fig. 10.1 Three-dimensional echocardiographic images of the normal heart displayed to demonstrate structures in an »anatomic« projection. In all images, superior structures are projected uppermost on the image and vice versa. **A** En face view of the atrial septum with the superior vena cava uppermost on the image. The border of the oval fossa is marked with asterisks (*). **B** En face view of the ventricular septum projected from the right ventricle. The inferior diaphragmatic border of the heart is marked with asterisks (*). **C** A view of the tricuspid valve is viewed from the ventricular apex. The inferior diaphragmatic border of the heart is marked with asterisks (*). The inferior, antero-superior and septal leaflets of the tricuspid valve are projected in an anatomically correct orientation. The arrowheads (<) indicate the ventricular septum. *SVC* superior vena cava, *IVC* inferior vena cava, *TV* tricuspid valve, *Ao* aorta, *RA* right atrium, *RVOT* right ventricular outflow tract, *LV* left ventricle, *SL* septal leaflet of the tricuspid valve, *ASL* antero-superior leaflet of the tricuspid valve, *IL* inferior leaflet of the tricuspid valve. [→Videos 10.1A–C]

10.3   Presentation of 3D echocardiographic images

Three dimensional echocardiography permits the projection of rendered images in practically any desired orientation. The unique cropping planes facilitate en face presentation of atrioventricular valves, semilunar valves, and septal structures. Recent work has addressed the optimal orientation and presentation of 3D echocardiographic views [13][14]. For imaging of septal structures such as the atrial septum and ventricular septum, there is a broad consensus as to the optimal mode of presentation. With respect to the orientation of atrioventricular valves, there are some differences between the published references [13][14] with some of the congenital groups who have published on this subject favoring an anatomic projection. Differences in approach might be explained by the patient groups involved. In the study of congenital heart defects, the relative position of different heart structures cannot be assumed so that an anatomic approach may be preferred. In these authors' view, presentation of images in an anatomic format makes the projection intuitive and also means that echocardiographic images are consistent with other imaging techniques such as computed tomography (CT) and magnetic resonance imaging (MRI) in terms of image orientation. Removal of any potential confusion with regard to left–right and supero-inferior relationships is essential to avoid diagnostic error with regard to cardiac morphology, particularly in the context of the malformed heart. This is particularly true for projections en face to cardiac structures which are not achievable using cross-sectional echocardiography (☐ Fig. 10.1).

A huge advantage of 3D echocardiography for the heart which is congenitally abnormal is that the raw data remains available for re-interrogation and can be cut in any desired imaging plane. By sequentially cropping through a 3D dataset, it is possible to convey the relationship of different cardiac structures in a simple and intuitive manner, rather than relying on predefined acquisition planes which cannot be retrospectively re-interrogated. In addition to being able to analyze a virtual heart by cropping through datasets retrospectively, different and novel projections of the heart can be displayed which are simply impossible using conventional echocardiographic techniques. An example of this is the »surgical« view of the atrioventricular valves, i.e. viewing the atrioventricular valves from the atrial aspect in keeping with how a surgeon would visualize these structures during an operation (☐ Fig. 10.2).

> Using 3D datasets different projections of the heart can be displayed which are simply impossible using conventional echocardiographic techniques.

10.4   Types of cardiac lesions which can be assessed using 3D echocardiography

The limitations of imaging congenital heart defects using 3D ultrasound are the same limitations which can be applied to all ultrasound techniques. Areas of the vasculature which are difficult to image using cross-sectional techniques will remain so using 3D echocardiography (e.g., imaging of the distal branch pulmonary arteries which are relatively inaccessible due to surrounding air-filled lung tissue). If cross-sectional imaging is of low quality due to factors such as poor acoustic windows or lack of co-operation in small children, then application of 3D techniques will result in poor quality ultrasound images. At our institution, 3D imaging has been applied to lesions where we feel there is a benefit in terms of understanding the morphology of the lesion or mechanism of abnormality (e.g. atrioventricular

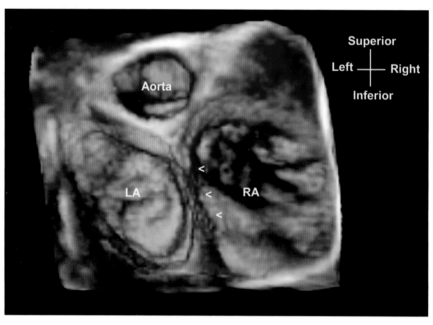

☐ **Fig. 10.2** This is a projection from the atrial side of the atrioventricular junction to demonstrate the normal relationships of the left atrium (*LA*), right atrium (*RA*), and aorta. The leaflets of the mitral valve and tricuspid valve can also be seen. The atrial septum is marked with the arrowheads (<). For congenitally malformed hearts, this projection is maintained, even if anatomic relationships differ from normal. [→Video 10.2]

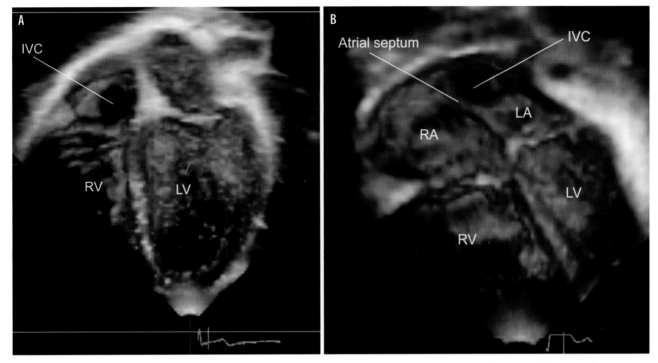

Fig. 10.3 Normal drainage of the inferior vena cava (*IVC*) to the right atrium in a 4-chamber projection (**A**). Abnormal drainage of the inferior vena cava to the left atrium (*LA*) in a child with an associated atrial septal defect (**B**). *RA* right atrium, *LV* left ventricle, *RV* right ventricle. [→Videos 10.3A,B]

valve regurgitation), which would translate into better information to plan surgical or catheter intervention. This is best demonstrated by images of different types of cardiac lesion.

10.4.1 Abnormalities of venous drainage

Abnormalities of venous drainage into the heart may be demonstrated readily by 3D echocardiography. An example is shown of the normal drainage of the inferior vena cava into the right atrium (■ Fig. 10.3A) and abnormal drainage of the inferior vena cava into the left atrium in a child with an associated atrial septal defect (■ Fig. 10.3B).

10.4.2 Atrial septal defects

Atrial septal defects have been widely studied by 3D echocardiography [15][16] to provide information on the size, location, and associated rims of such defects to aid selection of candidates for catheter closure of the atrial septal defect (■ Fig. 10.4A,B). Some authors [11][17][18] have used a transthoracic 3D approach to assist selection (■ Fig. 10.4A,B), but transesophageal 3D imaging of such defects is an alternative (■ Fig. 10.4C,D) which is preferred where acoustic windows are suboptimal or during catheter intervention [10][11][19]. Commonly, a transesophageal approach is used if transthoracic echocardiography does not provide sufficiently high quality images of the rims of the atrial septal defect. During interventional catheter closure of atrial septal defects, 3D echocardiography has proved particularly useful for assessing defects with multiple fenestrations when

decisions are made with regard to the number and size of devices which may need to be deployed to close large defects. Following the initial assessment of the actual defect size and site often using a full volume acquisition, a switch to a live 3D mode can then be used to guide the actual intervention, monitor the safe passage of catheters, and to assess device position before final release.

Aside from secundum atrial septal defects, other types of atrial septal defects such as sinus venosus defects may be studied. Real-time 3D echocardiography (RT3DE) not only allows one to image the morphology and location of the defect but also to identify associated lesions such as partial anomalous pulmonary venous drainage, which may be technically difficult to identify using cross-sectional techniques alone (■ Fig. 10.4E).

10.4.3 Ventricular septal defects

Three-dimensional echocardiography can be applied to all types of ventricular septal defects to provide complete information with regard to the size, location, and anatomic relationships (■ Fig. 10.5) [20][21][22][23][24]. The technique can be applied to infants with large ventricular septal defects, regardless of the location of the defect, and is particularly helpful where there are multiple or unusually shaped defects (■ Fig. 10.5A–D). In situations such as coronary cusp prolapse related to a ventricular septal defect then the technique can accurately delineate the anatomy of the aortic valve, the prolapsing cusp, and the relation to the ventricular septal defect (■ Fig. 10.5E, F) With the introduction of catheter closure of ventricular septal defects, the size and precise location of such defects such as their proximity to the tricuspid and aortic valves has assumed new importance [23].

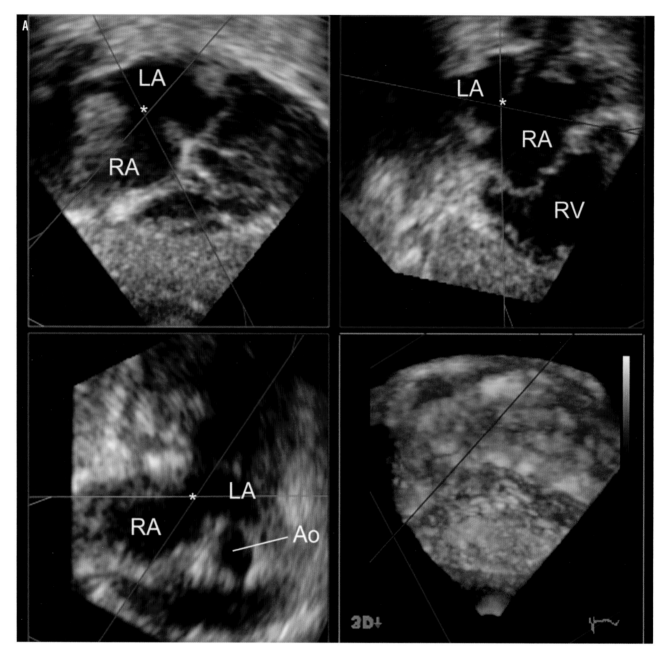

◘ **Fig. 10.4 A** Multiplanar reformatted image of an ASD (marked with *asterisk*) in a child. This technique is particularly good for delineating the rims of the ASD necessary for planning. The imaging planes can be set to produce en face views of the defect for sizing

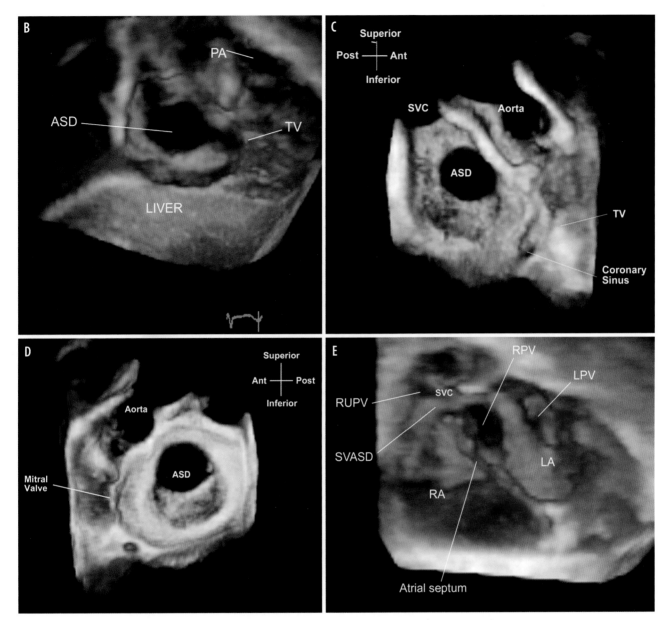

■ **Fig. 10.4** (continued) **B** Transthoracic 3D echocardiogram in a child taken from a subcostal projection. The relationships and size of the atrial septal defect (*ASD*) can be readily appreciated by this technique. The defect is imaged as though viewing the defect from the right atrium. **C** Transesophageal echocardiogram of a large secundum atrial septal defect (projection from the right atrium). This technique provides high definition imaging of the size and morphology of the defect. In this example, there is a large defect with a deficient aortic rim. The opening of the coronary sinus into the right atrium can also be visualized. **D** Transesophageal echocardiogram of the same atrial septal defect visualized from the LA. Thus, comprehensive imaging of ASD from either the right or left atrial aspect is achievable. **E** Subcostal transthoracic 3D echocardiogram of a sinus venosus atrial septal defect (*SVASD*). The defect is superior where the SVC meets the roof of the LA and RA. The right upper pulmonary vein (*RUPV*) is seen en face at the junction of the SVC with the atrial mass confirming anomalous drainage of this vessel. The left pulmonary veins (*LPV*) and the remaining right pulmonary veins (*RPV*) drain normally to the LA. *SVC* superior vena cava, *Ao* aorta, *TV* tricuspid valve, *PA* pulmonary artery, *LA* left atrium, *RA* right atrium, *RV* right ventricle. [→Videos 10.4A–D]

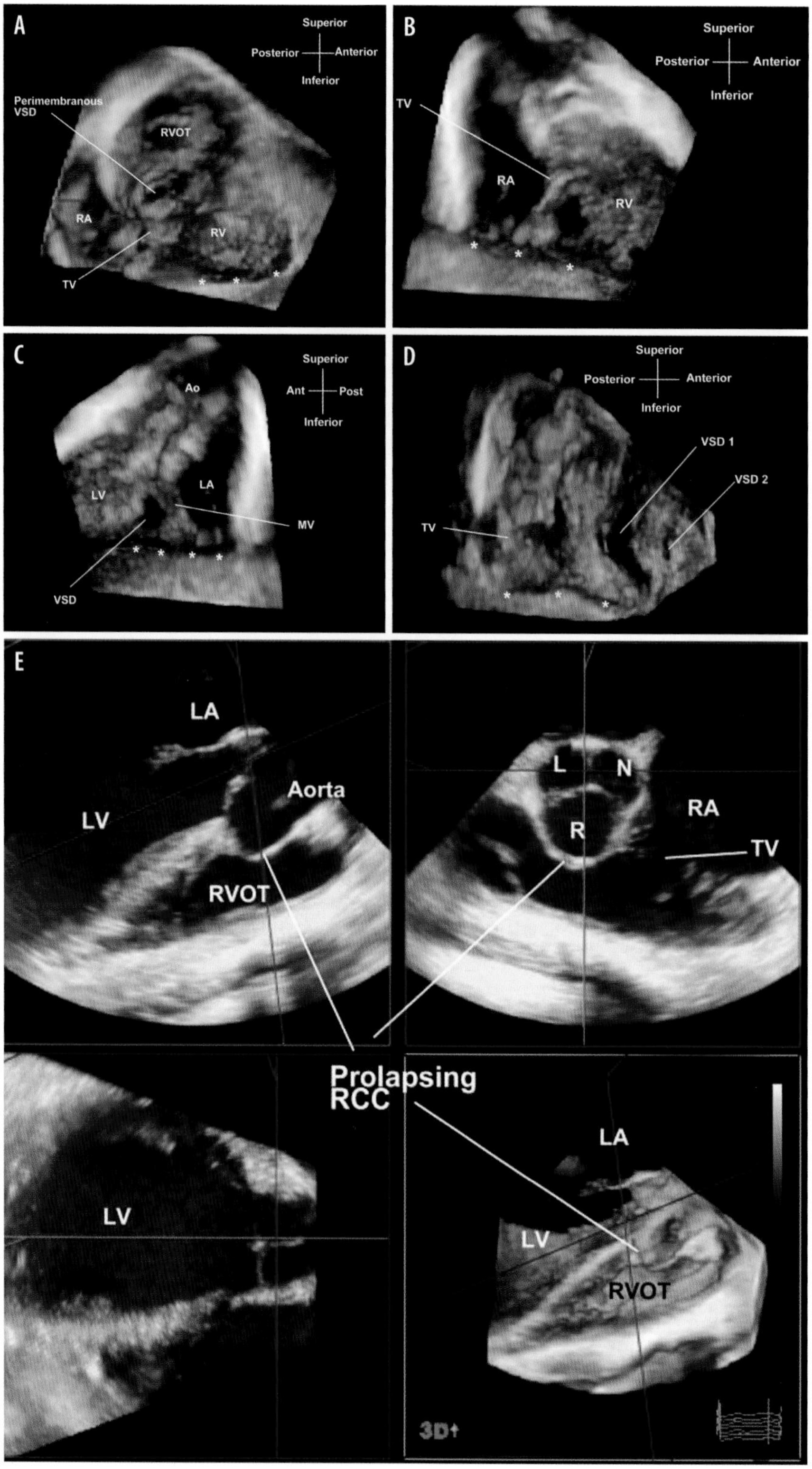

Fig. 10.5 Examples of ventricular septal defects. **A** Subcostal view of an infant with a perimembranous ventricular septal defect (*VSD*). Note that the tricuspid valve forms one of the margins of the VSD. **B** View of an inferiorly positioned muscular VSD viewed from the right ventricle (*RV*). **C** The same inferiorly positioned muscular VSD viewed from the left ventricle. **D** Multiple muscular midtrabecular and apical VSD projected from the right ventricular aspect. The shape of such defects is frequently irregular, 3D echocardiography facilitates accurate location and measurement. **E** Multiplanar reformatted and 3D rendered image (*lower right*) of a perimembranous VSD with prolapse of the right coronary cusp (*RCC*). The multiplanar technique permits accurate diagnosis of the prolapsing cusp to assist surgical planning

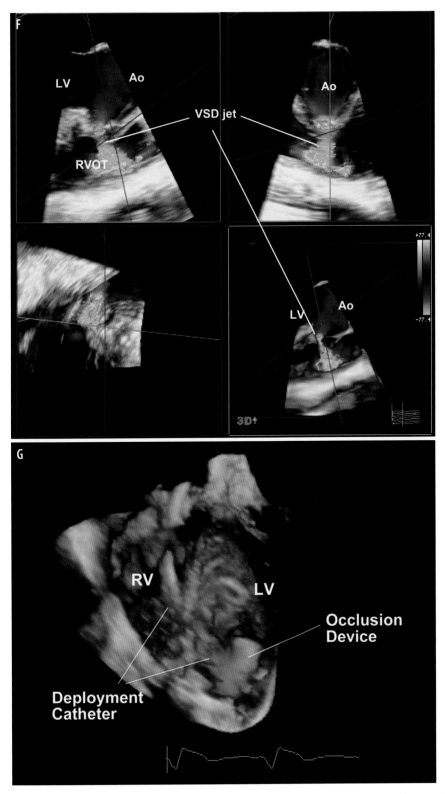

◻ **Fig. 10.5** (continued) Examples of ventricular septal defects. **F** Multiplanar reformatted imaging with the addition of color flow Doppler demonstrates the turbulent left-to-right flow across the ventricular septal defect, with analogous projections to **E. G** Live 3D echocardiography can be used to guide catheter occlusion of ventricular septal defects, in this case an apical muscular VSD. *TV* tricuspid valve, *RA* right atrium, *RVOT* right ventricular outflow tract, *LA* left atrium, *LV* left ventricle, *MV* mitral valve, *Ao* aorta, *L* left coronary cusp, *N* noncoronary cusp. [→Videos 10.5A–G]

Three-dimensional echocardiography is an ideal technique to make such assessments including measurement of the defect and its rims as well as live guidance of the occlusion procedure itself (■ Fig. 10.5G).

> Three-dimensional echocardiography is an ideal technique to assess the size and precise location of ventricular septal defects.

10.4.4 Atrioventricular valves

Atrioventricular valves are ideally suited to imaging by 3D techniques. Abnormalities of these valves have probably been assessed by 3D techniques more than any other. This provides comprehensive pre- and postoperative information with regard to valvular anatomy and function. A complete 3D assessment of atrioventricular (AV) valves typically involves all of the different 3D imaging modalities. Live 3D imaging can produce, for example, high quality short-axis views of the AV valves which include a »depth« of the valvular tissue, thus, facilitating the imaging of abnormalities such as clefts and double orifice morphologies. Full volume acquisition permits visualization of the entirety of the atrioventricular junction and the facility to visualize the AV valves from any desired plane using either multiplanar reformatted or 3D rendered projections. Such full volumes may also be acquired with color flow information. In practice, such color flow imaging allows precise localization of areas of valvular regurgitation so that operative repair may be planned accurately. This is particularly important in pediatric practice where replacement of atrioventricular valves may not be technically possible at all due to small patient size and even if technically feasible may represent a suboptimal result as prosthetic valves will not grow along with the child, thus, committing the child to serial valve replacements.

> Complete 3D assessment of atrioventricular valves typically involves all of the different 3D imaging modalities including color Doppler.

10.4.5 Atrioventricular septal defects

Atrioventricular septal defects (AVSDs) are characterized by a common atrioventricular junction. The size of the atrial and ventricular components of the defect are highly variable, ranging from large communications to non-existent communications. Three-dimensional echocardiography can demonstrate not only the anatomy of the atrioventricular connection and the anatomy of the valve leaflets (■ Fig. 10.6A) but also their attachments better than any other imaging technique [25][26][27]. Clinically important considerations include the anatomy of the left atrioven-

tricular valve, as well as the site and severity of atrioventricular valve regurgitation [28]. Detailed analysis of the angle of the atrioventricular valves to the ventricular septum has also been observed to correlate with outcome in terms of valvular function [29]. For unbalanced atrioventricular septal defects, the relative size of the left and right atrioventricular valves will also influence the approach including the feasibility of a biventricular repair (■ Fig. 10.6B,C).

10.4.6 Mitral valve abnormalities

Congenital and acquired abnormalities of the mitral valve are an extremely important group of lesions that can be imaged using a 3D echocardiographic approach to permit accurate delineation of the morphology which can be visualized from any chosen orientation to inform surgical repair. Images of the mitral valve can be relatively simply obtained from parasternal and apical views so that acquisition of high quality volumetric datasets is technically easy in the pediatric age range. A true cleft in the mitral valve [30][31][32] is demonstrated in ■ Fig. 10.7, including image orientation from both the ventricular and atrial aspects of the valve.

Three-dimensional echocardiography is able to project the chordal support apparatus of the mitral valve in addition to the valve leaflets. Cropping of the 3D volumetric dataset across the plane of the anterior mitral valve leaflet allows visualization of both the lateral and medial papillary muscles and the chordal support of the mitral valve in a single projection [33].

10.4.7 Ebstein's anomaly of the tricuspid valve

Ebstein's anomaly of the tricuspid valve is a lesion where the acquisition of 3D data greatly enhances the understanding of the abnormality [34][35]. This includes the displacement of the septal and inferior leaflets (■ Fig. 10.8A), the rotation of the plane of the tricuspid valve, and extension of attachments into the right ventricular outflow tract (■ Fig. 10.8B). This has proved to be of assistance in planning repair of the tricuspid valve in selected patients [34][35].

10.4.8 Atrioventricular junction

Abnormalities within the left atrium or at the left atrioventricular junction such as cor triatriatum (■ Fig. 10.9A,B) [36][37] and supramitral membrane (■ Fig. 10.9C,D) are readily imaged by 3D echocardiography. The use of both 3D rendered and multiplanar reformatted images assists in delineation of the anatomy in such cases.

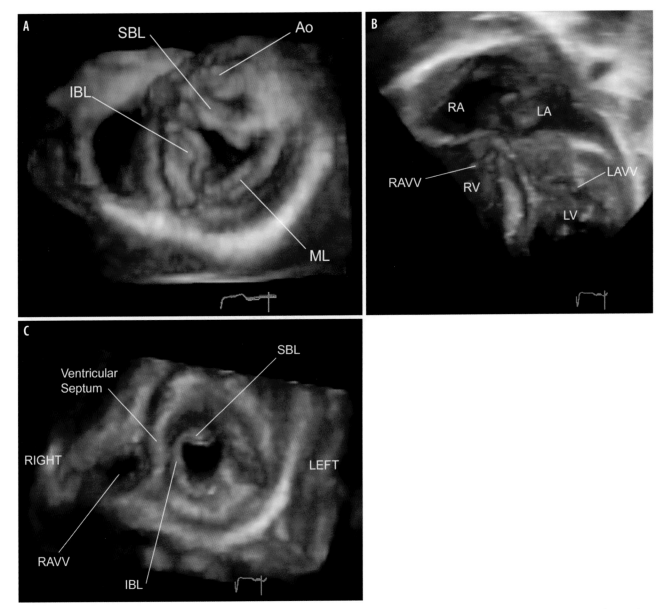

☐ **Fig. 10.6 A** This is an en face projection of the left atrioventricular valve viewed from the apex of the left ventricle in a patient with atrioventricular septal defect (*AVSD*). The trileaflet nature of the left atrioventricular valve can be clearly seen. **B** Apical 4-chamber view of an unbalanced AVSD with dominance of the left atrioventricular valve (*LAVV*) and left ventricle (*LV*). **C** En face projection of the atrioventricular junction viewed from the ventricular aspects demonstrating the hypoplasia of the right atrioventricular valve (*RAVV*) in a patient with AVSD. *SBL* superior bridging leaflet, *IBL* inferior bridging leaflet, *ML* mural leaflet of the left atrioventricular valve, *Ao* aorta, *LA* left atrium, *RA* right atrium, *RV* right ventricle. [→Videos 10.6A–C]

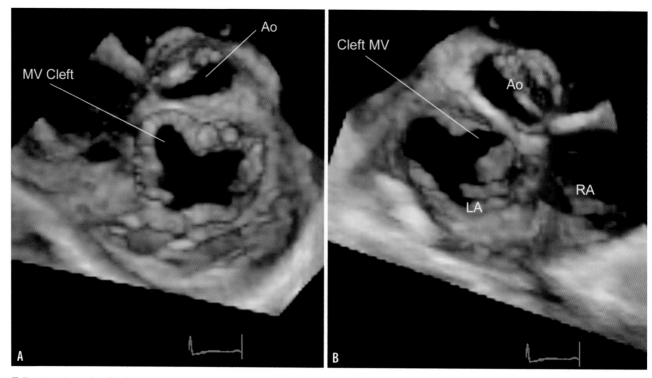

◘ Fig. 10.7 Examples of cleft mitral valve. **A** The 3D echocardiogram of a true cleft in the mitral valve (*MV*) demonstrating the orientation of the cleft towards the aorta (*Ao*). The valve is visualized from the ventricular side of the mitral valve. **B** The 3D echocardiogram of a true cleft of the mitral valve when imaged from the atrial aspect in a surgeon's view. *LA* left atrium, *RA* right atrium. [→Videos 10.7A,B]

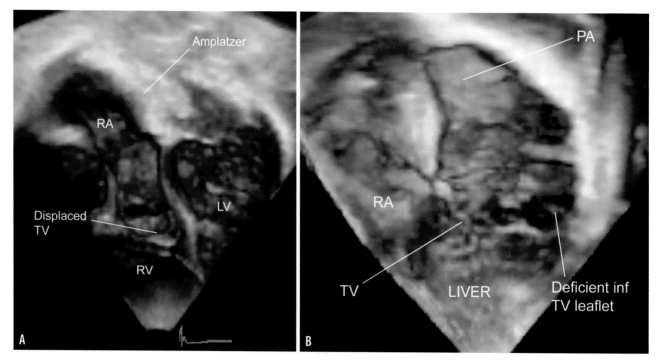

◘ Fig. 10.8 A Apical 4-chamber view of Ebstein's anomaly of the tricuspid valve (*TV*) demonstrating displacement of the septal leaflet of the TV which is characteristic of the lesion. In this patient an Amplatzer septal occluder, which has been used to close an associated atrial septal defect, is also visible. **B** Subcostal image of Ebstein's anomaly of the TV demonstrating the extent of attachments into the right ventricular outflow tract. In this example, there was severe deficiency of the inferior TV leaflet leading to severe TV regurgitation. *RA* right atrium, *PA* pulmonary artery, *RV* right ventricle. [→Videos 10.8A,B]

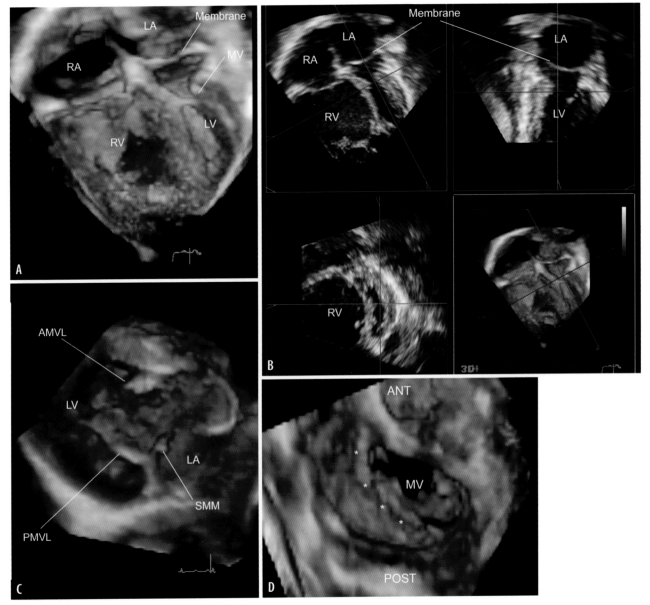

◘ Fig. 10.9 **A** The 4-chamber view of the cor triatriatum demonstrating clearly the anatomy of the obstructing membrane within the left atrium. **B** Multiplanar reformatted images of the same patient shown in **A** illustrating the ease with which the anatomic relations of the cor triatriatum can be demonstrated. **C,D** Parasternal long-axis view of a supramitral membrane (*SMM*) obtained by epicardial 3D echocardiography (**C**). Note that the SMM is immediately above the attachments of the mitral valve (*MV*), in contrast to the cor triatriatum where the obstructing membrane is on the pulmonary venous side of the left atrial appendage. **D** Epicardial 3D echocardiogram permitting visualization of a SMM (marked by asterisks) most prominent along the posterior aspect of the left atrioventricular junction. This view equates to the view that the surgeon will obtain at operation from the left atrium (*LA*). LV left ventricle, *LA* left atrium, *RA* right atrium, *RV* right ventricle, *AMVL* anterior mitral valve leaflet, *PVML* posterior mitral valve leaflet, *ANT* anterior, *POST* posterior. [→Videos 10.9A–D]

10.4.9 Complex anatomy

For many patients with congenital heart disease, a firm understanding of the spatial relationships of, for example, the ventricles and great arteries is essential to plan surgical intervention. Some groups of lesions such as double outlet right ventricle [38] and complex transposition of the great arteries lend themselves readily to interrogation by 3D echocardiographic techniques [36] [37]. In such patients, the development of small footprint high frequency matrix transducers has been a particularly important development because fundamental decisions with regard to type of repair are often made in infancy. In this clinical setting, high resolution imaging is essential to provide images of sufficient quality to assist surgical management. Examples shown include an infant with transposition of the great arteries, subpulmonary stenosis, and a ventricular septal defect (◘ Fig. 10.10A) and an infant with double outlet right ventricle in whom the anatomy of the great arteries and the relationship of these arteries to the ventricular septal defects can be visualized clearly (◘ Fig. 10.10B,C).

> In patients with complex congenital heart disease, high resolution 3D imaging is essential because fundamental decisions with regard to type of repair are often made in infancy.

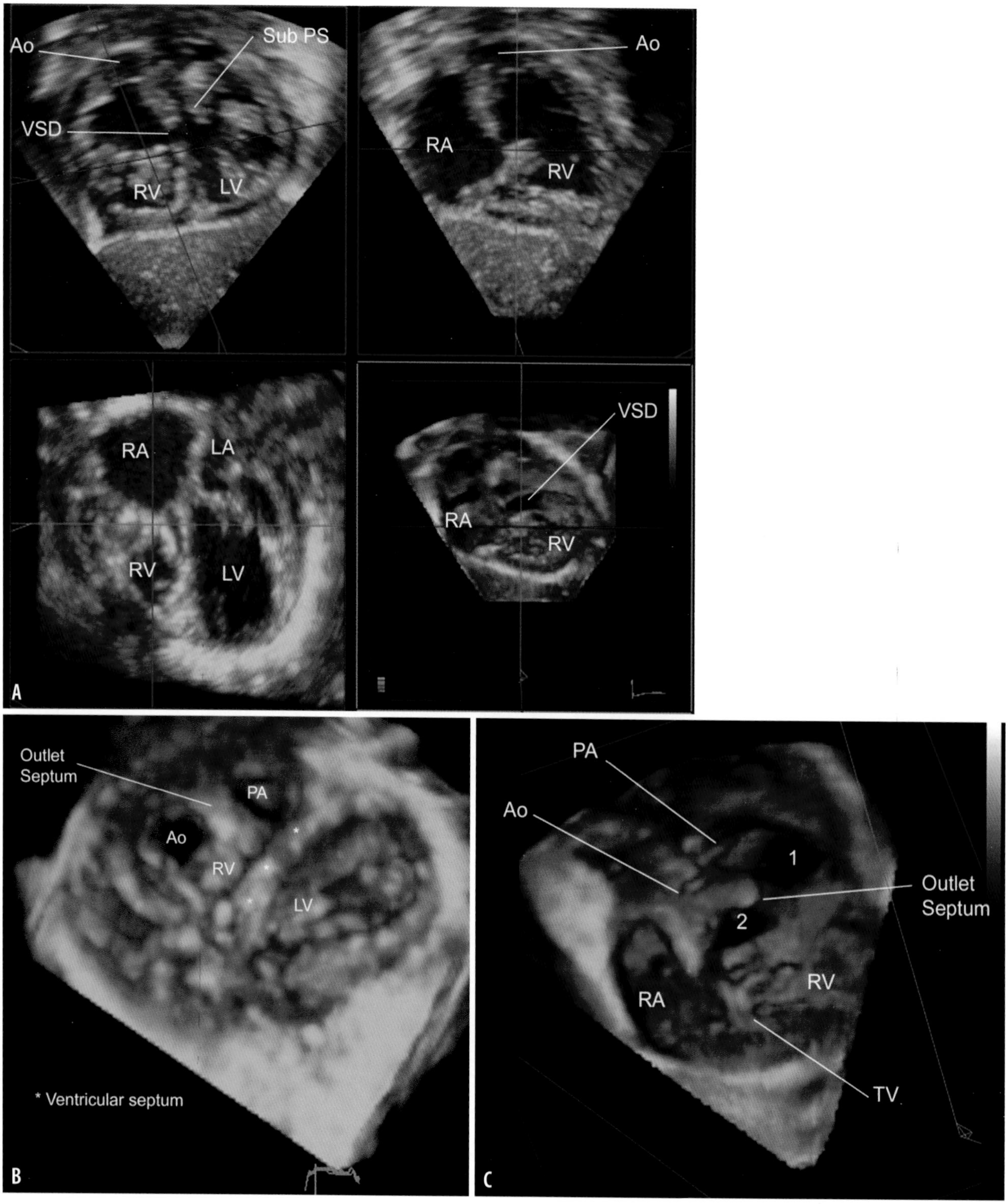

◘ Fig. 10.10 A Example of a patient with transposition of the great arteries, ventricular septal defect and subpulmonary stenosis. *Top left* There is a subcostal view showing the aorta (*Ao*) arising from the right ventricle (*RV*) and the pulmonary artery arising from the left ventricle with subpulmonary stenosis (*Sub PS*). *Top right* An oblique sagittal section through the right atrium (*RA*), tricuspid valve (*TV*), RV, and Ao is shown. *Bottom left* The cut along the plane of the 4-cham- ber view of the heart confirms the balanced relative size of the ventricles. *Bottom right* A rendered view of the ventricular septal defect (*VSD*) viewed from the right ventricular aspect is shown. **B,C** Example of double outlet right ventricle. **B** This projection looks towards the outlets of the heart from the ventricles. The ventricular septum can be visualized and confirms that both the aorta (*Ao*) and pulmonary artery (*PA*) arise from the right ventricle (RV). The muscular out- let septum separating the Ao and PA is also seen. **C** From the right ventricular aspect, the origin of the Ao and PA can be visualized. There are two ventricular septal defects (*1* and *2*) separated by a muscle bar which had not been diagnosed by conventional cross-sectional echocardiography. *LA* left atrium, *LV* left ven- tricle. [→Videos 10.10A–C]

10.5 Three-dimensional echocardiography during catheter intervention and surgery

10.5.1 Imaging during catheter intervention

During catheter interventions, the standard echocardiographic imaging technique is transesophageal echocardiography because of its obvious advantages in providing high-resolution, real-time imaging which can be obtained without interfering with the procedure itself. The transesophageal 3D technique is particularly suitable for near-field structures such as the atrioventricular valves and the atrial septum [39][40]. Thus, it is ideal for imaging during procedures such as device closure of atrial septal defects [11][19][41][42] and ventricular septal defects [43]. The 3D nature of the imaging means that catheter position can be visualized accurately and unique views of deployment of septal occluders can be obtained (◘ Fig. 10.11). Three-dimensional techniques are particularly useful for fenestrated atrial septal defects to ensure that catheters pass across the dominant defect rather than through small fenestrations and to optimize the size of device necessary for effective occlusion, including complex septal defects which require multiple devices to adequately cover the defect [44].

> ❯ The 3D nature of the imaging means that catheter position can be visualized accurately and unique views of deployment of septal occluders can be obtained.

10.5.2 Imaging during surgery

A 3D transesophageal approach as described above may be adopted for children of suitable size who are undergoing cardiac surgery to provide preoperative and postoperative information. An example is shown of a patient with both a supramitral membrane and subaortic stenosis in whom both pathologies can be visualized intraoperatively by interrogation of a single volumetric dataset (◘ Fig. 10.12). For smaller children (and prior to the development of the 3D transesophageal echocardiography probe) an epicardial approach could be employed. This is an approach which has been widely adopted at the authors' institution. The standard transthoracic pediatric 3D ultrasound probe is covered with an enclosed sterile plastic sheath and applied to the heart either before or after opening of the pericardium. The details of this technique have been published elsewhere [12]. This approach has proved extremely effective in obtaining high quality 3D images during surgery for example mitral valve chordal rupture (◘ Fig. 10.12).

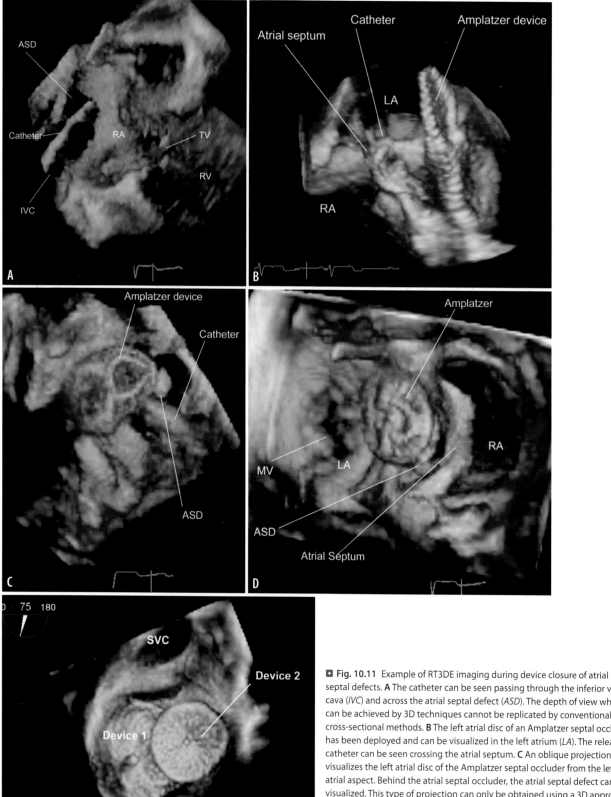

□ Fig. 10.11 Example of RT3DE imaging during device closure of atrial septal defects. **A** The catheter can be seen passing through the inferior vena cava (*IVC*) and across the atrial septal defect (*ASD*). The depth of view which can be achieved by 3D techniques cannot be replicated by conventional cross-sectional methods. **B** The left atrial disc of an Amplatzer septal occluder has been deployed and can be visualized in the left atrium (*LA*). The release catheter can be seen crossing the atrial septum. **C** An oblique projection visualizes the left atrial disc of the Amplatzer septal occluder from the left atrial aspect. Behind the atrial septal occluder, the atrial septal defect can be visualized. This type of projection can only be obtained using a 3D approach. **D** A projection from above the atrial septum allows one to look down towards the atrioventricular valves. The septal occluder can be visualized in position across the atrial septum. **E** Projection from the left atrium demonstrating the advantages of 3D echocardiography when multiple septal occluders are deployed. The relative position of the occluders, in this case visualized from the left atrium, can be appreciated. *TV* tricuspid valve, *RA* right atrium, *RV* right ventricle, *MV* mitral valve, *SVC* superior vena cava. [→Videos 11.11A–E]

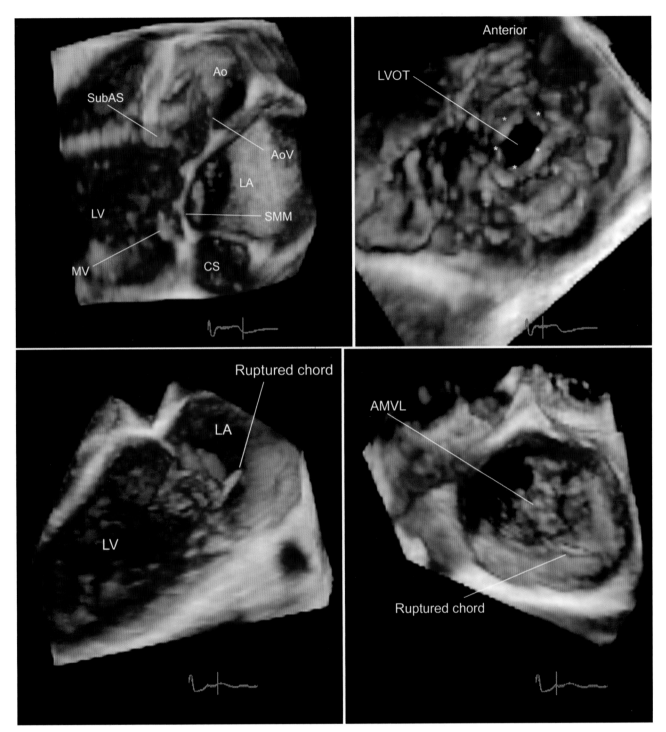

Fig. 10.12 Examples of intraoperative 3D echocardiography. *Top left* This projection is most akin to a conventional parasternal long-axis view and demonstrates a supramitral membrane (*SMM*) above the mitral valve (*MV*). There is a dilated coronary sinus (*CS*) due to an associated left superior vena cava. The region of subaortic stenosis is visualized (*Sub AS*). *Top right* This image of subaortic stenosis is demonstrated as viewed from the left ventricle (*LV*) looking into the left ventricular outflow tract (*LVOT*). The circumferential nature of the region of subaortic stenosis (marked by *asterisks*) is shown in a way which is not possible by conventional 2D techniques. *Bottom left* Epicardial 3D image of chordal rupture (*A2 leaflet*) from a projection akin to a parasternal long-axis view. The flail leaflet of the mitral valve and the ruptured chord are clearly visualized. *Bottom right* View of chordal rupture from a projection from the left atrium (*LA*) looking towards the mitral valve. The flail anterior mitral valve (*AMVL*) leaflet may be seen in the atrium during systole. *Ao* aorta, *SubAS* subaortic stenosis, *AoV* aortic valve, *Ao* aorta, * asterisks mark the circumferential subaortic stenosis. [→Videos 10.12A–D]

10.6   Role of RT3DE in the assessment of cardiac function in children

10.6.1 The left ventricle

Three-dimensional echocardiographic techniques now permit estimation of left ventricular end-diastolic, end-systolic volume, and ejection fraction using techniques which make far fewer assumptions of ventricular shape than conventional cross-sectional techniques. The technique adopted is identical to that used in adult practice which is described in detail in ▶ Chapter 3. Technical issues in this regard involve the faster heart rates in small children. For example, a newborn infant with a heart rate of 150 beats per minute will effectively have half the rate of sampling per cardiac cycle compared to an adult with a heart rate of 75 beats per minute. Patient co-operation is also a significant practical problem to ensure that there are no stitching artifacts related to patient movement. The resolution of the ultrasound system is also extremely important because the technique involves endocardial contour detection to quantitate movement of different cardiac segments. The introduction of a small footprint pediatric 3D probe with a frequency up to 7 MHz represents a significant advance in this regard.

Currently, there are no large, population-based reference ranges of left ventricular volumes in children, estimated by 3D echocardiography. Such data would have to be indexed for body size to take account of growth during childhood. However, recent data have provided some normal data, including comparison of different software analysis packages [45] and other imaging techniques [46][47]. When 3D echocardiography has been compared to other techniques such as MRI or ventriculography, there has been good agreement of left ventricular end-diastolic volume, end-systolic volume, and ejection fraction [48][49][50][51][52]. The observer variability has also been studied which was judged acceptable for clinical practice (±14% interobserver and ±9% intraobserver variability for left ventricular end-diastolic volume) [53]. Such agreement also appears acceptable for patients with abnormally shaped ventricles which is highly relevant to the population with congenital heart disease [54]. Left ventricular mass estimation has been reported, with 3D techniques giving estimations of left ventricular mass which were lower than cross-sectional techniques [55]. Despite the lack of population-based normal ranges of ventricular volumes, at the authors' institution 3D echocardiography has been used to track individual patient's progress, in the assessment of conditions such as dilated cardiomyopathy, myocarditis, and ischemic conditions such as anomalous origin of the left coronary artery. The segmental model of normal wall motion is shown in ◻ Fig. 10.13A as well as a video of a normal 3D study in a child (▶ Video 10.13A). This may be contrasted with the abnormal findings in an infant with an anomalous origin of the left coronary artery from the pulmonary artery which had led to myocardial infarction (◻ Fig. 10.13B).

> ❯ Despite the lack of population-based normal ranges of left ventricular volumes in children, 3D echocardiography has been used to track individual patient's progress.

The segmental model of the left ventricle, commonly used in adult practice, has been directly applied to children. Thus, information regarding regional wall motion and dyssynchrony is obtained in exactly the same way as in adult practice (▶ Chapters 3 and 5). Dyssynchrony is increasingly recognized as a potential problem in the pediatric as well as the adult population. Three-dimensional echocardiography has proved useful in quantitating such dyssynchrony [56][57]. Unique insights are being provided into disease states such as the relationship between the degree of dyssynchrony and systolic ventricular function [57][58] and the importance of ventriculoventricular interaction [56]. Recent studies have provided reference values of the normal range of dyssynchrony index derived from 3D echocardiography in children and adolescents [59][60].

10.6.2 The right ventricle

The right ventricle is a particular challenge to assess echocardiographically due to its complex shape. The right ventricle is wrapped around the left ventricle with an inlet portion which has a completely different anatomic orientation from the outlet. Software which has been developed to model the volume of the left ventricle has been based around a central axis from the mitral valve to the cardiac apex. The right ventricle does not have such a central axis and so software which has been designed for the left ventricle cannot be used to measure right ventricular volume. Aside from modeling the shape of the right ventricle, there is a technical challenge in obtaining a single 3D volumetric dataset which incorporates the inlet, trabecular, and outlet portions of the right ventricle. The outlet is a particular challenge due to its anterior position just behind the chest wall. Nonetheless, published work has demonstrated that calculation of right ventricular volumes and ejection fraction is feasible and correlates reasonably well with other techniques such as MRI [61][62]63].

However, recent data have consistently shown that 3D echocardiography produces lower RV volumes than MRI [64][65][66][67][68]. One software program (RV-Function©, Tomtec, Munich, Germany) has been designed specifically to assess the right ventricle. Analysis by this method is semiautomated utilizing a real-time 3D volumetric dataset. This involves manual landmark setting within the software package coupled with automatic contour detection. This provides information on right ventricular end-diastolic volume, end-systolic volume, and ejection fraction. An example of such an analysis in a child with hypoplastic left heart syndrome is shown in ◻ Fig. 10.13C. One reason why 3D echocardiography might produce lower RV volumes than MRI relates to the difficulty of incorporating the whole RV in the echocardiographic volume. Recently, RV volume estimation has been achieved using »knowledge-based reconstruction« which utilizes a series of 2D images obtained from different sonographic projections and a tracked ultrasound probe. Initial results have shown good agreement with volumes obtained by MRI [67][69].

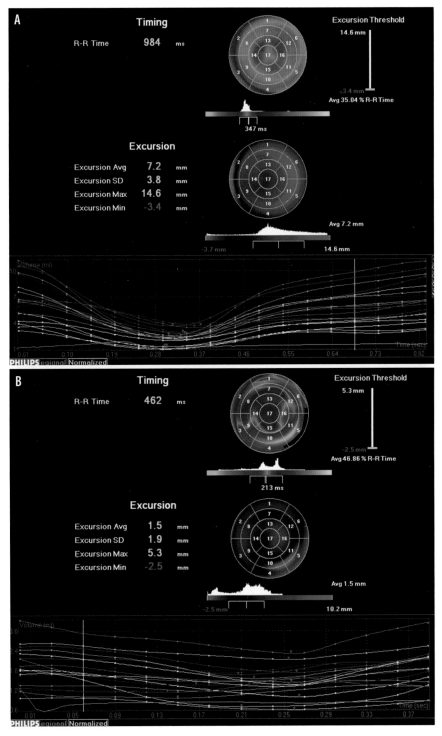

Fig. 10.13 A Assessment of left ventricular function. This is a normal study from a child demonstrating the application of the standard 17-segment model of the left ventricle. The *upper panel* represents the timing of different segments in reaching the minimum volume and *the lower panel* represents the excursion of the different segments when related to the central axis of the left ventricle (▶ Chapter 3). The waveforms in the lower part of the image are the volumes of different segments of the heart during the cardiac cycle. The *red triangles* mark the time at which the minimum systolic volume is reached. In this example these triangles are tightly grouped indicating a high degree of synchrony. **B** Assessment of left ventricular function. This image is from an infant who presented with anomalous origin of the left coronary artery from the pulmonary artery (*PA*) leading to myocardial ischemia and infarction. The *upper panel* and *lower panels* confirm the abnormal timing and excursion of the myocardium. There is paradoxical movement of the inferior and lateral myocardial segments, consistent with myocardial infarction. The *red triangles* in the lower waveforms are far more widely spread than normal indicating a lack of synchrony in motion of the myocardium

□ **Fig. 10.13** (continued) **C** Assessment of right ventricular function. The patient in this example has hypoplastic left heart syndrome. The right ventricle (*RV*) has been modeled to demonstrate the tricuspid and pulmonary valves (shown in *grey*) and the right ventricle itself (*green*). The analysis permits computation of ventricular volumes and ejection fraction. The right ventricle has no central axis to gauge segmental motion and currently no information is provided with regard to synchrony. *TV* tricuspid valve. [→Videos 10.13A–C]

10.7 Conclusion

Three-dimensional echocardiography has shown itself to be a technique which can be applied to children with structural and functional cardiac abnormalities. It is providing new information and perspectives on cardiac morphology and function which are increasing our understanding of disease states and assisting in tailoring appropriate surgical and medical therapies. The noninvasive and repeatable nature of the technique coupled with good acoustic windows in smaller patients mean that it is ideally suited to the pediatric age range. Further enhancements in rapidity of acquisition, spatial resolution, temporal resolution, and software analyses of the raw 3D datasets are likely to enhance its usefulness even further.

References

1. Simpson JM, Miller O (2011) Three-dimensional echocardiography in congenital heart disease. Arch Cardiovasc Dis 104:45–56
2. Takuma S, Zwas DR, Fard A et al (1999) Real-time, 3-dimensional echocardiography acquires all standard 2-dimensional images from 2 volume sets: a clinical demonstration in 45 patients. J Am Soc Echocardiogr 12:1–6
3. Arbeille P, Eder V, Casset D et al (2000) Real-time 3-D ultrasound acquisition and display for cardiac volume and ejection fraction evaluation. Ultrasound Med Biol 26:201–208
4. Roelandt J, Salustri A, Mumm B, Vletter W (1995) Precordial three-dimensional echocardiography with a rotational imaging probe: methods and initial clinical experience. Echocardiography 12:243–252
5. Salustri A, Spitaels S, McGhie J et al (1995) Transthoracic three-dimensional echocardiography in adult patients with congenital heart disease. J Am Coll Cardiol 26:759–767
6. Dall'Agata A, Cromme-Dijkhuis AH, Meijboom FJ et al (1999) Use of three-dimensional echocardiography for analysis of outflow obstruction in congenital heart disease. Am J Cardiol 83:921–925
7. Espinola-Zavaleta N, Vargas-Barron J, Keirns C et al Three-dimensional echocardiography in congenital malformations of the mitral valve. J Am Soc Echocardiogr 15:468–472
8. Simpson JM (2008) Real-time three-dimensional echocardiography of congenital heart disease using a high frequency paediatric matrix transducer. Eur J Echocardiogr 9:222–224
9. Martin-Reyes R, Lopez-Fernandez T, Moreno-Yanguela M et al (2009) Role of real-time three-dimensional transoesophageal echocardiography for guiding transcatheter patent foramen ovale closure. Eur J Echocardiogr 10:148–150
10. Budts W, Troost E, Voigt JU (2008) Optimising device imaging in atrial septal closure by three-dimensional transoesophageal echocardiography. Heart 94:1110
11. Acar P, Massabuau P, Elbaz M (2008) Real-time 3D transoesophageal echocardiography for guiding Amplatzer septal occluder device deployment in an adult patient with atrial septal defect. Eur J Echocardiogr9: 822–823
12. Rawlins DB, Austin C, Simpson JM (2006) Live three-dimensional paediatric intraoperative epicardial echocardiography as a guide to surgical repair of atrioventricular valves. Cardiol Young 16:34–39

13. Simpson J, Miller O, Bell A et al (2012) Image orientation for three-dimensional echocardiography of congenital heart disease. Int J Cardiovasc Imaging 28:743–753

14. Lang RM, Badano LP, Tsang W et al (2012) EAE/ASE recommendations for image acquisition and display using three-dimensional echocardiography. Eur Heart J Cardiovasc Imaging 13:1–46

15. Faletra FF, Nucifora G, Ho SY (2011) Imaging the atrial septum using real-time three-dimensional transesophageal echocardiography: technical tips, normal anatomy, and its role in transseptal puncture. J Am Soc Echocardiogr 24:593–599

16. Pushparajah K, Miller OI, Simpson JM (2010) 3D echocardiography of the atrial septum: anatomical features and landmarks for the echocardiographer. JACC Cardiovasc Imaging3:981–984

17. van den Bosch AE, Ten Harkel DJ, McGhie JS et al (2006) Characterization of atrial septal defect assessed by real-time 3-dimensional echocardiography. J Am Soc Echocardiogr 19:815–821

18. Xie MX, Fang LY, Wang XF et al (2006) Assessment of atrial septal defect area changes during cardiac cycle by live three-dimensional echocardiography. J Cardiol 47:181–187

19. Roberson DA, Cui W, Patel D et al (2011) Three-dimensional transesophageal echocardiography of atrial septal defect: a qualitative and quantitative anatomic study. J Am Soc Echocardiogr 24:600–610

20. Chen FL, Hsiung MC, Nanda N et al (2006) Real time three-dimensional echocardiography in assessing ventricular septal defects: an echocardiographic-surgical correlative study. Echocardiography 23:562–568

21. Mehmood F, Miller AP, Nanda NC et al (2006) Usefulness of live/real time three-dimensional transthoracic echocardiography in the characterization of ventricular septal defects in adults. Echocardiography 23:421–427

22. van den Bosch AE, Ten Harkel DJ, McGhie JS et al (2006) Feasibility and accuracy of real-time 3-dimensional echocardiographic assessment of ventricular septal defects. J Am Soc Echocardiogr 19:7–13

23. Acar P, Abadir S, Aggoun Y (2007) Transcatheter closure of perimembranous ventricular septal defects with Amplatzer occluder assessed by real-time three-dimensional echocardiography. Eur J Echocardiogr 8:110–115

24. Bassil R, Acar P, Abadir S et al (2006) [New approach to perimembranous ventricular septal defect by real-time 3D echocardiography]. Arch Mal Coeur Vaiss 99:471–476

25. van den Bosch AE, Ten Harkel DJ, McGhie JS et al (2006) Surgical validation of real-time transthoracic 3D echocardiographic assessment of atrioventricular septal defects. Int J Cardiol 112:213–218

26. van den Bosch AE, van Dijk VF, McGhie JS et al (2006) Real-time transthoracic three-dimensional echocardiography provides additional information of left-sided AV valve morphology after AVSD repair. Int J Cardiol 106:360–364

27. Hlavacek AM, Crawford FA, Jr., Chessa KS, Shirali GS (2006) Real-time three-dimensional echocardiography is useful in the evaluation of patients with atrioventricular septal defects. Echocardiography 23:225–231

28. Takahashi K, Mackie AS, Thompson R et al (2012) Quantitative real-time three-dimensional echocardiography provides new insight into the mechanisms of mitral valve regurgitation post-repair of atrioventricular septal defect. J Am Soc Echocardiogr 25:1231–1244

29. Bharucha T, Sivaprakasam MC, Haw MP et al (2008) The angle of the components of the common atrioventricular valve predicts the outcome of surgical correction in patients with atrioventricular septal defect and common atrioventricular junction. J Am Soc Echocardiogr 21:1099–1104

30. Kuperstein R, Feinberg MS, Carasso S et al (2006) The added value of real-time 3-dimensional echocardiography in the diagnosis of isolated cleft mitral valve in adults. J Am Soc Echocardiogr 19:811–814

31. Abadir S, Dulac Y, Taktak A, Acar P (2005) Images in cardiology: cleft mitral valve assessed by transthoracic real time three dimensional echocardiography. Heart 91:1632

32. Sinha A, Kasliwal RR, Nanda NC et al (2004) Live three-dimensional transthoracic echocardiographic assessment of isolated cleft mitral valve. Echocardiography 21:657–661

33. Valverde I, Rawlins D, Austin C, Simpson JM (2012) Three-dimensional echocardiography in the management of parachute mitral valve. Eur Heart J Cardiovasc Imaging 13:446

34. Acar P, Abadir S, Roux D, et al (2006) Ebstein's anomaly assessed by real-time 3-D echocardiography. Ann Thorac Surg 82:731–733

35. Vettukattil JJ, Bharucha T, Anderson RH (2007) Defining Ebstein's malformation using three-dimensional echocardiography. Interact Cardiovasc Thorac Surg 6:685–690

36. Mercer-Rosa L, Fedec A, Gruber P, Seliem M (2006) Cor triatriatum sinister with and without left ventricular inflow obstruction: visualization of the entire supravalvular membrane by real-time three-dimensional echocardiography. Impact on clinical management of individual patient. Congenit Heart Dis 1:335–339

37. Vogel M, Simpson JM, Anderson D (2008) Live three-dimensional echocardiography of cor triatriatum in a child. Heart 94:794

38. Pushparajah K, Barlow A, Tran VH et al (2013) A systematic three-dimensional echocardiographic approach to assist surgical planning in double outlet right ventricle. Echocardiography 30:234–238

39. Balzer J, Kelm M, Kuhl HP (2009) Real-time three-dimensional transoesophageal echocardiography for guidance of non-coronary interventions in the catheter laboratory. Eur J Echocardiogr 10:341–349

40. Nomoto K, Hollinger I, DiLuozzo G, Fischer GW (2009) Recognition of a cleft mitral valve utilizing real-time three-dimensional transoesophageal echocardiography. Eur J Echocardiogr 10:367–369

41. Balzer J, Kuhl H, Franke A (2008) Real-time three-dimensional transoesophageal echocardiography for guidance of atrial septal defect closures. Eur Heart J 29:2226

42. Morgan GJ, Casey F, Craig B, Sands A (2008) Assessing ASDs prior to device closure using 3D echocardiography. Just pretty pictures or a useful clinical tool? Eur J Echocardiogr 9:478–482

43. Charakida M, Qureshi S, Simpson JM (2013) 3D echocardiography for planning and guidance of interventional closure of VSD. JACC Cardiovasc Imaging 6:120–123

44. Ojala T, Rosenthal E, Nugent K et al. (2013) Live 3-dimensional echocardiography to guide closure of residual atrial septal defects after percutaneous closure. J Am Coll Cardiol: Cardiovascular Imaging 6:523–525

45. Seguela PE, Hascoet S, Brierre G et al (2012) Feasibility of three-dimensional transthoracic echocardiography to evaluate right ventricular volumes in children and comparison to left ventricular values. Echocardiography 29:492–501

46. Friedberg MK, Su X, Tworetzky W et al (2010) Validation of 3D echocardiographic assessment of left ventricular volumes, mass, and ejection fraction in neonates and infants with congenital heart disease: a comparison study with cardiac MRI. Circ Cardiovasc Imaging 3:735–742

47. Laser KT, Bunge M, Hauffe P et al (2010) Left ventricular volumetry in healthy children and adolescents: comparison of two different real-time three-dimensional matrix transducers with cardiovascular magnetic resonance. Eur J Echocardiogr 11:138–148

48. Riehle TJ, Mahle WT, Parks WJ et al (2008) Real-time three-dimensional echocardiographic acquisition and quantification of left ventricular indices in children and young adults with congenital heart disease: comparison with magnetic resonance imaging. J Am Soc Echocardiogr 21:78–83

49. Poutanen T, Ikonen A, Jokinen E et al (2001) Transthoracic three-dimensional echocardiography is as good as magnetic resonance imaging in measuring dynamic changes in left ventricular volume during the heart cycle in children. Eur J Echocardiogr 2:31–39

50. Pouleur AC, le Polain de Waroux JB, Pasquet A et al (2008) Assessment of left ventricular mass and volumes by three-dimensional echocardiography in patients with or without wall motion abnormalities: comparison against cine magnetic resonance imaging. Heart 94:1050–1057

51. Lu X, Xie M, Tomberlin D et al (2008) How accurately, reproducibly, and efficiently can we measure left ventricular indices using M-mode, 2-dimensional, and 3-dimensional echocardiography in children? Am Heart J 155:946–953

52. Iino M, Shiraishi H, Ichihashi K et al (2007) Volume measurement of the left ventricle in children using real-time three-dimensional echocardiography: comparison with ventriculography. J Cardiol 49:221–229

53. Baker G, Flack E, Hlavacek A et al (2006) Variability and resource utilization of bedside three-dimensional echocardiographic quantitative measurements of left ventricular volume in congenital heart disease. Congenit Heart Dis 1:309–314

54. Soriano BD, Hoch M, Ithuralde A et al (2008) Matrix-array 3-dimensional echocardiographic assessment of volumes, mass, and ejection fraction in young pediatric patients with a functional single ventricle: a comparison study with cardiac magnetic resonance. Circulation 117:1842–1848

55. Poutanen T, Jokinen E (2007) Left ventricular mass in 169 healthy children and young adults assessed by three-dimensional echocardiography. Pediatr Cardiol 2007;28:201–207

56. Raedle-Hurst TM, Mueller M, Rentzsch A et al (2009) Assessment of left ventricular dyssynchrony and function using real-time 3-dimensional echocardiography in patients with congenital right heart disease. Am Heart J 157:791–798

57. Baker GH, Hlavacek AM, Chessa KS et al (2008) Left ventricular dysfunction is associated with intraventricular dyssynchrony by 3-dimensional echocardiography in children. J Am Soc Echocardiogr 21:230–233

58. Friedberg MK, Silverman NH, Dubin AM, Rosenthal DN (2007) Mechanical dyssynchrony in children with systolic dysfunction secondary to cardiomyopathy: a Doppler tissue and vector velocity imaging study. J Am Soc Echocardiogr 20:756–763

59. Cui W, Gambetta K, Zimmerman F et al (2010) Real-time three-dimensional echocardiographic assessment of left ventricular systolic dyssynchrony in healthy children. J Am Soc Echocardiogr 23:1153–1159

60. Ten Harkel AD, Van Osch-Gevers M, Helbing WA (2009) Real-time transthoracic three dimensional echocardiography: normal reference data for left ventricular dyssynchrony in adolescents. J Am Soc Echocardiogr 22:933–938

61. Grison A, Maschietto N, Reffo E et al (2007) Three-dimensional echocardiographic evaluation of right ventricular volume and function in pediatric patients: validation of the technique. J Am Soc Echocardiogr 20:921–929

62. Tamborini G, Brusoni D, Torres Molina JE et al (2008) Feasibility of a new generation three-dimensional echocardiography for right ventricular volumetric and functional measurements. Am J Cardiol 102:499–505

63. Lu X, Nadvoretskiy V, Bu L et al (2008) Accuracy and reproducibility of real-time three-dimensional echocardiography for assessment of right ventricular volumes and ejection fraction in children. J Am Soc Echocardiogr 21:84–89

64. van der Zwaan HB, Helbing WA, McGhie JS et al (2010) Clinical value of real-time three-dimensional echocardiography for right ventricular quantification in congenital heart disease: validation with cardiac magnetic resonance imaging. J Am Soc Echocardiogr 23:134–140

65. Crean AM, Maredia N, Ballard G et al (2011) 3D Echo systematically underestimates right ventricular volumes compared to cardiovascular magnetic resonance in adult congenital heart disease patients with moderate or severe RV dilatation. J Cardiovasc Magn Reson 13:78

66. Grewal J, Majdalany D, Syed I et al (2010) Three-dimensional echocardiographic assessment of right ventricular volume and function in adult patients with congenital heart disease: comparison with magnetic resonance imaging. Journal of the American Society of Echocardiography 23:127–133

67. Dragulescu A, Grosse-Wortmann L, Fackoury C, Mertens L (2012) Echocardiographic assessment of right ventricular volumes: a comparison of different techniques in children after surgical repair of tetralogy of Fallot. European Heart Journal–Cardiovascular Imaging 13:596–604

68. Khoo NS, Young A, Occleshaw C et al (2009) Assessments of right ventricular volume and function using three-dimensional echocardiography in older children and adults with congenital heart disease: comparison with cardiac magnetic resonance imaging. J Am Soc Echocardiogr 22:1279–1288

69. Dragulescu A, Grosse-Wortmann L, Fackoury C et al (2011) Echocardiographic assessment of right ventricular volumes after surgical repair of tetralogy of fallot: clinical validation of a new echocardiographic method. Journal of the American Society of Echocardiography 24:1191–1198

Cardiac tumors and sources of embolism

Björn Plicht

T. Buck et al. (Hrsg.), *Three-dimensional Echocardiography*,
DOI 10.1007/978-3-642-36799-1_11, © Springer-Verlag Berlin Heidelberg 2014

Cerebral or peripheral embolism is a frequent indication for echocardiographic studies to rule out a cardiac mass or any other potential source of embolism. Behind the diagnosis »cardiac mass« is a broad spectrum of pathologies that must be taken into account: primary or secondary cardiac tumors are rare clinical conditions but are a significant cause of morbidity and mortality, while intracardiac thrombi are more frequent. Other potential cardiac sources of embolism are patent foramen ovale, degenerative valvular alterations, endocarditis, or aortic pathologies.

Conventional two-dimensional (2D) transesophageal echocardiography has been demonstrated to discriminate between conditions with a high risk for embolization (atrial thrombus, mobile aortic thrombi, patent foramen ovale (PFO) with interatrial septum aneurysm, atrial myxoma, valvular vegetations) and a lower risk for embolization (spontaneous echo contrast, reduced flow velocities within the left atrial appendage, PFO without IAS aneurysm, mitral valve prolapse, plaques, and ulceration of the aorta) [1][2].

With the unique advantage of providing en face views of cardiac structures by real-time 3D echocardiography (RT3DE), the true dimensions of cardiac masses and their orientation to other cardiac structures can be displayed in an anatomically realistic manner [3][4]. Moreover, morphologic patterns of intracardiac masses like mobility, surface structure, and deformation may improve their identification. Volumetry of cardiac masses has been shown to improve risk estimation and therapy monitoring [5]. All these advantages are assisting the communication between cardiologist and surgeon when planning surgical therapy [6][7].

Current recommendations by the European Association of Echocardiography (EAE) for echocardiography use in the diagnosis and management of cardiac sources of embolism see an additional benefit of the new 3D imaging modalities, particular in the characterization of intracardiac tumors [8].

> Using real-time 3D echocardiography the true dimensions of cardiac masses and their orientation to other cardiac structures can be displayed in an anatomically realistic manner.

11.1   Sources of embolism

11.1.1 Cardiac and vascular thrombi, spontaneous echo contrast

Thrombus formation is one of the most common causes for stroke [9]. Usually predisposing factors can be found like valvular heart disease which leads to atrial dilation, atrial fibrillation, wall motion abnormalities post myocardial infarction, or thrombophilia.

Spontaneous echo contrast (SEC) is often found in patients with dilated atria due to valvular heart disease and/or atrial fibrillation. It represents aggregation of the cellular components of blood in the conditions of blood stasis or low-velocity blood flow [10]. As a lower risk factor for embolization SEC, however, indicates a high risk for thrombus formation especially in the left atrial appendage (LAA). Evidence of SEC should motivate a closer search for manifest thrombus formation. Live 3D echocardiography is able to display formation and dissolution of SEC during a heart cycle as shown in ☐ Fig. 11.1; however, it is not clear yet whether this offers any advantage over conventional 2D transthoracic echocardiography (TTE). In this case, live 3D echocardiography also detected thrombus formation in the left atrium (☐ Fig. 11.2).

As described in a case series by Duncan et al. [11], RT3D TTE was found to be helpful in the evaluation of left ventricular thrombi, particularly in identifying the exact point of attachment and the delineation of absence or presence of focal echolucent areas indicative for clot lysis, which may have a potential therapeutic and prognostic implication (☐ Fig. 11.3). The success of thrombolytics and anticoagulants can be monitored by 3D sizing of masses based on RT3DE datasets which was demonstrated in a study by Sinha et al. [12], where the reduction of left ventricular thrombus size was assessed in serial RT3D TTE examinations under heparin administration.

Anwar et al. [13] compared 2D TTE with RT3D TTE using 2D TEE for reference demonstrating higher detection rate of LA and LAA thrombi with RT3DE (Kappa 2D TEE vs. 3D TTE 0.9; Kappa 2D TTE vs. 3D TTE between 0.21 and 0.45). Recently, Marek et al. demonstrated an additional value for RT3D TEE for discrimination of LAA thrombi and identification of muscular trabeculae [14]. Beside improved detection of LA thrombi, RT3DE can be helpful in the discrimination and localization of multiple masses in the LA atrium as illustrated in . Fig. 11.4. As a rare and impressive finding, ☐ Fig. 11.5 illustrates the representation of a ball thrombus in the RA by RT3DE.

For the examination of LAA for thrombi, RT3D TEE provides a direct view into the LAA, thereby, permitting improved anatomic assessment of the often irregular shape of the LAA (☐ Fig. 11.6). By displaying two simultaneous orthogonal planes using the matrix array transducer, the acquisition of a live 3D dataset can be planned. A RT3D TEE color Doppler dataset might be helpful in identifying a flow pattern within the LAA. Mizuguchi et al. [15] demonstrated that the use of RT3D TEE helped to revise the false diagnosis of a LAA thrombus which was correctly diagnosed to be the septum of a bilobular appendage. A recent study defined morphologic and functional parameters derived from RT3D datasets in a larger collective, even LAA ejection fraction, which not surprisingly is reduced in the presence of atrial fibrillation [16].

Beyond diagnostic use, RT3DE imaging of the atrial level and LAA may play an important role in guiding and monitoring interventional LAA occlusion, similar to the benefit observed in other interventions [17] especially when transseptal puncture is performed (see ▶ Chapter 12) [18]. As a possible complication of LAA occlusion, thrombus formation on the Amplatzer Cardiac Plug (St. Jude Medical, St. Paul, MN, USA) has recently been described, especially in patients with reduced left ventricular function [19]. In some cases the central screw of the device seemed to be the origin of the thrombus. Extension and mobility of the thrombus can be ideally demonstrated by RT3D imaging (☐ Fig. 11.7).

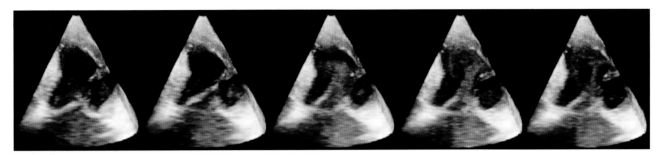

Fig. 11.1 Series of RT3D TTE images illustrating massive spontaneous echo contrast traveling through the mitral valve and its resolution in the left ventricle in the same patient as shown in Fig. 12.2. In contrast to the 2D pictures provided by the xPlane views shown in Fig. 12.2, live 3D visualization provides the impression of a cloud of smoke dissolving in the left ventricle. [→Video 11.1]

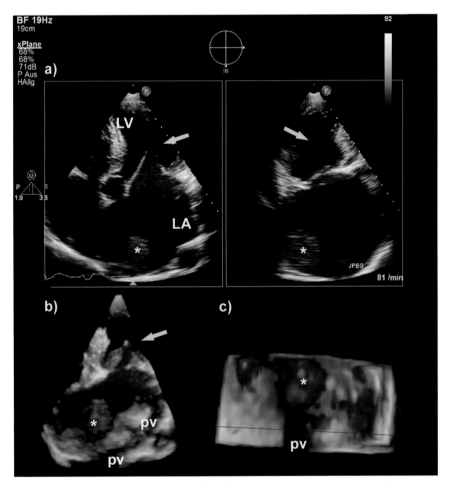

Fig. 11.2 Thrombus formation (*) within an extremely enlarged left atrium (*LA*) with spontaneous echo contrast passing through the mitral valve in the same patient as shown in Fig. 12.1. **a** The 2D xPlane view provides simultaneous detection of the thrombus location within the LA in two perpendicular views. **b,c** The spatial relation of the thrombus to the pulmonary veins (*PV*) could only be revealed by RT3DE imaging which enabled a direct view to the surfaces of the LA roof. By choosing an angulated perspective into the LA both PVs could be displayed, while a direct view from the mitral valve to the roof of the LA gives an impression of the extension of the thrombus. *LV* left ventricle. [→Videos 11.2a–c]

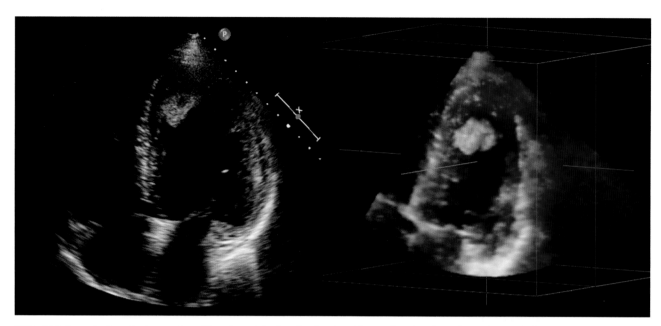

Fig. 11.3 Example of a patient presenting with stroke and clotting disorder where 2D transthoracic echocardiography unveiled an apical thrombus within the LV which was confirmed by histology after embolization into the right lower limb. The 2D echocardiography shows the cut plane through the thrombus demonstrating an inhomogeneous structure, while the whole extension was difficult to assess due to mobility of the structure. RT3D TTE presents the full extension, shape, and mobility of the thrombus. [→Videos 11.3a,b]

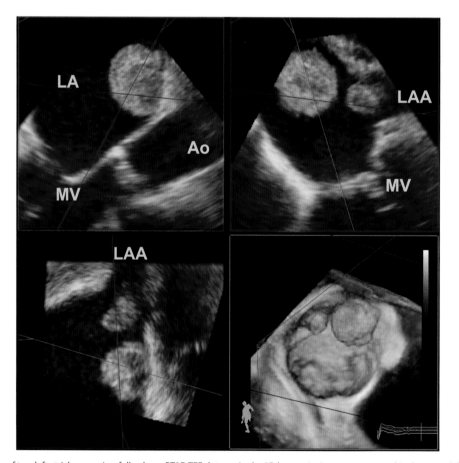

Fig. 11.4 Illustration of two left atrial masses in a full volume RT3D TEE dataset. In the 2D long-axis view as represented in the *upper left panel* of the multiplanar representation (*MPR*), the mass might be considered as to be a myxoma. However, with the detection of the second mass growing out of the left atrial appendage (*LAA; upper right and lower left panel*) with the typical appearance of a left atrial appendage thrombus, both masses are most likely thrombi. The location of the two thrombi can be clearly appreciated in the 3D image with the smaller thrombus sitting in the left atrial appendage and the larger thrombus sitting on the anterior left atrial wall. *LA* left atrium, *MV* mitral valve, *Ao* aorta. [→Video 11.4]

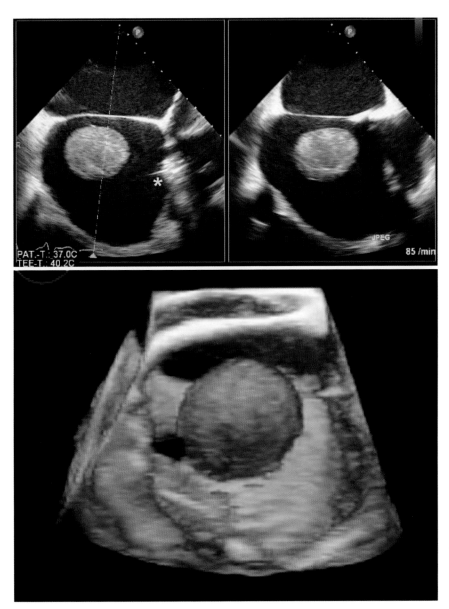

☐ Fig. 11.5 Example of a ball thrombus in the right atrium in a 72-year-old patient with mechanical tricuspid valve prosthesis (*asterisk*) and severely dilated right atrium. The *upper image* shows visualization of the thrombus in two simultaneous orthogonal views using xPlane mode demonstrating the thrombus is not attached to any wall. RT3D TEE image (*below*) provides full spatial capture of the thrombus moving freely through the right atrial cavity but mainly bouncing from the interatrial septum (*IAS*) motion up and down between the IAS and tricuspid valve prosthesis. [→Video 11.5A,B]

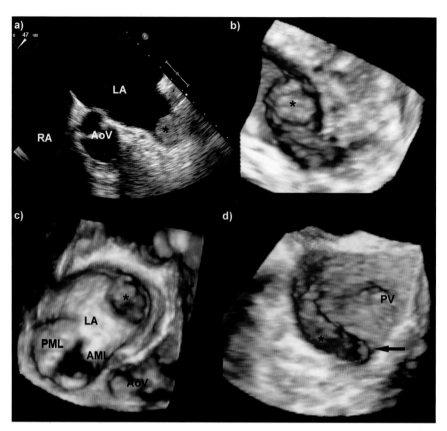

◘ Fig. 11.6 Example of a large thrombus within the left atrial appendage (*LAA*) in a patient with mitral stenosis and permanent atrial fibrillation. **a** Transesophageal 2D image showing thrombus within the LAA (*asterisk*). **b** Live 3D view demonstrating the full extension of the thrombus filling the LAA. **c** RT3DE full volume dataset with a view from the left atrium (*LA*) to the mitral valve and LAA: the LAA with the thrombus (*asterisk*) lies antero-lateral to the mitral valve with the posterior (*PML*) and anterior leaflet (*AML*). **d** Slight rotation of the dataset reveals the anatomic relation of the LAA with the thrombus (*asterisk*) to the upper left pulmonary vein (*PV*). The *arrow* highlights the entrance of the LAA. *AoV* aortic valve. [→Videos 11.6a–d]

RT3DE is also very helpful in identifying the origin of a thrombus as demonstrated in ◘ Fig. 11.8, where 2D TEE was not definite in identifying whether the thrombus was adherent to a cardiac structure or a central venous catheter. Mechanical heart valves are also prone to thrombosis with the consequence of functional failure. Faletra et al. [20] reported a case of thrombosis of a mechanical mitral valve prosthesis with sequential 3D studies during thrombolysis therapy demonstrating a comprehensive evaluation of number, location, and size of thrombi and their evolution. The example shown in ◘ Fig. 11.9 illustrates different perspectives for the evaluation of a thrombosed aortic valve prosthesis using RT3D TEE showing the whole extension of mobile and fixed thrombotic material.

> ❯ Beside identifying the exact location and origin of a thrombus, RT3DE provides monitoring of the size of thrombi during thrombolytic therapy.

Evaluation of the ascending and descending aorta sometimes reveals intraluminal thrombi (◘ Fig. 11.10) or severe plaque formation as the possible source of embolism. RT3D TTE has been shown to clearly visualize the extension and adherence of aortic wall thrombi and plaques [21]. Beyond this, RT3D TEE provides high-resolution en face views to the intimal surface of the aortic wall (◘ Fig. 11.11).

11.1.2 Patent foramen ovale

With an incidence of more than 20% in the general population, the patent foramen ovale (PFO) with characteristic intermittent right-to-left shunt over the interatrial septum (IAS) is a common finding [22]. It becomes clinically relevant after occurrence of a stroke event especially when associated with an interatrial septum aneurysm (◘ Fig. 11.12) [23]. Several published cases demonstrated in-transit thrombi moving across PFO in RT3D TEE [24][25], confirming the concept of being a source of embolism.

A recent study by Monte et al. [26] demonstrated the usefulness of RT3D TTE in the detection of PFO compared to 2D echocardiography. Particularly RT3D TEE enables a unique en face view of the entire interatrial septum which allows identification of the morphology and exact location of the right-to-left shunt. In the example presented in ◘ Fig. 11.13, the flap-like opening of the septum secundum could be clearly identified. Especially in complex anatomies like multiple PFO openings or long tunnels RT3D TEE is superior to 2D TEE [27].

To acquire a direct 3D view toward the IAS, the TEE probe should be adjusted to show a conventional 2D short-axis view of the aortic valve with the IAS near the transducer. Activation of the live 3D zoom mode and narrowing the 3D sector in the two

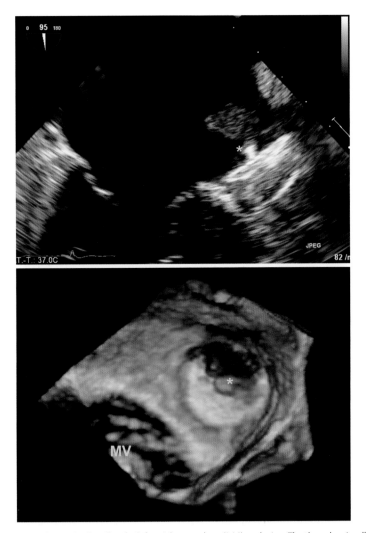

■ **Fig. 11.7** Thrombus formation on an Amplatzer Cardiac Plug for left atrial appendage (*LAA*) occlusion. The thrombus is adherent to the central screw (*asterisk*) of the device. The *upper figure* shows a 2D cut plane through the central screw with the mass connected to it, while the *lower figure* gives an idea of thrombus extension and anatomic correlation of the LAA occluder to the mitral valve (*MV*). [→Video 11.7a,b]

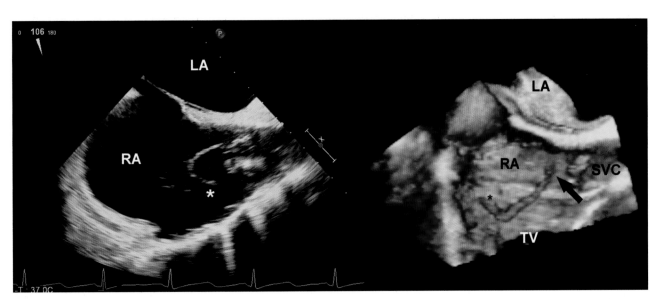

■ **Fig. 11.8** Example of the detection of a filiform thrombus (*asterisk*) in the right atrium (*RA*) prior to transseptal puncture. *Left* In the 2D TEE image, the origin of the thrombus remains uncertain. *Right* RT3D TEE reveals that the thrombus (*asterisk*) is attached to the right atrial wall but not to a central venous catheter (not displayed). *LA* left atrium, *TV* tricuspid valve, *SVC* superior vena cava. [→Videos 11.8a,b]

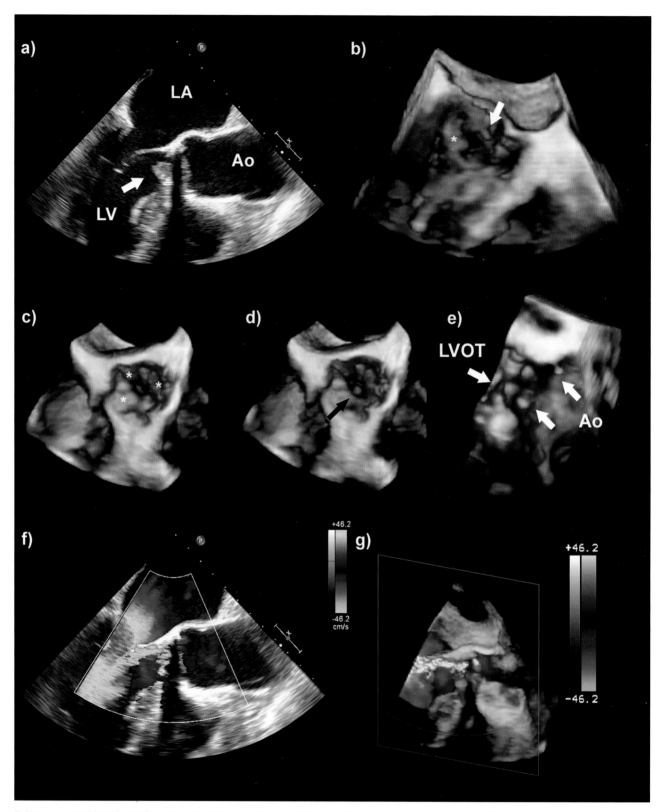

❑ **Fig. 11.9** Acute thrombosis of a mechanical aortic valve prosthesis (*AVP*) in a patient undergoing urologic surgery with insufficient anticoagulation.
a The 2D transesophageal long-axis view shows a thrombus mass attached to the AVP. **b** RT3DE view from the left ventricular outflow tract toward the AVP showing a thrombotic mass (*asterisk*) on the AVP and mobile structures moving into the LVOT (*white arrow*). **c** Live 3D dataset showing a view from the aortic root to the AVP with multiple thrombus formations (*asterisk*) with one mobile thrombotic structure prolapsing through the valve (*arrow*) shown in **d**.
e Cropping the aortic roof reveals a view to the AVP with the presentation of multiple mobile thrombotic masses (*white arrows*). **f, g** The 2D and RT3D color Doppler data sets showing mild-to-moderate aortic regurgitation through the thrombosed AVP. *LA* left atrium, *LV* left ventricle, *Ao* aorta, *LVOT* left ventricular outflow tract. [→Videos 11.9a–c,e–g]

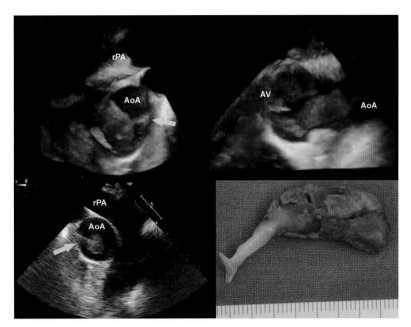

◘ Fig. 11.10 Example of a 22-year-old male presenting after sudden major stroke who had a blunt chest trauma in his history years ago. *Bottom left* Initial 2D TEE detected a mobile mass within the ascending aorta (*AoA*) with pedunculated adherence (*arrow*). *Top* RT3D TEE clearly visualized the relationship between the aortic valve and the mass as well as shape and size of the mass and its adherence to the aortic wall (*arrow*). *Lower right* Immediate surgery revealed a large thrombus attached to damaged endothelium probably due to the prior chest trauma. *rPA* right pulmonary artery. [→Videos 11.10a–c]

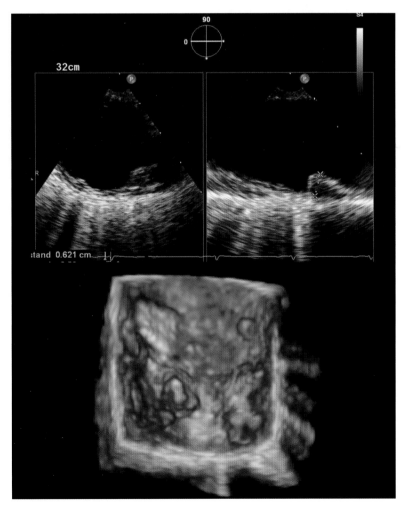

◘ Fig. 11.11 Example of severe atherosclerotic plaque formation in the descending aorta. While in the 2D xPlane view (*top*), the plaques are visualized in two orthogonal views for cross-sectional assessment, RT3D TEE provides a direct en face view to the surface of the aortic wall providing an anatomically realistic representation of a »crater landscape« caused by aortic atherosclerosis (*bottom*). [→Videos 11.11a,b]

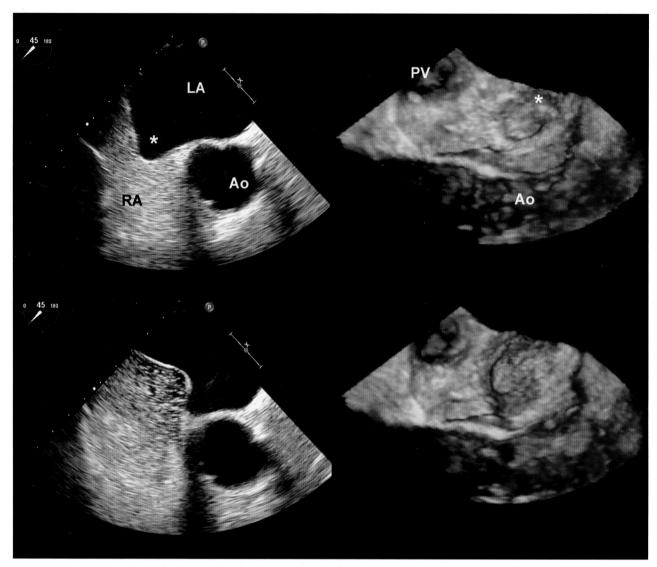

◘ Fig. 11.12 Example of an interatrial septum (*IAS*) aneurysm. The upper 2D and RT3D TEE images are representing the IAS (*asterisk*) bulged toward the right atrium (*RA*) which is fully filled with contrast bubbles. *Upper right* The RT3DE view from the left atrium (*LA*) toward the IAS shows the fossa ovalis (*asterisk*) and its anatomic relation to the aortic root (*Ao*) and a right pulmonary vein (*PV*). *Bottom* After the Valsalva maneuver, the IAS bulges towards the LA. No contrast passage across the IAS could be detected. [→Videos 11.12a,b]

simultaneous orthogonal 2D views to the region of interest provides a high frame rate RT3DE image. Then a longer loop should be acquired by adjusting the heart cycles to be recorded up to 20 cycles in order to visualize contrast agent flush without and with a Valsalva maneuver. In RT3DE, the IAS itself sometimes appears very thin and translucent, with even a complete dropout artifact mimicking an ASD in some cases (see example in ▶ Chapter 2.6.2). By adjusting the gain settings, slightly better visualization can be achieved accompanied by an increase of gain artifacts in other regions of the sector. In these cases, the use of right heart contrast agents can help to show the distinct anatomy of the IAS as the surface boundary between the contrast-filled right atrium and the left atrium. In addition, a combination of both 2D and RT3D TEE imaging can help differentiate dropout artifacts from a true ASD.

> In the RT3DE en face view to the IAS, the IAS itself sometimes appears very thin and translucent, with even a complete dropout artifact mimicking an ASD in some cases.

11.1.3 Infective endocarditis

Two-dimensional transesophageal echocardiography is currently the gold standard for the detection of vegetations as a cause of infective endocarditis with excellent specificity and sensitivity [28]. Experience on the value of RT3DE for diagnosis of endocarditis is limited so far in the literature. Liu et al. [29] described superior specificity (100% vs. 88.2%) of RT3D TTE in the detection of vegetations compared to conventional 2D TTE, but with similar sensitivity (91.6%). However, RT3D TEE has been

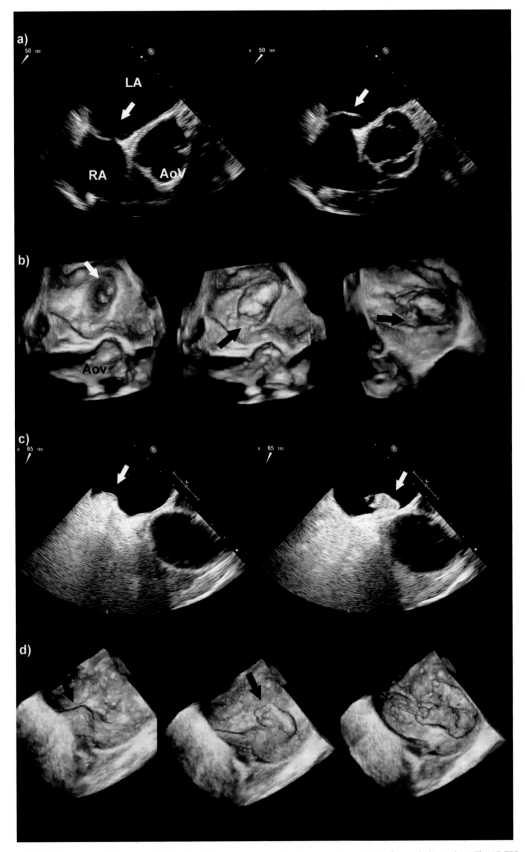

◘ **Fig. 11.13** Example of a large patent foramen ovale (PFO) with spontaneous contrast passage in a patient after embolic stroke. **a** The 2D TEE shows an interatrial septum (*IAS*) aneurysm (*white arrow*) in aortic valve (*AoV*) short-axis view. **b** In live 3D zoom images, the complete IAS is shown with the fossa ovalis bulging towards the RA (*left, white arrow*) and detection of the PFO when the IAS is bulging towards the LA (*black arrow*). **c** 2D TEE proved the PFO by demonstration of IAS bulging toward the LA (*left, arrow*) with contrast passage across the IAS (*right, arrow*). **d** Live 3D zoom provided a 3D view of the entire LA space showing the IAS bulging (*left, arrow*) and the cloud of contrast bubbles passing through the IAS. *RA* right atrium. [→Videos 11.13a–d]

demonstrated to improve management of infective endocarditis due to better visualization of infective complications like chordal rupture, leaflet perforation, or abscess formation (◼ Fig. 11.14) [30][31][32], especially in complicated cases like prosthetic valve endocarditis [33]. Single vegetations can be accurately sized by volumetry using available 3D software [5].

A major advantage of RT3DE's three-dimensional demonstration of infective complications like abscess formation is that it significantly improves communication between the cardiologist and cardiac surgeon in the operating room, as described by Jungwirth et al. for mitral valve reconstruction [7]. When planning surgery for infective endocarditis, RT3DE en face views of the mitral or aortic valve combined with 2D cross-sectional views provides detailed information of the structure and destruction of the valve for decision-making on valve repair (see examples in ▶ Fig. 7.22 and ▶ Fig. 7.46 in Chapter 7).

Due to the irregular and fast motion of vegetations, volume datasets acquired in the live 3D mode (see ▶ Chapter 2) are the most informative because of the relatively high spatial and temporal resolution with the avoidance of stitch artifacts (◼ Fig. 11.15). As a potential limitation, live 3D TEE volumes might be too narrow to encompass the entire mitral valve. In addition, a broad full volume should also be recorded to obtain an overview of the region of interest for the detection of abscesses with potential communication with surrounding cardiac structures (◼ Fig. 11.16). Intracardiac implants, like pacemaker and defibrillator probes, should be displayed using the same techniques.

> RT3DE en face views of the mitral or aortic valve combined with 2D views provide detailed information of the structure and destruction of the valve for decision making on valve repair.

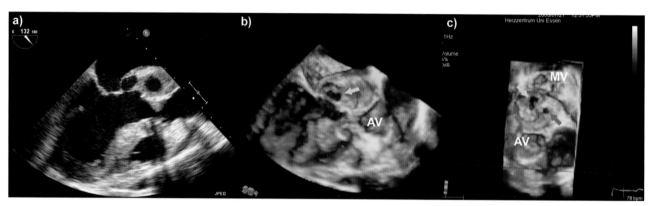

◼ **Fig. 11.14** Aortic root abscess due to *Staphylococcus aureus* endocarditis of an aortic valve bioprosthesis. **a** Two-dimensional TEE detected the extension and location of the abscess in a long-axis view and demonstrated communication to the left ventricular outflow tract (*arrow*). **b** Full volume RT3DE revealed the volume of the cavity and the exact position of the communication (*arrow*) in a slightly rotated modified long-axis view. **c** By cropping the dataset from its top (*blue plane*) to demonstrate the anatomic relation to the aortic (*AV*) and mitral valve (*MV*), a second communication (*red arrow*) from the abscess to the left ventricle was unexpectedly revealed. [→Videos 11.14a–c]

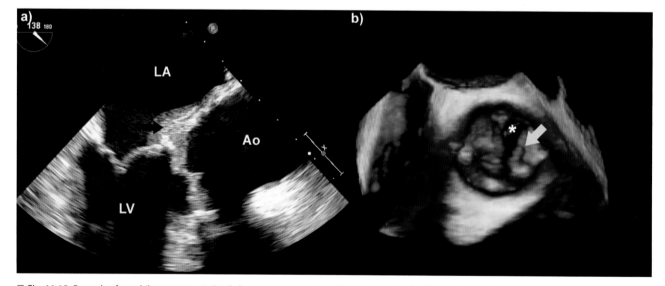

◼ **Fig. 11.15** Example of a mobile vegetation in *Staphylococcus aureus* endocarditis of an aortic valve bioprosthesis. **a** The 2D TEE long-axis view shows thickening of the prosthesis leaflets as well as thickening of the fibrous trigonum suspicious of an aortic root abscess (*arrow*). **b** The RT3D TEE en face view from the aortic root to the prosthesis reveals a mobile vegetation (*arrow*) attached at the valve and a large defect of one leaflet (***). *LA* left atrium, *LV* left ventricle, *Ao* aorta [→Videos 11.15a,b]

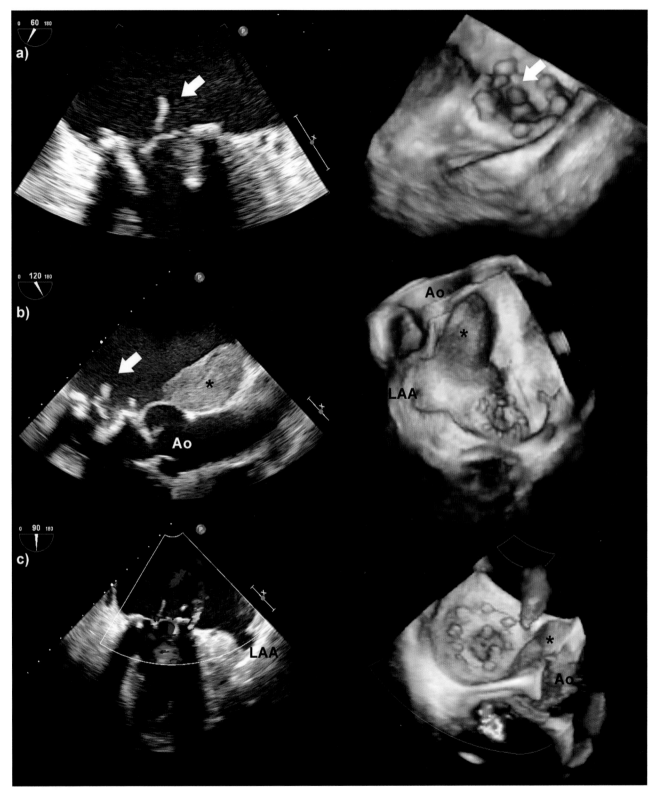

☐ **Fig. 11.16** Example of 2D and RT3DE examinations in a patient with bioprosthetic mitral valve replacement and with acute spondylodiscitis presenting with major embolic stroke, recurrent fever, and elevated inflammation markers. **a** The 2D TEE and live 3D zoom images of the bioprosthesis showing a mobile vegetation as a sign of infective endocarditis attached to one leaflet (*arrow*). **b** The 2D TEE showed spontaneous echo contrast and a large thrombus formation at the anterior wall of the severely enlarged left atrium (*LA*). The 2D cross-sectional view could clearly detect thrombus layering (*) due to appositional growth. The RT3DE full volume dataset showing nearly the entire left atrium, however, revealed the whole extent of the thrombus. **c** The 2D and RT3DE representations of a small anterolateral paravalvular leakage as a cause of endocarditis with additional detection of trace valvular regurgitation. *Ao* aorta, *LAA* left atrial append-age. [→Videos 11.16a–f]

11.2   Primary cardiac tumors

The prevalence of primary cardiac tumors is between 0.001% and 0.3% based on autopsy data [34]. More than 75% of the tumors were benign—nearly half of them being myxomas.

The initial clinical presentation can be an embolic event, symptoms of valve obstruction, or conduction disturbances; however, most are diagnosed incidentally. Identification of the etiology of the tumor by echocardiography might be challenging even for the most experienced examiners. RT3D TEE provides improved assessment of size, shape, and location of the tumor as well as its mobility and the exact site and extent of adherence to other cardiac structures as described by Plana et al. [3].

RT3D color Doppler echocardiography might be useful in the evaluation of tumor vascularization as well as flow acceleration around the mass due to flow obstruction (◘ Fig. 11.17).

> ⟩ RT3DE has been demonstrated to provide accurate anatomic visualization as well as improved identification of the spatial relation of a myxoma to the interatrial septum.

11.2.1 Primary benign cardiac tumors

■ **Myxoma**

In the rare condition of primary cardiac tumors, myxoma is the most common, representing 50% of all benign cardiac tumors. Myxomas can occur in hereditary syndromes, but 93% are nonhereditary myxomas. Typically, patients are referred to echocardiography after a cerebral or peripheral embolic event; in rare cases, patients show clinical signs of valvular obstruction [35] which can be verified by color Doppler as demonstrated in the example of a giant left atrial myxoma shown in ◘ Fig. 11.17.

Although myxoma can be connected to any endocardial area, they are commonly attached to the left-sided interatrial septum and the fossa ovalis. Usually connected to the endocardium by a pedicle, myxoma can also occur with a broad base. RT3DE has been demonstrated to provide accurate anatomic visualization as well as improved identification of the spatial relation of a myxoma to the interatrial septum [35][36][37]. Butz et al. [35] described an improvement in evaluation of obstructive effects on ventricular in- or outflow by using RT3D TEE. Myxomas captured in 3D datasets can be sliced tomographically to identify structural patterns, including cysts, necrosis, hemorrhage, or calcification, which can be characteristically found inside myxomas. Mehmood et al. [36] described that isolated echolucent areas consistent with hemorrhage/necrosis in the tumor mass point towards myxoma in contrast to closely packed echolucencies which are more likely to be found in hemangioma. While in histological specimen myxomas are usually well vascularized, blood flow within the tumor is difficult to prove by echocardiography. Nevertheless, acquisition of a RT3DE color Doppler dataset to a sufficiently low pulse repetition frequency might detect vascularization inside the tumor which makes a thrombus unlikely. However, 2D color flow mapping is likely to be superior in this context.

To include the entire myxoma as well as surrounding cardiac structures, acquisition of a RT3DE dataset in full volume mode (see ► Chapter 2) is required in most cases. Although initial reports demonstrated RT3D TTE to be useful in the identification of myxoma [36], a recent report of RT3D TEE assessment has shown superior visualization of tumor characteristics and identification of spatial relationships [35], which can be important when planning the surgical procedure [38|.

■ **Papillary fibroelastoma**

In autopsy studies, 10% of benign cardiac tumors are papillary fibroelastomas representing the second largest entity after myxomas. Usually they are incidental findings with a characteristic appearance as small, mobile masses with a stippled edge, with shimmer or vibration at the tumor–blood interface [39]. In larger tumors, a speckled appearance can be found [40]. Finger-like projections can produce the impression of a sea anemone (◘ Fig. 11.18). Commonly fibroelastomas are attached to the endocardium either on the aortic or left ventricular side of the aortic valve or neighboring endocardium. Fibroelastomas attached to the aortic valve often appear like infectious vegetations or Lambl's excrescences, which makes differentiation challenging. Beside the advantages of RT3DE described for the identification of myxomas, live RT3DE provides a clear improvement in spatial assessment [40], particularly for the detection of the precise site of attachment [40][41].

■ **Hemangioma**

Cardiac hemangiomas, which present 5–10% of all benign cardiac tumors, are often clinically insignificant, exist unrecognized, or are diagnosed incidentally. Hemangiomas can be found in any cardiac location. They vary in size between less than 1 cm and more than 8 cm and are pedunculated, noncalcified but hyperdense [42]. Recent reports have shown the additive value of RT3DE in the detection and characterization of hemangioma, for example, RT3DE detects more extensive and closely packed echolucencies [36] and an intensive vascularization compared to myxoma [37].

■ **Rhabdomyoma**

Rhabdomyomas are the most common primary cardiac tumor in children. They represent myocardial hamartomas and are associated with tuberous sclerosis in up to 50% of cases [43]. Usually rhabdomyoma show regression or will disappear within the third trimester of pregnancy or postnatally [44]. These tumors are usually characterized by multiple masses, with a pedunculated or spherical intramural shape, and they most commonly involve the ventricular myocardium where they appear echodense [45]. The size of the tumors may vary from miliary nodules measuring less than 1 mm up to masses with a diameter of 10 cm. When occurring intramurally, a circumscribed ventricular wall thickening of the left and/or right ventricle with regional wall motion abnormality can be found (◘ Fig. 11.19). RT3DE imaging and offline qualitative analysis of data allows detailed visualization of the mass, revealing an irregular multilobed architecture with inhomogeneous echogenicity and a torsional–dyskinetic movement during systole [45].

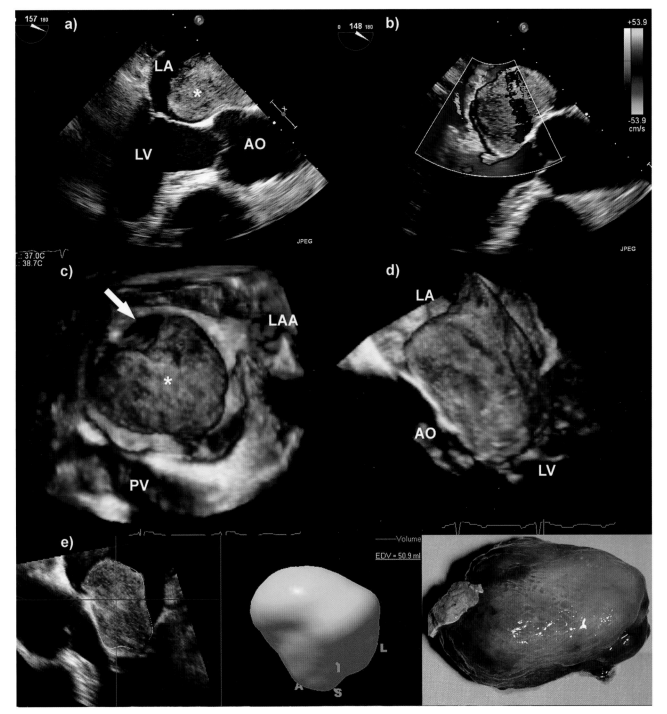

□ **Fig. 11.17** Example of 2D and RT3DE representations of a left atrial (*LA*) myxoma (*asterisk*), adherent to the inferior fossa ovalis. **a** The 2D TEE cross-sectional view providing important information about tumor structure. **b** The 2D TEE color Doppler reveals mitral valve obstruction by the myxoma during diastole. **c** Full volume RT3DE provided clear visualization of the tumor's whole extension, shape, and surface structure from a surgeon's view [anterior aortic root (*AO*) and lateral left atrial appendage (*LAA*)]. The *arrow* pointing to the remaining obstructed funnel towards the mitral valve (as detected by color Doppler in **b**). **d** RT3DE image demonstrating mitral valve obstruction by the tumor mass. **e** RT3DE volumetry of the tumor provided a volume of 50.9 ml. The resected histologic specimen on the right with a jelly-like shiny surface of a benign myxoma compared very well in shape and appearance with representation by RT3DE in **d**. *LV* left ventricle, *PV* pulmonary vein. [→Videos 11.17a–d]

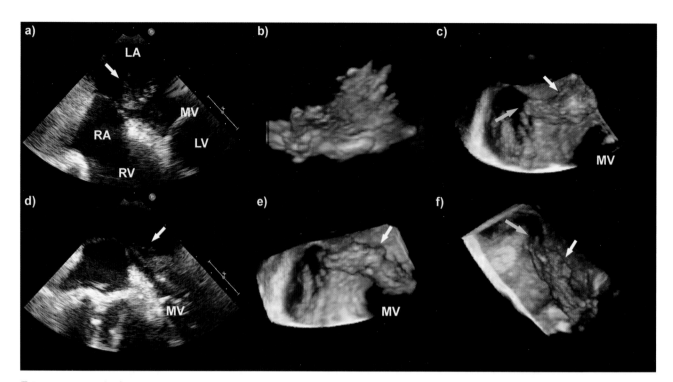

◘ Fig. 11.18 Example of 2D and RT3D TEE representations of a fibroelastoma in an uncommon location attached to the interatrial septum as an incidental finding in a male patient. **a** 2D TEE detection of the mass (*white arrow*) in the left atrium (*LA*). **b** Live 3D dataset with clear visualization of the fragile structure of the fibroelastoma with characteristic finger-like excrescences. **c** Live 3D image revealed that the mass was attached to the interatrial septum, which appeared translucent because of dropout artifact. **d** The 2D TEE showed diastolic prolapse of the mass toward the mitral valve. **e** Live 3D projection of the mass' prolapse toward the mitral valve. **f** A slight rotation of the live 3D image clearly displayed the origin of the mass (*yellow arrow*). *MV* mitral valve, *RA* right atrium, *LV* left ventricle, *RV* right ventricle. [→Videos 11.18a–c,e]

▪ Fibroma

Cardiac fibroma is the second most common cardiac tumor in children. However, although being a congenital neoplasm, 15% of cardiac fibromas were found in adolescents and adults. Common clinical manifestations in patients with cardiac fibromas are heart failure, arrhythmias, and sudden death. Cardiac fibromas are usually located within the myocardium of the ventricles and the interventricular septum. The lateral wall of the left ventricle is most commonly involved but in rare cases the free right lateral wall can be affected [46]. The size of the tumors is rather large and varies between 2 and 5 cm. In the echocardiographic evaluation, a cardiac fibroma appears as a noncontractile solid mass often attached to the left ventricular septum which is well demarcated from the surrounding myocardium by multiple calcifications.

Yang et al. [47] demonstrated RT3D TEE to offer better delineation of spatial relationship to adjacent structures in a case of a fibroma located in the left atrium with subtotal obstruction of the entrance of the right pulmonary veins. The characteristic inner calcific foci of the fibroma were well defined within multiple 3D tomographic planes.

11.2.2 Primary malignant tumors

Nearly all primary malignant cardiac tumors are sarcomas, being angio- or rhabdomyosarcomas in more than 50% of cases, whereas histiosarcomas, osteosarcomas, and leiomyosarcomas are less common. At the time of initial diagnosis, 50% of these tumors have already metastasized [48].

Histiocytomas, osteosarcomas, and leiomyosarcomas usually affect the left atrium, while angiosarcomas might affect the right atrium or the pericardium [49]. Direct infiltration of the cardiac wall or pericardial effusion is an indicator for malignancy. In contrast to benign myxomas, sarcomas often originate from the roof of the left or right atrium. RT3DE has been demonstrated to be of additive value in identifying the origin of the tumor and infiltration of neighboring cardiac structures. In RT3DE studies, angiosarcomas appeared as a mass of mixed echogenicity, predominantly cystic with fluid and some hyperechoic densities consistent with a vascular tumor [50]. Identification of infiltration of cardiac structures (e.g., heart valves or venous structures) should be the subject of a comprehensive RT3DE examination.

Primary cardiac lymphoma is a very rare condition [51] and mostly found in immunosuppressed patients [52]. It often appears as an immobile, sometimes polypoid mass, predominantly in the right atrium, commonly combined with malignant pericardial effusion. The cardiac walls may be infiltrated, showing thickening associated with wall motion abnormalities in the affected regions. Larger tumor masses can lead to relevant valve obstruction [53].

> ❯ Identification of infiltration of cardiac structures (e.g., heart valves or venous structures) should be the subject of a comprehensive RT3DE examination.

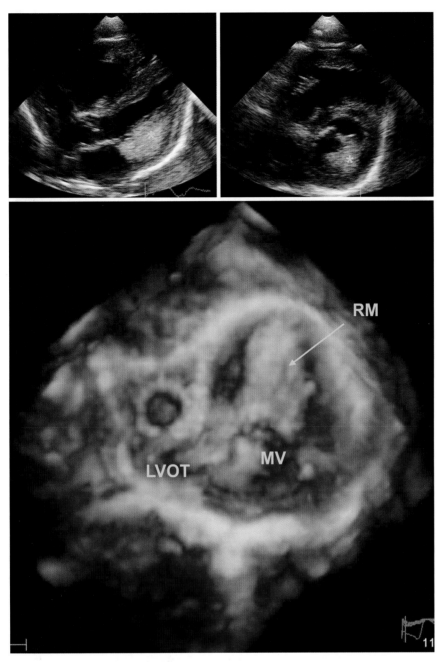

■ Fig. 11.19 Rhabdomyoma in a newborn on his first day involving the inferior wall of the left ventricular myocardium as demonstrated in the 2D cut planes of the *upper panels*. The tumor (*asterisk*) appears as an echo thick mass. The 3D reconstruction allows en face visualization of the tumor embedded in the healthy myocardium which nearly disappears in comparison to the echo thickness of the rhabdomyoma. The tumor vanished several weeks later. *RM* rhabdomyoma, *LVOT* left ventricular outflow tract, *MV* mitral valve. (Courtesy of Dr. U. Neudorf, Pediatric Cardiology, University Clinic, Essen, Germany) [→Videos 11.19a–c]

11.3   Secondary cardiac tumors and metastases

As shown in autopsy studies, cardiac metastases of malignant tumors are much more frequent than primary cardiac tumors. They can be found in up to 3% of patients with malignomas, but detection in vivo is very rare [54]. Malignant melanomas are frequently seeded into the heart (50%), followed by bronchial and mamma carcinoma and lymphoma/leukemia (30% each). They are often associated with a malignant, often sanguineous pericardial effusion. Other clinical appearances can be rhythm disturbances, e.g., AV node blockade or ventricular arrhythmias.

> Tomographic slicing of cardiac metastases represented in RT3DE color Doppler datasets might be useful for detection of tumor perfusion.

Small or myocardial metastases may be difficult to detect. The use of contrast agents may improve the detection rate when demonstrating the irregular vascularization of the metastatic tissue. Tomographic slicing of cardiac metastases represented in RT3DE color Doppler datasets might be useful for detection of tumor perfusion as demonstrated in a patient with a metastasis of an adenocarcinoma (◨ Fig. 11.20). RT3DE can be also used to obtain accurate 3D volumetry of a metastasis (◨ Fig. 11.21) as well as estimating the volume of a malignant pericardial effusion [55]. To discriminate between genuine cardiac metastasis or tumor infiltration from outside the heart, RT3DE can be used to determine the origin of the mass (◨ Fig. 11.22).

While primary cardiac lymphoma is rare, 16–28% of the patients with disseminated lymphoma show cardiac involvement [56]. ◨ Fig. 11.23 shows an example of a secondary cardiac lymphoma where RT3DE shows cardiac involvement with a tumorous mass within the interatrial septum and growth into both right and left atrium leading to possible obstruction of the mitral valve.

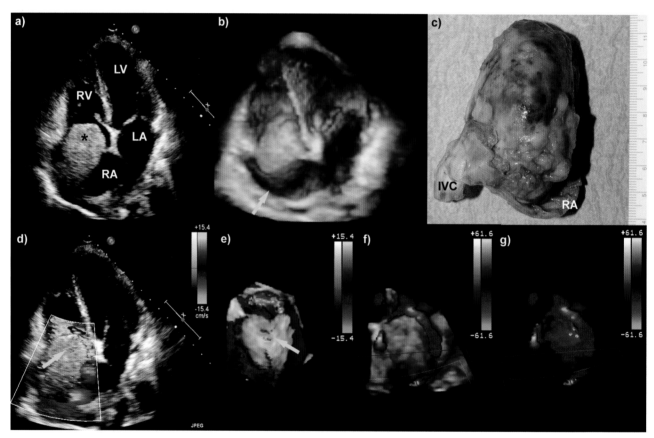

◨ **Fig. 11.20** The 2D and RT3DE representations of a right atrial mass in a 67-year-old woman with known cholangiocarcinoma and metastases in lung and liver. The mass was leading to tricuspid valve obstruction with superior vena cava syndrome. During surgical resection, the tumor was found be adherent to the right atrial roof with growth into the superior vena cava and histologically classified as a metastasis of adenocarcinoma. **a** The 2D TTE 4-chamber view showing the tumor mass (*asterisk*) in the right atrium (*RA*). **b** Acquisition of a RT3DE full volume dataset improved identification of the tumor origin from the posterior RA wall where the inferior vena cava (*IVC*) is entering (*arrow*). **c** Pathologic specimen presenting a peduncle to the IVC and a piece of the adherent RA wall. **d** By reducing the Nyquist velocities, flow within the tumor can be displayed indicating perfusion (*arrow*). Turbulent flow around the tumor indicates the stenotic effect of the tumor when obstructing the tricuspid valve. **e** Evidence of perfusion in the RT3DE color Doppler dataset (*arrow*). **f** RT3DE color Doppler flow around the tumor with and without the tissue information (**g**). *LA* left atrium, *RV* right ventricle, *LV* left ventricle. [→Videos 11.20a,b,d,f]

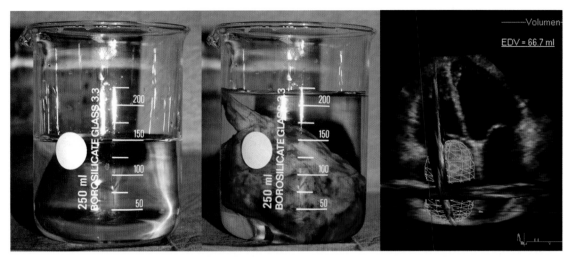

Fig. 11.21 RT3DE volumetry of the same tumor shown in Fig. 11.20 compared to the true volume. *Right* Preoperative RT3DE volumetry of the tumor provided a volume of 66.7 ml. Volume measurement of the excised tumor including the peduncle to the IVC as the volume difference of a water-filled beaker with (230 ml, *middle*) and without (150 ml, *left*) the tumor resulted in a volume of 80 ml

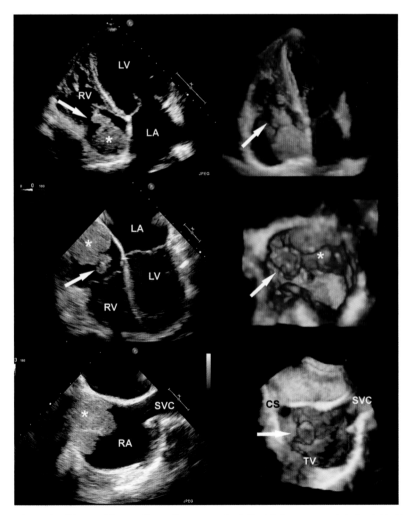

Fig. 11.22 Hepatocellular carcinoma in a 75-year-old man with continuous growth via the inferior vena cava into the right atrium (*RA*). *Top left* The 2D TTE 4-chamber view shows the tumor (*asterisk*) in the RA with a mobile structure attached to the tumor surface which is most likely an apposition thrombus (*arrow*). *Top right* The RT3D TTE provides additional information about the tumor attachment and extension as well as the spatial relation of the thrombus formation to the tricuspid valve. *Middle left* The 2D TEE provided high-resolution cross-sectional image of the tumor's inner structure. *Middle right* Live 3D zoom provided a view from the right ventricle (*RV*) through the tricuspid valve into the RA onto the tumor (*asterisk*) with the mobile mass (*arrow*). *Bottom left* The 2D TEE bicaval view clearly demonstrated the tumor growing out of the inferior vena cava. *Bottom right* In addition, the RT3DE full volume allowed simultaneous presentation of superior vena cava (*SVC*), tricuspid valve in the background (*TV*), and the entrance of the coronary sinus (*CS*) and their close spatial relationship to the tumor. *LV* left ventricle, *LA* left atrium. [→Videos 11.22a–f]

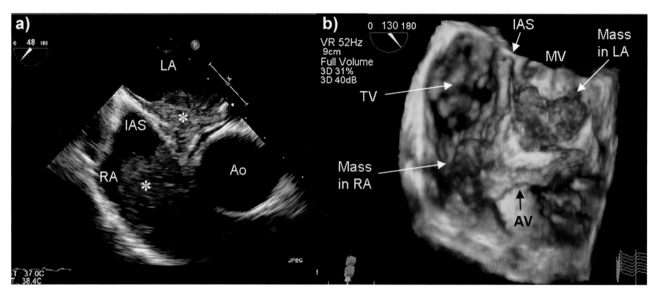

◘ Fig. 11.23 Example of 2D and RT3D TEE representation of secondary cardiac involvement of a non-Hodgkin lymphoma in a young man. **a** The 2D echocardiographic short-axis view at the level of the aortic root (*Ao*) showed a mass (*asterisk*) within the interatrial septum (*IAS*) with severe growth into the right atrium (*RA*) and left atrium (*LA*). **b** The RT3DE full volume dataset provided a direct view from the roof of both atria toward the interatrial septum and both the mitral (*MV*) and tricuspid valve (*TV*) which revealed the true extension of the tumor mass and its anatomical relation to the TV, MV, and Ao. *AV* aortic valve. [→Video 11.23]

References

1. Hart RG (1992) Cardiogenic embolism to the brain. Lancet 339:589–594
2. Edwards LC III, Louie EK (1994) Transthoracic and transesophageal echocardiography for evaluation of cardiac tumours, thrombi, and valvular vegetations. Am J Cardiac Imaging 8:45–48
3. Plana JC (2009) Added value of real-time three-dimensional echocardiography in assessing cardiac masses. Curr Cardiol Rep 11:205–209
4. Reddy VK, Faulkner M, Bandarupalli N et al (2009) Incremental value of live/real time three-dimensional transthoracic echocardiography in the assessment of right ventricular masses. Echocardiography 26:598–609
5. Asch FM, Bieganski SP, Panza JA, Weissman NJ (2006) Real-time 3-dimensional echocardiography evaluation of intracardiac masses. Echocardiography 23:218–224
6. Müller S, Feuchtner G, Bonatti J Müller L et al (2008) Value of transeophageal 3D echocardiography as an adjunct to conventional 2D imaging in preoperative evaluation of cardiac masses. Echocardiography 25: 624–631
7. Jungwirth B, Mackensen GB (2008) Real-time 3-dimensional echocardiography in the operating room. Semin Cardiothoracic Vasc Anesth 12: 248–264
8. Pepi M, Evangelista A, Nihoyannopoulos P et al (2010)Recommendations for echocardiography use in the diagnosis and management of cardiac sources of embolism: European Association of Echocardiography (EAE) (a registered branch of the ESC). Eur J Echocardiogr 11:461-476
9. Pearson AC, Labovitz AJ, Tatineni S, Gomez CR (1991) Superiority of transesophageal echocardiography in detecting cardiac source of embolism in patients with cerebral ischemia of uncertain etiology. J Am Coll Cardiol 17:66–72
10. Merino A, Hauptman P, Badimon L et al (1992) Echocardiographic »smoke« is produced by an interaction of erythrocytes and plasma proteins modulated by shear forces. J Am Coll Cardiol 20:1661–1668
11. Duncan K, Nanda NC, Foster WA et al (2006) Incremental value of live/ real time three-dimensional transthoracic echocardiography in the assessment of left ventricular thrombi. Echocardiography 23:68–72
12. Sinha A, Nanda NC, Misra V et al (2004) Morphological assessment of left ventricular thrombus by live three-dimensional transthoracic echocardiography. Echocardiography 21:749–753

13. Anwar AM, Nosir YFM, Ajam A, Chamsi-Pasha H (2010) Central role of real-time three-dimensional echocardiography in the assessment of intracardiac thrombi. Int J Cardiovasc Imaging 26:519–526
14. Marek D, Vindis D, Kocianova E (2013) Real time 3-dimensional transesophageal echocardiography is more specific than 2-dimensional TEE in the assessment of left atrial appendage thrombosis. Biomedical papers of the Medical Faculty of the University Palacky, Olomouc, Czechoslovakia 157:22–6
15. Mizuguchi KA, Burch TM, Bulwer BE et al (2009) Thrombus or bilobar left atrial appendage? Diagnosis by real-time three-dimensional transesophageal echocardiography. Anesth Analg 108:70–72
16. Chen O-, Wu W-C, Jiang Y et al (2012) Assessment of the morphology and mechanical function of the left atrial appendage by real-time three-dimensional transesophageal echocardiography. Chin Med J 125:3416–3420
17. Silvestry FE, Kerber RE, Brook MM et al (2009) Echocardiography-guided interventions. J Am Soc Echocardiogr 22:213–231
18. Chierchia GB, Capulzini L, de Asmundis C et al (2008) First experience with real-time three-dimensional transesophageal echocardiography-guided transseptal in patients undergoing arial fibrillation ablation. Europace 10:1325–1328
19. Plicht B, Konorza TFM, Kahlert P et al (2013) Thrombus formation on the Amplatzer Cardiac Plug after left atrial appendage occlusion. J Am Coll Cardiol Cardiovascular Interventions 6:606–613
20. Faletra FF, Moschovitis G, Auricchio A (2009) Sequential three-dimensional live transesophageal echocardiography examinations showing progressive dissolution of thrombi on prosthetic mitral valve. Eur Heart J 30:1476
21. Bainbridge D (2005) 3-D imaging for aortic plaques assessment. Sem Cardiothorac Vasc Anesth 9:163–165
22. Hausmann D, Mugge A, Becht I, Daniel WG (1992) Diagnosis of patent foramen ovale by transesophageal echocardiography and association with cerebral and peripheric embolic events. Am J Cardiol 70:668–672
23. Overell JR, Bone I, Lees KR (2000) Interatrial septal abnormalities and stroke: a meta-analysis of case-control studies. Neurology 55:1172–1179
24. Sattiraju S, Masri SC, Liao K, Missov E (2012) Three-dimensional transesophageal echocardiography of a thrombus entrapped by a patent foramen ovale. Ann Thorac Surg 94:e101–102

25. Ramani GV, Kligerman S, Lehr E (2012) Multimodality imaging of thrombus in transit crossing a patent foramen ovale. J Am Coll Cardiol 59:e19

26. Monte I, Grasso S, Licciardi S, Badano LP (2010) Head-to-head comparison of real-time three-dimensional transthoracic echocardiography with transthoracic and transesophageal contrast echocardiography for the detection of patent foramen ovale. Eur J Echocardiogr 11:245–249

27. Rana BS, Shapiro LM, McCarthy KP, Ho SY (2010) Three-dimensional imaging of the atrial septum and patent foramen ovale anatomy: defining the morphological phenotypes of patent foramen ovale. Eur J Echocardiogr 11:i19–25

28. Erbel R, Rohmann S, Drexler M et al (1988) Improved diagnostic value of echocardiography in patients with infective endocarditis by transoesophageal approach. A prospective study. Eur Heart J 9:43–53

29. Liu YW, Tsai WC, Lin CC et al (2009) Usefulness of real-time three-dimensional echocardiography for diagnosis of infective endocarditis. Scand Cardiovasc J 6:1–6

30. Hansalia S, Biswas M, Dutta R et al (2009) The value of live/real time three-dimensional transesophageal echocardiography in the assessment of valvular vegetations. Echocardiography 26:1264–1273

31. Sadat K, Joshi D, Sudhakar S et al (2012)Incremental role of three-dimensional transesophageal echocardiography in the assessment of mitral-aortic intervalvular fibrosa abscess. Echocardiography 29:742–744

32. Sedgwick JF, Burstow DJ (2012) Update on echocardiography in the management of infective endocarditis. Curr Infect Dis Rep 14:373–380

33. Maffè S, Zenone F, Dellavesa P et al (2012) Usefulness of three-dimensional transthoracic echocardiography in particular clinical settings: a case of aorto-cavitary fistula in periprosthetic aortic valve abscess. Echocardiography29:E141-144

34. Reynen K (1995) Cardiac myxomas. N Engl J Med 333:1610–1617

35. Butz T, Scholtz W, Körfer J et al (2008) Prolapsing left atrial myxoma: preoperative diagnosis using a multimodal imaging approach with magnetic resonance imaging and real-time three-dimensional echocardiography. Eur J Echocardiogr 9:430–432

36. Mehmood F, Nanda NC, Vengala S et al (2005) Live three-dimensional transthoracic assessment of left atrial tumors. Echocardiography 22:137–143

37. Khairnar P, Hsiung MC, Mishra S et al (2011) The ability of live three-dimensional transesophageal echocardiography to evaluate the attachment site of intracardiac tumors. Echocardiography 28:1041–1045

38. Tolstrup K, Shiota T, Gurudevan S et al (2011) Left atrial myxomas: correlation of two-dimensional and live three-dimensional transesophageal echocardiography with the clinical and pathologic findings. J Am Soc Echocardiogr 24:618–624

39. Klarich KW, Enriquez-Sarano M, Gura GMet al (1997) Papillary fibroelastoma: echocardiographic characteristics for diagnosis and pathologic correlation. J Am Coll Cardiol 30:784–790

40. le Tourneau T, Pouwels S, Gal B et al (2008) Assessment of papillary fibroelastomas with live three-dimensional transthoracic echocardiography. Echocardiography 25:489–495

41. Parthenakis F, Nyktari E, Patrianakos A et al (2009) Asymptomatic papillary fibroelastoma of the aortic valve in a young woman – a case report. Cardiovascular Ultrasound 7:43–47

42. Kojima S, Suiyoshi M, Suwa S et al (2003) Cardiac hemangioma: a report of two cases and review of the literature. Heart Vessels 18:153–156

43. Grebenc ML, Rosado de Christenson ML et al (2000) Primary cardiac and pericardial neoplasms: radiologic-pathologic correlation. Radiographics 20:1073–1110

44. Chadha R, Johnson JA, Fuitman D et al (2011) A rare case of cardiac rhabdomyomas in a dizygotic twin pair. J Obstet Gynaecol Can 33:854–857

45. Motto A, Ballo P, Bocelli A et al (2006) Echocardiographic history of an asymptomatic congenital cardiac tumor. No changes in mass dimensions during a 14-year follow-up. Circulation 114: e591–e593

46. Teis A, Sheppard MN, Alpendurada F (2011) Unusual location for a large cardiac fibroma. Circulation 124:1481–1482

47. Yang HS, Arabia FA, Chaliki HP et al (2008) Left atrial fibroma in Gardner syndrome. Circulation 118:e692–e696

48. Reynen K, Daniel WG (1997) Malignant primary tumors of the heart. Z Kardiol 86:598–607

49. Chalhoub E, Mattar BI, Shaheen W, Schulz TK (2012) Cardiac angiosarcoma presenting with tamponade. Intern Med. 2012;51:2905–2907

50. Yang HS, Sengupta S, Umland MM et al (2008) Primary cardiac angiosarcoma evaluated with contrast two-dimensional and real-time three-dimensional echocardiography. Eur J Echocardiogr 9:733–738

51. Burke A (2008) Primary malignant cardiac tumors. Semin Diagn Pathol 25:39–46

52. Holladay AO, Siegal RJ (1992) Cardiac malignant lymphoma in acquired immune deficiency syndrome. Cancer 70:2203–2207

53. Kawamura T, Sakaguchi T, Nishi H et al (2013) Successful treatment of a large primary cardiac lymphoma by surgical resection combined with chemotherapy: report of a case. Surg Today 43:1066–1070

54. Rafajlovski S, Tatic V, Ilic S, Kanjuh V (2005) Frequency of metastatic tumors in the heart. Vojnosanit Pregl 62:915–920

55. Hernandez CM, Singh P, Hage FG et al (2009) Live/real time three-dimensional transthoracic echocardiographic assessment of pericardial disease. Echocardiography 26:1250–1263

56. Zielenska M, Kaczmarek K, Tylkowski M (2008) Predictors of left ventricular thrombus formation in acute myocardial infarction treated with successful primary angioplasty with stenting. Am J Med Sci 335:171–176

Monitoring and guiding cardiac interventions and surgery

Harald P. Kühl, Andreas Franke, Thomas Buck

T. Buck et al. (Hrsg.), *Three-dimensional Echocardiography*,
DOI 10.1007/978-3-642-36799-1_12, © Springer-Verlag Berlin Heidelberg 2014

Recent advances in a number of surgical and catheter-based therapeutic approaches in cardiology have allowed less invasive treatment with a better prognosis even in complex cases. These techniques include electrophysiological examination and ablation, surgical and transcatheter mitral valve repair as well as transfemoral aortic valve implantation, and percutaneous closure of atrial appendage, septal defects, and paravalvular leaks.

Most of these interventions require precise preinterventional imaging and patient selection. Most of them also need guiding during as well as monitoring of the result immediately after the procedure. Thus, there is a clear need for periinterventional imaging techniques that should optimally be performed in the cardiac catheterization laboratory or the operating room. Echocardiography as a technique that can be easily installed in the catheterization lab or operating room and that is harmless and repeatable has been recommended to be the optimal method for real-time visualization of cardiac structures and interventional tools [1].

> With the advent of transesophageal RT3DE, providing superior image quality, true online spatial orientation during catheter-based interventions became possible.

Early after becoming commercially available, transthoracic three-dimensional (3D) echocardiography was used to monitor endomyocardial biopsies and transcatheter septal closures in children [2][3]. Although, transthoracic real-time 3D echocardiography (RT3DE) can be useful for periinterventional monitoring in adult patients with good image quality (see example of ventricular septal defect (VSD) occlusion below), it is limited by its impaired image quality in the majority of patients in a supine position. With the advent of transesophageal RT3DE, providing superior image quality, true online spatial orientation during catheter-based interventions became possible. However, moderate sedation or even general anesthesia is necessary to allow longer duration of transesophageal echocardiography (TEE) application.

Other imaging techniques have been used to monitor and guide catheter-based interventions, such as intracardiac echocardiography (ICE) during patent foramen ovale (PFO) and atrial septal defect (ASD) closure or electrophysiological examinations [4][5]. However, these techniques are invasive and always limited regarding their image plane orientation. This is mainly due to the fact that the imaging probe lies within the right atrium and may interfere with diagnostic and interventional catheters [6]. The relatively recent availability of transnasal echocardiography may provide another imaging technique for use during these procedures [7].

Thus, because of its advantages in periinterventional imaging, echocardiography grew more and more into the catheterization lab and became an indispensible part of transcatheter interventions for valvular and structural heart disease, as probably the most important development in the field of echocardiography in recent time. This is mirrored by the development of new dedicated echocardiography systems, new software solutions to fuse and synchronize angiographic and echocardiographic image information ▶ Section 12.3.5), and importantly the treatment of this new clinical application in a recent EAE/ASE recommendation [1].

12.1   Method

Basic principles and clinical application of the RT3D TEE technique and different imaging modalities have been explained in detail in ▶ Chapter 2 (see ▶ Fig. 2.15). With respect to guiding and monitoring of interventions, the modalities used need to provide online or live 3D imaging. Thus, 3D acquisition techniques as live 3D mode, zoomed live 3D, or even live full volume (one-beat full volume) are normally preferred. Compared to this, intraoperative monitoring and guiding is less dependent on live imaging, so gated full volume 3D datasets providing higher spatial and temporal resolution can be used more frequently. General recommendations for 3D image acquisition, image orientation and display have been recently published [8].

> With respect to guiding and monitoring of interventions, the modalities used need to provide online or live 3D imaging.

However, despite image acquisition and display, using RT3DE during surgical or interventional procedures is similar to the application in the echo lab as covered in the previous chapters, there are important differences pertaining to the setup and work flow of the echocardiographic examination. Today both the operating room and the catheterization lab are not designed to provide room for the echocardiographic system and the echocardiographer. As a consequence, in most places the echocardiographer and the system have to be squeezed into the procedure room in such a way to be close enough to the head of the patient to manipulate the TEE probe while at the same time taking care not to collide with the rotating C-arm of the x-ray system. In addition, equally important, the position of the echocardiography system must allow the monitor to be oriented such that the surgeon or interventionalists can watch it during the procedure for guiding and monitoring. Finally, particularly in the catheterization lab, the echocardiographer has to be protected from radiation as it has been shown that the echocardiographer near the x-ray tube has the highest x-ray exposition of the entire team. From these practical aspects, important implications arise for the future planning of catheterization labs. Some include miniaturization of echocardiography systems, steering the TEE probe from the catheterization table using a robot arm, and, of course, displaying the echo images on the monitor of the x-ray system (see ▶ Section 12.3.5), some of which have already been realized.

12.2   Intraoperative monitoring and guiding

The use of RT3DE has been demonstrated to be feasible and provide important information particularly during valve surgery [9][10]. Recent studies showed superior agreement of intraoperative RT3DE en face views of pathologic mitral valves and surgical findings compared to two-dimensional (2D) TEE assessment (▶ Chapter 7, Fig. 7.11) [9][10]. Hien et al. [11] found significant superiority of RT3D TEE over 2D TEE particularly for identification of mitral valve prolapse in scallops A2, P1, and P2 and for chordal rupture in scallops A2 and P2. Furthermore, RT3D TEE was found to be particularly accurate in the detection of leaflet clefts. Intraoperative 3D visualization of the mitral valve, showing its exact pathology in dynamic motion, provides critically important information to the surgeon before and during the operation (□ Fig. 12.1). This is because the surgeon can normally assess the mitral valve only in a static and unloaded condition and has a very limited field of view during minimally invasive repair. In a recent study [12], intraoperative RT3D TEE was also found to accurately predict complexity of mitral valve repair mainly based on multisegment pathology, prolapsing height, and posterior leaflet angle. A comprehensive overview of the intraoperative application of RT3D TEE during cardiac surgery with valuable advice on specific requirements for image display and orientation for various heart structures and surgical procedures was provided by Vegas et al. [13].

> ❯ Intraoperative 3D visualization of the mitral valve, showing its exact pathology in dynamic motion, provides critically important information to the surgeon during the operation.

However, the value of intraoperative RT3DE lies not only in the accurate representation of aortic or mitral valve pathologies but even more in the demonstration of the surgical result immediately after valve repair (□ Fig. 12.2 and □ Fig. 12.3). For instance, without RT3DE, the surgeon can test the competence of the repaired valve using the water testing maneuver, which only mimics a nonphysiologic loading condition of the valve and, therefore, is often unreliable (□ Fig. 12.3). RT3DE, compared to 2D echocardiography, provides an anatomic and realistic visual-

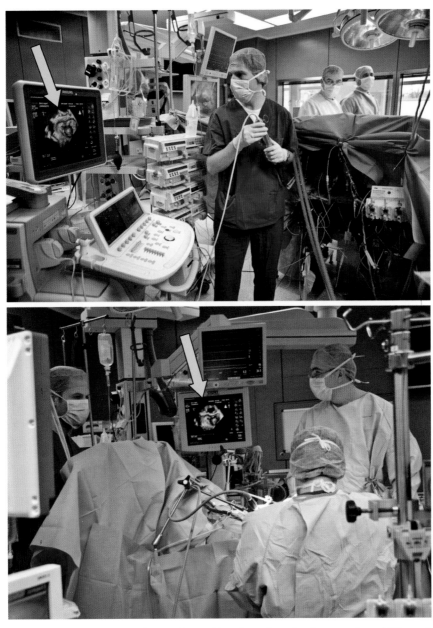

□ **Fig. 12.1** Intraoperative 3D echocardiography setting at the West German Heart Center Essen. *Top* A transesophageal 3D image (*arrow*, in this case the surgeon's view to the mitral valve with a large P2 flail leaflet) is shown on the 3D echocardiography system. *Bottom* On a separate monitor (*arrow*) the surgeon (*sitting*) can view the 3D image of the mitral valve during continual physiologic motion during minimally invasive repair

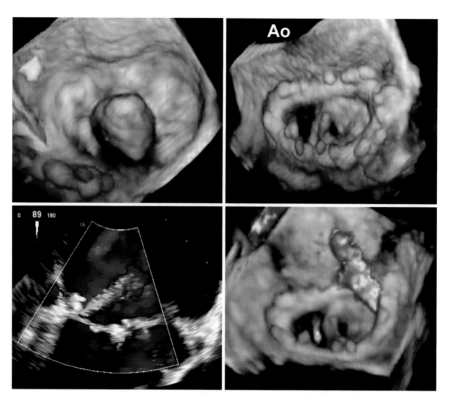

☐ Fig. 12.2 Example of intraoperative RT3DE monitoring of mitral valve (*MV*) repair in a patient with P2 prolapse. *Top left* En face view of a large P2 prolapse directly prior to repair. *Top right* En face view of the repaired valve with an annuloplasty ring. *Bottom left* 2D color Doppler echocardiography revealing a postero-medial regurgitant jet directly after restoring cardiovascular circulation. *Bottom right* RT3D color Doppler clearly shows a mild to moderate regurgitant jet which is located postero-medial directly at the inner edge of the annuloplasty ring. Based on the echocardiographic findings, it was decided that revision of the repair was not necessary. *Ao* aorta. [→Videos 12.2A–D]

izthation of the repaired valve immediately after restoration of circulation and under physiologic loading conditions. This allows detection of valvular or paravalvular regurgitation using RT3DE color Doppler and allows the surgeon to make a decision on re-repair or valve replacement (☐ Fig. 12.3) [14][15][16]. Intraoperative RT3DE even has the potential to allow 3D simulation of the planned surgical procedure as demonstrated for virtual decision-making on the optimal annuloplasty ring size during mitral valve repair [17].

12.3 Periinterventional monitoring and guiding

12.3.1 Transcatheter closure of PFO and ASD

Transcatheter device closure of interatrial communications has become an established technique for the prevention of paradoxical embolism in patients with PFO. It has also become an effective alternative treatment to surgery for selected patients with secundum-type ASDs that are associated with significant left-to-right shunting.

Most centers use both fluoroscopy and 2D TEE for guiding and monitoring septal defect closures, especially in ASDs where correct estimation of the defect size and its surroundings are crucial for procedural success. While conventional 2D TEE requires mental reconstruction of the spatial anatomy of septal

defects, particularly in cases of complex multifenestrated ASDs (► Fig. 9.8 and ► Fig. 9.9 in Chapter 9), 3D techniques provide unique anatomic views, such as direct en face visualization of an ASD, thus, making accurate determination of size, shape, dynamics, and number of the shunt lesion possible (see details in ► Chapter 9). Seo et al. [18] recently explored the effect of ASD shape on the maximal ASD diameter measured by RT3D TEE compared to balloon sizing and proposed a formula to determine the device size.

Transthoracic RT3DE has also been used to monitor ASD closures in infants from a subcostal window, which resulted in decreased fluoroscopy time [19]. In adults, image quality of transthoracic imaging is normally not sufficient to adequately guide closing procedures of interatrial communications.

Real-time 3D TEE is feasible and provides fast and complete information regarding the appropriate deployment and position of the device with regard to the surrounding structures in both ASD and PFO closure [20][21][22][23][24][25][26]. It serves as a complementary imaging modality to conventional 2D image planes throughout the whole interventional procedure [27].

> Unique anatomic RT3DE en face view of an ASD provides crucial information concerning size, shape, and tissue rim during interventional closure procedures.

After passage of the exchange wire and a first guiding catheter through the PFO or the ASD, RT3DE is able to show the position of the wire tip (☐ Fig. 12.4) and in many cases helps to position

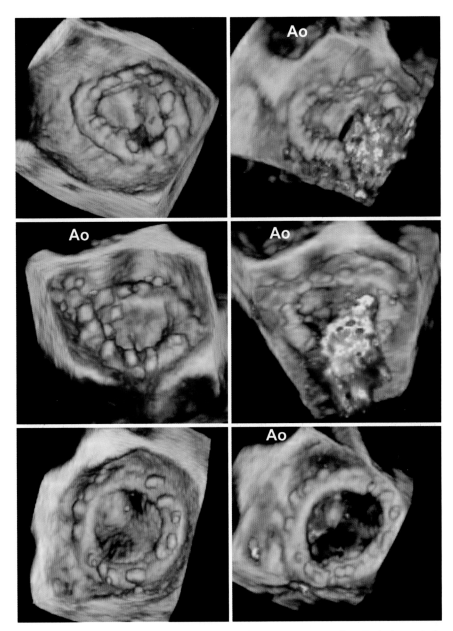

◨ **Fig. 12.3** Intraoperative monitoring using RT3DE in a patient with relevant mitral regurgitation 5 years after mitral valve repair. *Top row* Intraoperative RT3DE finding before mitral valve re-repair with postero-medial regurgitation. *Middle row* Intraoperative RT3DE revealed again postero-medial insufficiency immediately after re-repair despite the water test showing valve competence (▶ Surgical report). *Bottom row* Intraoperative RT3DE finding after bioprosthetic mitral valve replacement. *Ao* aorta [→Videos 12.3A–F]

Surgical report: »… *The mitral valve showed a thickened anterior and retracted posterior leaflet with postero-medial leakage. Because the coaptation area of both leaflets looked sufficient, a 28 mm Sorin ring was implanted after excision of the old ring. Subsequent water testing showed complete competence of the valve. However, 3D TEE control examination showed renewed postero-medial insufficiency. As a consequence, the valve was now excised with sparing of the posterior leaflet and the attached valve apparatus and afterwards implantation of a 29 mm Perimount bioprosthesis.…*«

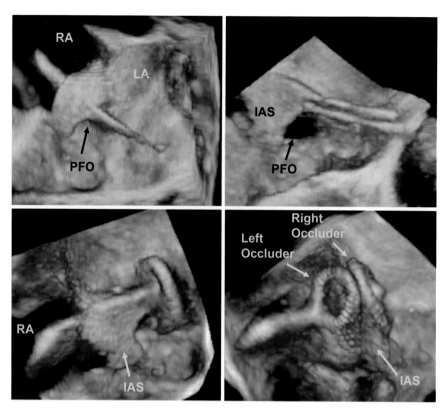

□ Fig. 12.4 RT3DE monitoring and guiding during percutaneous patent foramen ovale (*PFO*) occluder implantation. *Top left* Passage of the guide wire from the right atrium (*RA*) through the PFO into the left atrium (*LA*). *Top right* Introduction of the 9-French delivery catheter into the LA via the PFO. Note the presentation of the interatrial septum (*IAS*) which is tented by the catheter. *Bottom left* Opening of the left-sided occluder within the left atrium. *Bottom right* Finally, opening of the right-sided occluder within the right atrium catching the interatrial septum between the two parts of the occluder. [→Videos 12.4A–D]

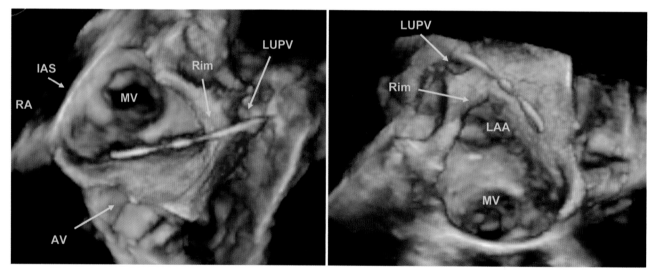

□ Fig. 12.5 Guide wire crossing the interatrial septum (*IAS*) and navigated into the left upper pulmonary vein (*LUPV*). *RA* right atrium, *LA* left atrium, *MV* mitral valve, *AV* aortic valve, *LAA* left atrial appendage. [→Videos 12.5A,B]

the wire correctly in the left upper pulmonary vein instead of the left atrial appendage (◘ Fig. 12.5). This is important to avoid potential perforation of the left atrial appendage during the interventional procedure. The location of the delivery catheter into the left upper pulmonary vein can also be monitored easily as well as the position of its tip after withdrawal from the pulmonary vein into the left atrial cavity (◘ Fig. 12.6) [24]. In this case, the TEE probe is located in a high esophageal position and directed toward the left atrial appendage and the pulmonary vein ostium. The wire position can be best monitored in a large one-beat full volume (low temporal resolution, wide overview) or a more focused live 3D zoom volume with increased temporal resolution.

As already mentioned in ▶ Chapters 9 and 10, the most relevant perspective of an ASD is the orthogonal en face view demonstrating its complete circumference (◘ Fig. 12.6). This advantage of 3D echocardiography becomes even more important during interventional ASD closures, because knowledge about size, shape, and tissue rim are crucial [23][24][26]. If there

is suspicion of a multifenestrated ASD, RT3D TEE is of great value to determine number and exact location of each individual ASD and their anatomic relation to each other (see ▶ Fig. 9.8 and ▶ Fig. 9.9 in Chapter 9) for planning and guiding transcatheter closure [28]. The best 3D images can be achieved when starting with a 40° rotation of the 2D image plane and then switching to the live 3D zoom mode. The 3D images from a left atrial perspective towards the PFO or ASD provide the best visualization of the spatial anatomy, whereas the right atrial aspect in many cases interferes with artifacts from the catheter or device. However, this perspective can be useful for confirmation of the tissue rim size and to provide guidance during crossing of a defect, if this proves difficult.

In the next step, unfolding of the left atrial occluder disk by advancing it outside the sheath into the left atrium can be monitored (◘ Fig. 12.4). Both the delivery catheter and left atrial occluder disk are then pulled back towards the interatrial septum. This step can easily be monitored and guided using 3D images not only in PFO closure procedures (◘ Fig. 12.4) but also in more

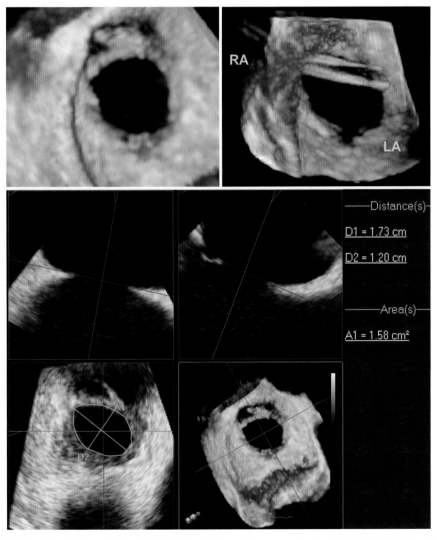

◘ Fig. 12.6 *Top left* RT3DE en face view of a large atrial septal defect prior to intervention, perspective from the left atrial side. *Top right* Same en face view with the 9-French delivery catheter passing the ASD into the left atrium (*LA*). *Below* The 3D sizing of the ASD maximal dimensions (see ▶ Chapter 9). *RA* right atrium. [→Videos 12.6A,B]

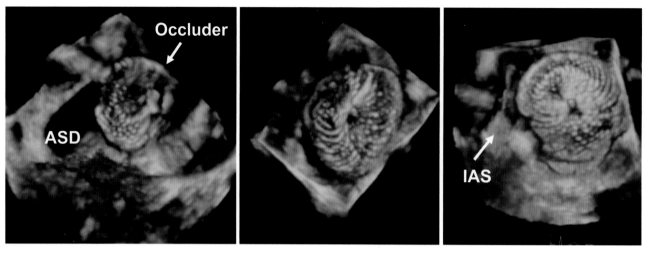

■ **Fig. 12.7** Left atrial disk of an ASD occluder (Amplatzer™ ASD Occluder) unfolded in the left atrium (*left*). Pullback of the occluder towards the interatrial septum (*IAS*), the left atrial disk now being in contact with the septum (*middle* and *right*). Note the high image resolution showing the wire mesh structure of the device

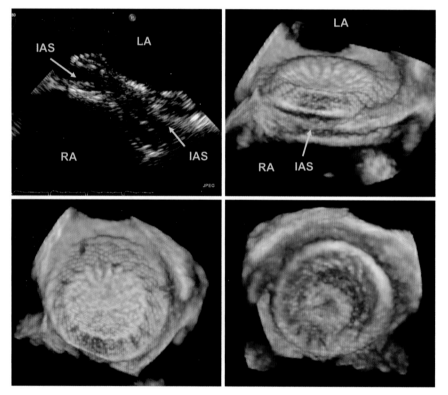

■ **Fig. 12.8** Comparison of detection of correct capture of the IAS between the left and right atrial occluder disk (21 mm Occlutech™ ASD occluder) using 2D echocardiography (*top left*) versus RT3DE visualization. Note that the thin IAS is not only visible between the two occluder disks (*top right*), but the RT3DE en face view also allows the sealing of the ASD around the entire occluder circumference from left atrial perspective (*bottom left*) and right atrial perspective (*bottom right*) to be ensured. [→Videos 12.8A–D]

complex ASD closures (◘ Fig. 12.7) even without simultaneous fluoroscopy. The advantage of RT3DE imaging is the ability to visualize the complete circumference of the occluder and the septal defect [23].

Subsequently, the right atrial disk is deployed by further withdrawal of the sheath and the correct alignment of the occluder and septum, controlled by 2D or RT3D TEE imaging. RT3DE images can be limited in visualizing the right atrial surface due to artifacts caused by the device itself. However, 3D images are extremely helpful and sensitive to demonstrate whether the device has grasped the septal rim over its complete circumference (see thin septal tissue in ◘ Fig. 12.4 and ◘ Fig. 12.8) [23][26]. Once the operator is satisfied with its position, the device is finally released.

Due to the comprehensive nature of 3D data, it is also easier to determine the result of the intervention – the extent and location of residual shunts can be visualized and if necessary a transcatheter repair be planned [29]. ◘ Fig. 12.9 shows a complex case of a multifenestrated ASD with two partially overlapping occluder devices after a first procedure and a residual shunt in a third defect. Moreover, initial studies have shown that the use of RT3D TEE might significantly reduce radiation exposure during

the procedure [30]. This is clearly due to the higher confidence of the operator in the echocardiographic images and its ability to show clinically relevant information which might allow fluoroscopy to be replaced in the future.

As a novel application, a dedicated software solution called EchoNavigator improves the transcatheter intervention of structural heart disease (SHD) like ASD or PFO closure by intelligent synchronization of x-ray and RT3D TEE images for improved navigation of device catheters as described in more detail below (▶ Section 12.3.5).

12.3.2 Transcatheter closure of VSD

Transcatheter device closure is an accepted therapeutic approach for congenital VSDs and has also recently been applied increasingly to post-AMI (acute myocardial infarction) VSDs. The majority of reports of echocardiographic periinterventional monitoring and guiding are, therefore, available in younger patients with congenital VSDs. Usually the procedure is performed under fluoroscopic control and 2D TEE monitoring. However, Acar et al. [31] demonstrated the added value of 3D echocardio-

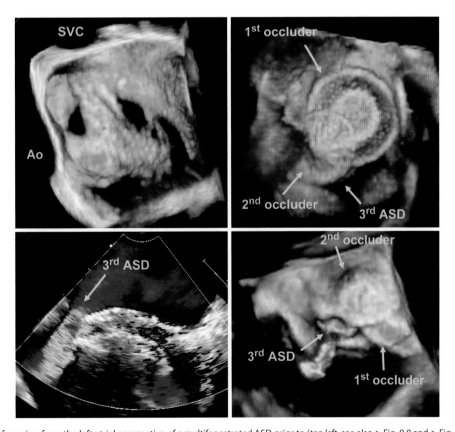

◘ **Fig. 12.9** RT3DE en face view from the left atrial perspective of a multifenestrated ASD prior to (*top left*, see also ▶ Fig. 9.8 and ▶ Fig. 9.9 in Chapter 9) and immediately after implantation of a 16 mm Amplatzer™ ASD occluder (*1st*) in the superior–posterior defect and a 23/25 mm Occlutech™ PFO occluder (*2nd*) in the smaller superior–anterior defect (*top right*). Note the displacement of the ASDs after occluder implantation. Both 2D echocardiography (*bottom left*) and RT3D show the remaining inferior ASD (*3rd*), but RT3DE allows superior anatomic orientation of the remaining defect in relation to the two occluders (*bottom right*). The decision was made to close the remaining defect in a second procedure. *SVC* superior vena cava, *Ao* aorta. [→Videos 12.9A–D]

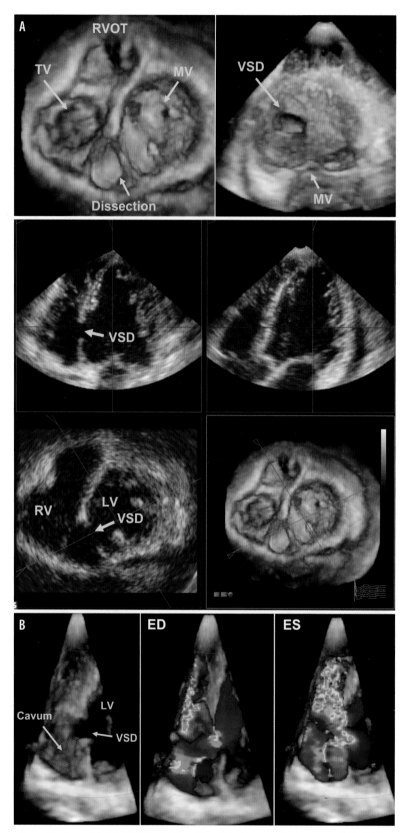

☐ **Fig. 12.10 A** Illustrative case of a ventricular septal defect (*VSD*) with dissection of the interventricular septum (*IVS*) which occurred 4 days after posterior myocardial infarct. *Top left* Transthoracic RT3DE apical view toward the IVS, tricuspid valve (*TV*), mitral valve (*MV*), and right ventricular outflow tract (*RVOT*). The posterior part of the IVS is split into two layers with a cavum between them. *Top right* The RT3DE en face view from the left ventricle to the VSD. *Bottom* Multiplane representation of the VSD within the 3D dataset. **B** RT3DE color Doppler dataset of the patient with post myocardial infarct VSD shown in **A**. *Left* RT3DE volume with color suppressed showing a view toward the IVS cavum and VSD. *Middle* The 3D color Doppler end-diastolic (*ED*) blood flow (*blue*) from the left ventricle (*LV*) through the VSD into the IVS cavum. *Right* End-systolic (*ES*) blood flow (*red*) from the LV through the VSD and through an apical communication towards the right ventricle

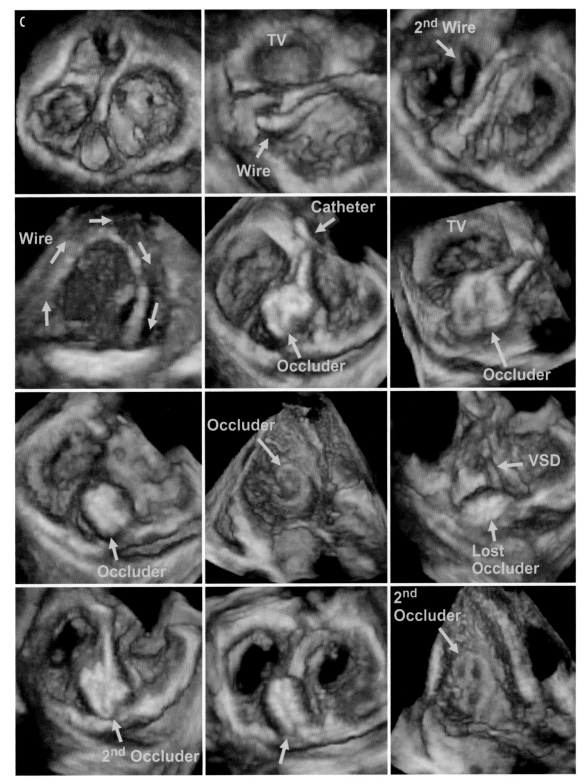

⬛ **Fig. 12.10** (continued) **C** Periinterventional monitoring and guiding using transthoracic RT3DE of occluder implantation into the VSD shown in **A** and **B**. *Top left* Preinterventional finding as demonstrated in **A**. *Top middle* Monitoring of the guide wire entering retrogradely from the left ventricular outflow tract (*LVOT*) through the LV and through the VSD into the IVS cavum. *Top right* Second guide wire entering antegradely through the TV into the right ventricle (*RV*). *2nd row left* Monitoring of the guide wire position entering from the RV through the apical IVS into the IVS cavum and through the VSD into the LV. *2nd row middle and right* Guiding of the occluder (16 mm Amplatzer ASD occluder) into the VSD. Both occluder disks are unfolded but still attached to the catheter. *3rd row left* Monitoring of optimal occluder position within the VSD after release from the catheter. *3rd row middle* The RT3DE en face view from the LV to the left ventricular occluder disk. *3rd row right* Loss of the occluder, most likely because the occluder size was too small when compared to the defect size. *Bottom left* Guiding of second occluder (20 mm Amplatzer ASD occluder) into the VSD. *Bottom middle* Monitoring of optimal position of the second occluder (*arrow*) within the VSD after release from the catheter. *Bottom right* Final result showing the second occluder in an en face view from the left ventricle to the IVS. Right below the second occluder the first occluder is shining through the thin IVS. [→Videos 12.10A(a,b), B(a,b), C(a–l)]

graphic visualization of muscular VSDs and surrounding structures for planning the device closure and monitoring the result using reconstructive 3D echocardiography. More recently, they reported the use of RT3D TTE for more accurate preinterventional sizing of perimembranous VSDs compared to conventional 2D TEE [32].

Compared to congenital VSD, an acquired VSD commonly occurs as a mechanical complication of AMI and is associated with very high morbidity and mortality. Transmural tissue necrosis causes a dynamic defect of the interventricular septum. Rarely, intramural extension with dissection of the interventricular septum may occur (◘ Fig. 12.10A, B) [33]. Transcatheter closure of a postinfarct VSD has been reported as an alternative approach in patients at too high risk for surgical repair [34]. Experiences so far in about 130 reported cases yielded a device implantation success rate of 85%. The usefulness of RT3D TEE to provide detailed assessment of the defect orifice and to guide the closure procedure has been recently reported by Halpern et al. [35]. In addition to accurate evaluation of a VSD's size and shape as the basis for the decision of what size of device to use, RT3DE provides accurate guidance for catheter manipulations in both acquired and congenital VSDs [36]. It is also used for accurate positioning and deployment of the occluder device (◘ Fig. 12.10C).

12.3.3 Transcatheter aortic valve implantation

Percutaneous balloon valvuloplasty followed by transcatheter implantation of a stent-based aortic valve prosthesis for the treatment of aortic stenosis has become a feasible and established procedure in patients at too high risk for conventional surgical therapy [37][38][39]. As in other percutaneous interventions, there is a need for precise imaging of cardiac structures, delivery catheters, and valve implants. The important role of 2D echocardiography identifying patients suitable for transcatheter aortic valve implantation (TAVI), as well as monitoring and guiding the intervention has been elaborated [1][40][41][42].

Two-dimensional echocardiography is particularly useful in determining the aortic annular diameter as the basis for prosthesis sizing, guiding the positioning of the prosthesis during implantation, and finally monitoring the function of the implanted prosthesis, including possible valvular and paravalvular regurgitation [1]. However, 2D echocardiography is limited to cross-sectional long-axis and short-axis views of the outflow tract and aortic valve; therefore, spatial orientation and understanding of the valve pathology and the dynamic processes during TAVI are lacking. Compared to this, RT3DE has been demonstrated to provide superior spatial orientation of the entire outflow tract before and during the TAVI procedure [24, 43]. As the aortic annulus is more elliptic than circular, recent studies demonstrated RT3DE to provide more accurate estimates of the aortic annular size. Janosi et al. [44] described significant differences in aortic annular diameters obtained by 2D TTE, 2D TEE, and RT3D TEE, but found the lowest interobserver variability for measurements made by RT3D TEE. In addition, RT3D TEE measurements of

aortic annular dimensions provided significant asymmetry with a long diameter of 2.40±0.39 cm and a short diameter of 2.13±0.44 cm [44].

As an important clinical implication the differences in aortic annular sizing by the three echocardiographic techniques led to significant differences in the decision on transcatheter heart valve size, with the largest heart valve sizes suggested from RT3D TEE measurements [44]. Comparing estimates of circular areas of aortic annulus and left ventricular outflow tract (LVOT) using 2D TEE and RT3D TEE and planimetered areas obtained from RT3D TEE, RT3D TEE planimetered annular and LVOT areas showed the smallest underestimation and the best agreement with multislice computed tomography (MSCT) which was used for reference [45]. The clinical importance of superior accuracy of RT3D TEE for measuring aortic annular dimensions has also been demonstrated for predicting the appearance of paravalvular regurgitation after transcatheter aortic valve implantation [46][47]. Comparing 2D TEE and RT3D TEE estimates of aortic annular area, only mismatch between RT3D TEE planimetered aortic annular area and prosthesis area was found to be an independent predictor of paravalvular regurgitation [46]. And similar to Janosi et al. [44], other groups [46][48] found that using RT3D TEE planimetered aortic annular area changed the decision on aortic valve prosthesis size to a larger size in a reasonable number of patients. Thus, incorporating the additional benefits of RT3D TEE in a systematic echocardiographic protocol combined with a 3D aortic valve prosthesis sizing strategy has been found to contribute to the excellent outcome of transcatheter aortic valve implantation [49].

> ❯ RT3DE has recently demonstrated to provide superior spatial orientation of the entire outflow tract before and during the TAVI procedure.

As an additional important advantage of RT3DE over 2D echocardiography, RT3DE is required for accurate determination of the distance between the ostium of the left coronary artery (LCA) and the aortic annulus which lies in the coronal plane and cannot be acquired by 2D imaging (▸ Fig. 8.13.B) [1]. A recent report suggested that the distance should be at least 14 mm to prevent LCA occlusion and myocardial infarction at the time the valve prosthesis is inflated and the bulky native valve leaflets are crushed towards the aortic wall [50]. Current guidelines recommend annulus-to-left main distances of >10 or >11 mm depending on 23 mm or 26 mm balloon-expandable valves [1]. Thus, the RT3DE long-axis view of the outflow tract provides detailed visualization of the LCA ostium and the aortic valve as a complementary technique to angiographic assessment (◘ Fig. 12.11, ◘ Fig. 12.12, ◘ Fig. 12.13). Because direct measurements in 3D images have not been available until recently, and new imaging modalities providing 3D image measurements have not been validated yet, the distance between the LCA ostium and aortic annulus must be estimated using a grid superimposed to the image (◘ Fig. 12.12). A new automated 3D algorithm to model and quantify aortic root dimensions from RT3D TEE data has recently been shown to be feasible and accurately measure annulus dimensions, leaflet dimensions, and annulus-to-left main ostium distance [51].

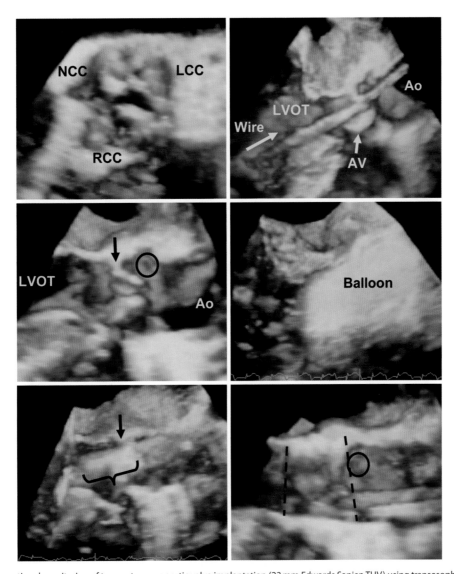

Fig. 12.11 Periinterventional monitoring of transcutaneous aortic valve implantation (23 mm Edwards Sapien THV) using transesophageal RT3DE. *Top left* En face view from the aorta to the severely calcified aortic valve with a small stenotic aortic valve opening area. *Top right* Position of the guide wire within the left ventricular outflow tract (*LVOT*) and passing through the aortic valve into the aorta. *Middle left* Long-axis view to the aortic valve with detection of the distance of LCA ostium (*circle*) to the aortic annulus (*arrow*). *Middle right* Inflation of the valvuloplasty balloon. *Bottom left* Guiding of optimal placement of the aortic valve prosthesis mounted on the balloon catheter (*parenthesis*) in relation to the aortic annulus (*arrow*). *Bottom right* Final position of the implanted aortic valve prosthesis with detection of the close proximity of the prosthesis (*dashed lines*) and the LCA ostium (*circle*). *NCC* noncoronary cusp, *LCC* left coronary cusp, *RCC* right coronary cusp, *Ao* aorta, *AV* aortic valve. [→Videos 12.11A–F]

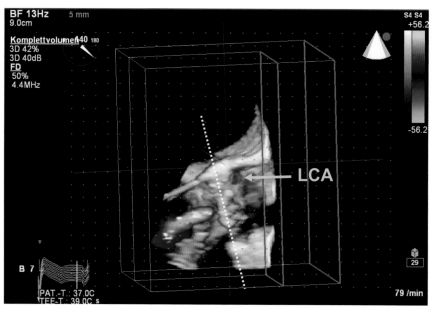

■ **Fig. 12.12** Estimation of distance between left coronary artery (*LCA*) ostium and aortic annulus (*dashed line*) using a 5 mm grid superimposed on the 3D image. The distance was estimated to be approximately 7 mm

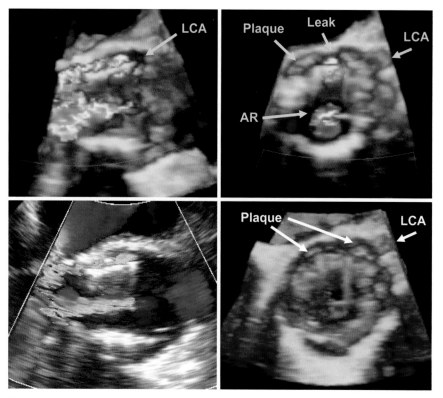

■ **Fig. 12.13** Result immediately after percutaneous aortic valve implantation demonstrated by RT3DE. *Top left* RT3DE color Doppler long-axis view shows the position of the valve prosthesis (26 mm, Edwards-SAPIEN™, Edwards Lifesciences), which is extremely close to the left coronary artery (*LCA*) ostium. There is also paravalvular flow as well as mild central aortic regurgitation (*AR*). *Top right* RT3DE color Doppler short-axis view showing the LCA as well as the small para-valvular leakage and the central aortic regurgitation. Note that the paravalvular leak occurs between the calcific plaques from the native aortic valve scallops squeezed between the prosthesis and the aortic wall (see also *bottom right*). *Bottom left* The 2D color Doppler long-axis view. Note that the 2D image cannot show the LCA ostium and the prosthesis cross-section because the LCA ostium lies behind the image plane. [→Videos 12.13A–D]

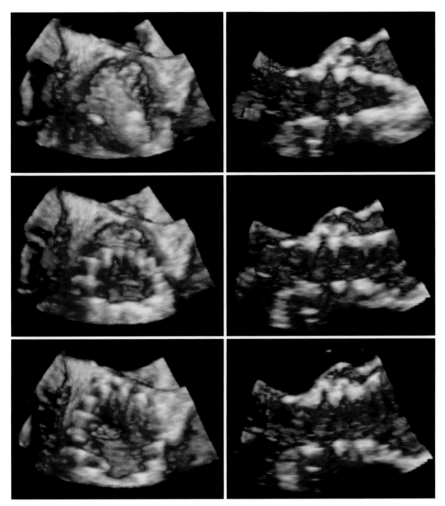

⬛ Fig. 12.14 Monitoring of the progressive expansion (*top to bottom*) of a CoreValve™ aortic valve prosthesis by RT3DE from an aortic short-axis perspective (*left*) and long-axis perspective (*right*). [→Videos 12.14A,B]

During implantation of the prosthesis, RT3DE using the live 3D mode allows continuous monitoring of the dynamic process of prosthesis inflation (⬛ Fig. 12.14). Immediately after prosthesis inflation, RT3DE provides unique visualization of the implanted prosthesis and assessment of prosthesis function. Most importantly, RT3DE can visualize the distal end of a balloon-expanded prosthesis in relation to the LCA ostium (⬛ Fig. 12.11 and ⬛ Fig. 12.13) and the presence and location of valvular and paravalvular leaks (⬛ Fig. 12.13) [1][52]. In addition, RT3DE is useful to demonstrate the calcified plaque material of the bulky native valve leaflets squeezed between the prosthesis and the aortic wall which can be the cause of paravalvular regurgitation (⬛ Fig. 12.13) or even aortic rupture [53].

12.3.4 Percutaneous mitral valve intervention

Percutaneous catheter-based approaches for mitral valve interventions in patients with severe mitral regurgitation (MR) have been developed as an alternative therapeutic option for patients at too high risk for conventional surgical mitral valve repair because of old age, severe heart failure, or comorbidities [1][54]. Of all the techniques, two have gained the most attention recently: percutaneous mitral valve repair, which is adopted from the surgical Alfieri »edge-to-edge« technique, and percutaneous mitral annuloplasty via the coronary sinus [55]. The role of RT3DE for periinterventional monitoring and guiding of the two procedures is described in the following two sections.

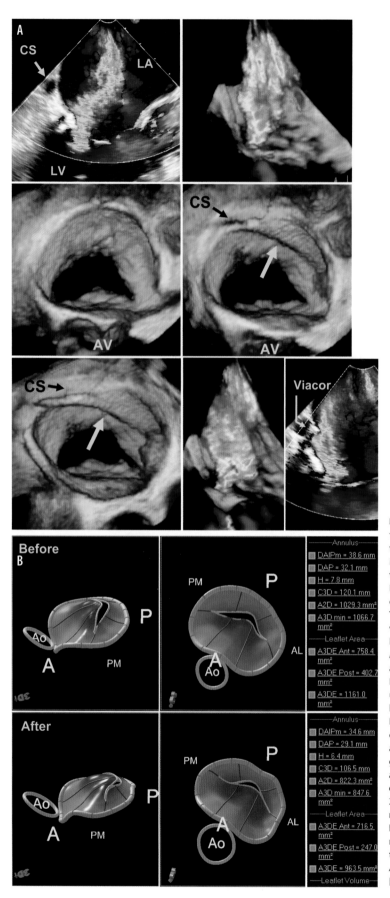

■ **Fig. 12.15** **A** Monitoring of percutaneous mitral annuloplasty (PTMA™ device, Viacor Inc.) using RT3DE in a patient with functional mitral regurgitation (*MR*). *Top left* The 2D color Doppler image showing severe MR before intervention. Note the location of the coronary sinus (*CS*). *Top right* RT3DE color Doppler representing the MR jet. *Middle left* RT3DE en face view of the mitral valve from a left atrial perspective. *Middle right* The 3D view showing deformation of the posterior left atrial wall after insertion of the first PTMA rod into the flexible multi-lumen catheter lying within the coronary sinus (*arrow*). *Bottom left* Final result with maximum deformation of posterior left atrial wall after insertion of all three PTMA rods. *Bottom right* RT3DE color Doppler demonstrating mitral regurgitation of unchanged severity most likely because of the distant superior location of the coronary sinus relative to the mitral annulus. Note the representation of the annuloplasty device within the coronary sinus (*arrow*) (see ■ Fig. 12.19 for further interventional management). **B** Quantitative 3D analysis of mitral valve geometry before (*top*) and after (*bottom*) percutaneous mitral annuloplasty (MVQ 7.0, Philips Medical Systems). Note the decrease of the anterior–posterior diameter from 32.1 mm to 29.1 mm corresponding to a deformation of 3 mm. Also the mitral valve area decreased from 1029.3 mm² to 822.3 mm². However, as shown in **A** deformation of the mitral annulus was not sufficient to lead to satisfactory reduction of mitral regurgitation. *AV* aortic valve, *LA* left atrium, *LV* left ventricle, *A* anterior, *Ao* aorta, *P* posterior, *PM* postero-medial, *AL* antero-lateral. [→Videos 12.15A(a–g)]

■ **Percutaneous mitral annuloplasty**

The anatomic proximity of the coronary sinus to the posterior mitral annulus led to the hypothesis that mitral annuloplasty could be performed percutaneously by placing a device in the coronary sinus and causing anterior displacement of the posterior annulus. This facilitates improved mitral leaflet coaptation [56]. To date, several different annuloplasty devices (introduced into the coronary sinus), such as the MONARC™ device (Edwards Lifesciences, Irvine, CA, USA), the CARILLON™ device (Cardiac Dimensions, Kirkland, WI, USA), and the PTMA™ device (Viacor Inc., Wilmington, MA, USA), have been implanted in patients with promising success [55]. The importance of meticulous echocardiographic assessment before and during percutaneous mitral annuloplasty has been described in detail by Kahlert et al. [57]. Particularly, the variable location of the coronary sinus in relation to the mitral annulus is a critical determinant for the procedure success. Recently, the complementary value of 3D visualization using RT3D TEE for periinterventional monitoring during percutaneous mitral annuloplasty has been demonstrated [24][57]. By offering a 3D en face view of the left atrium and the mitral valve, RT3D TEE provides unique continuous visualization of the annuloplasty device and deformation of the posterior left atrial wall during the intervention (◘ Fig. 12.15). In addition, based on RT3DE datasets before and after annuloplasty, changes in the geometry of the mitral valve apparatus can be quantified using dedicated 3D analysis software [24].

❯❯ Based on RT3DE datasets before and after annuloplasty, changes in the geometry of the mitral valve apparatus can be quantified using dedicated 3D analysis software.

■ **Percutaneous mitral valve repair**

Percutaneous mitral valve repair is a novel interventional valve procedure aiming to reduce the severity of mitral regurgitation (MR) in selected patients with advanced mitral insufficiency who are poor candidates for open-heart surgery. Adopting the surgical edge-to-edge technique initially developed by Alfieri et al. [58], the anterior and posterior mitral valve leaflets are coapted by means of a clip device, thereby, creating a double-orifice valve [55][59]. The clip device is delivered to the mitral valve via percutaneous femoral venous transseptal access. It is aligned above the mitral valve and advanced across the mitral orifice before grasping and coapting the leaflets. Although the procedure is performed in the cardiac catheterization laboratory under fluoroscopic control, TEE is the most important technique for guiding the different steps of the intervention [1]. These include the transseptal puncture, alignment of the clip device in the left atrium, and leaflet grasping. As mentioned, the percutaneous mitral valve repair technique is basically an echocardiographically guided interventional procedure. The initial descriptions for selecting appropriate patients and monitoring the procedure were based on 2D TEE [60]. However, because of the unique spatial orientation and 3D visualization, RT3D TEE has become indispensible in identifying 3D mitral valve pathology as well as monitoring and guiding the different complex steps of the interventional procedure [1][24][57][61][62]. The benefits of RT3DE imaging during the MitraClip procedure will be further increased by the

recently introduced EchoNavigator tool enabling integration and synchronization of x-ray and 3D echocardiographic information for improved guiding of the device catheter as described more detailed in ► Section 12.3.5. This is supported in a structured analysis by Altiok et al. [63] who reported RT3D TEE to be advantageous over 2D TEE guiding in 9 of 11 steps during the procedure with RT3D TEE guidance, resulting in greater operator confidence to adequately perform the procedure. This was confirmed by findings of other investigators who also found combined 2D TEE and RT3D TEE imaging to result in shorter procedural time compared to 2D TEE guidance alone [64]. Furthermore, RT3D TEE has been shown to provide unique information about functional and morphologic changes induced by percutaneous mitral valve repair with the remaining vena contracta area being of particular importance for patient outcome [65]. Thus, the EchoNavigator tool is a promising solution to further improve and ease the technically challenging MitraClip procedure.

■ **Selecting patients for percutaneous mitral valve repair**

RT3D TEE has been demonstrated to play an important role in selecting patients with appropriate mitral apparatus morphology for transcatheter mitral valve repair [1][8][66][67]. Beside general criteria in patient selection like severe comorbidity and high perioperative risk, several morphologic criteria for successful repair have also been defined [1]. In principle, percutaneous mitral valve repair is a suitable technique for both organic (or primary) and functional (or secondary) MR mechanisms where RT3D TEE can provide important information as described in detail in ► Chapter 7. Specific anatomic criteria postulated for percutaneous mitral valve repair are a coaptation length of ≥2 mm and a coaptation height of ≤11 mm in patients with functional MR, and a flail height or gap of <10 mm and a flail width of <15 mm in patients with flail leaflet [59]. In addition, both leaflets, particularly the posterior leaflet, should be of appropriate length (≥10 mm) and without thickening, plaques or calcification which could prevent successful grasping. Also, as clipping of the two leaflets causes restriction of leaflet opening, the mitral valve opening area should be ≥4 cm^2 prior to the procedure [59]. Recently, Altiok et al. [65] showed that using RT3D TEE analysis the maximum diastolic mitral valve area decreased from 6.0±2.0 cm^2 to 2.9±0.9 cm^2 after the procedure.

■ **Guiding percutaneous mitral valve repair**

In contrast to the percutaneous ASD and PFO closure procedures described above where a guide wire passes the interatrial septum through a preexisting orifice (PFO or ASD), a transseptal puncture needs to be performed under echocardiographic guidance during percutaneous mitral valve repair. The correct puncture site (posterior–superior aspect of the fossa ovalis) is of great importance and is a prerequisite for the correct positioning of the clip device in the left atrium. Identification of the correct puncture site is best performed using two orthogonal simultaneous 2D TEE long-axis and short-axis views of the interatrial septum using the real-time 3D xPlane mode displaying the tenting of the interatrial septum caused by 3D the puncture needle (◘ Fig. 12.16). Compared to 2D images, the RT3DE en face view

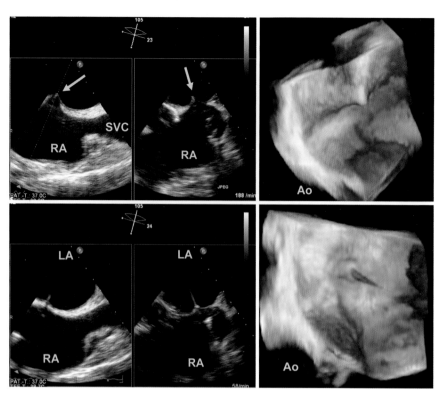

◘ Fig. 12.16 Monitoring and guiding of transseptal puncture using RT3DE. *Top left* The 2D TEE images in the RT3DE xPlane mode demonstrate the optimal puncture site of the interatrial septum immediately before transseptal puncture. The *arrows* point to the tenting of the interatrial septum evoked by the puncture needle. *Top right* RT3DE provides even better representation of the IAS tenting by the puncture needle. *Bottom left* RT3DE xPlane visualization of the needle penetrating the IAS. *Bottom right* RT3DE en face view of the IAS showing the exact location of the transseptal puncture. *RA* right atrium, *LA* left atrium, *SVC* superior vena cava, *Ao* aorta. [→Videos 12.16A–C]

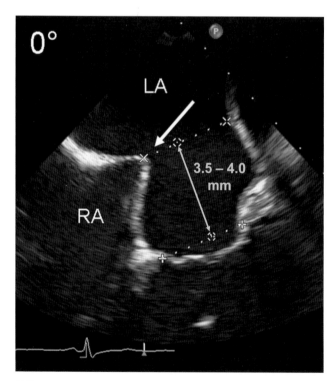

◘ Fig. 12.17 Measurement of distance between the transseptal puncture site and mitral annulus before percutaneous edge-to-edge mitral valve repair. *LA* left atrium, *RA* right

to the interatrial septum provides a more anatomic realistic orientation of the puncture site in relation to the neighboring structures (◘ Fig. 12.16) which can make an important difference [68][69]. Sufficient height of 3.5–4.0 cm from the mitral valve annular plane to the interatrial puncture site should be achieved to enable the clip delivery system an optimal range of movement [1]. A puncture site too far from the mitral valve (>4.0 cm) may prevent sufficient movement of the clip on the left ventricular side of the mitral valve, whereas a puncture site too close (<3.5 cm) to the mitral valve may inhibit steerability of the clip arm (◘ Fig. 12.17).

> RT3DE en face view to the interatrial septum provides an anatomically realistic orientation of the transseptal puncture site in relation to neighboring structures.

After successful transseptal puncture, RT3DE is helpful in navigating the guide wire through the left atrium into the left upper pulmonary vein (◘ Fig. 12.5). Next, a steerable guiding catheter and dilator are advanced through the septum. RT3D TEE displays the correct position and spatial orientation of the guide catheter relative to the mitral valve (◘ Fig. 12.18) [61].

The clip delivery device is subsequently advanced through the guide catheter into the left atrium. Using fluoroscopic and echocardiographic guidance, the clip is steered until axially aligned and centered over the origin of the regurgitant jet. During

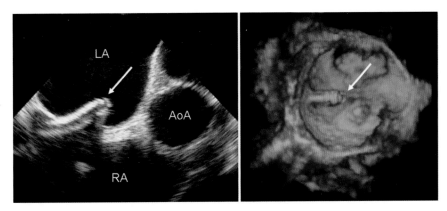

Fig. 12.18 *Left* The 2D TEE image of the guide catheter (*arrow*) penetrating the interatrial septum. *Right* RT3D TEE image showing the guide catheter (*arrow*) protruding into the left atrium. The improved spatial orientation allows for better steering of the clip in the left atrium and towards the mitral valve. *LA* left atrium, *RA* right atrium, *AoA* ascending aorta

advancement and steering of the rigid clip in the left atrium, meticulous care needs to be taken to avoid laceration of the lateral atrial wall or the aortic root. At all times during this complex procedure, RT3D TEE gives a superb overview of the spatial orientation and exact position of the clip in the left atrium. RT3DE monitoring of the individual steps of percutaneous mitral valve repair (with closure of the transseptal puncture hole by ASD occluder implantation at the end of the procedure) is illustrated in ■ Fig. 12.19. Compared to RT3DE imaging, guidance of the steering arm using 2D TEE imaging requires cumbersome switching between different 2D views.

After correct positioning of the clip in the left atrium, the clip is opened to extend the two arms (■ Fig. 12.20). These arms need to be aligned perpendicular to the line of coaptation of the mitral valve. Because the coaptation line is never straight, RT3D TEE can easily be used to display the actual position of the arms relative to it and for monitoring changes during adaptive maneuvers (■ Fig. 12.19) [24][57][61][62][70].

> ❯ RT3DE visualization of the clip device allows ideal monitoring of perpendicular alignment of the clip to the coaptation line of the mitral valve.

Subsequently, the clip is advanced into the left ventricle. Importantly, no change in the orientation of the clip arms relative to the coaptation line of the mitral valve is allowed at this stage. Using RT3D TEE, the correct position of the clip arms in the left ventricle can be easily monitored from a left atrial as well as left ventricular perspective (■ Fig. 12.21).

Grasping of both the anterior and posterior mitral leaflets and monitoring of correct leaflet insertion is primarily performed under 2D TEE guidance (■ Fig. 12.21) because of the high temporal and spatial resolution required for this step. RT3D TEE is very helpful in confirming the correct position of the closed clip and the correct shape of the double orifice situation of the mitral valve prior to clip release [61]. Before release of the clip RT3D TEE color Doppler provides superior information of the clipping effect on location, size and direction of the MR jet or multiple jets. Based on this information the clip might be positioned differently.

After release, RT3D TEE shows an en face view onto the double orifice mitral valve from the atrial and left ventricular aspect (■ Fig. 12.19). RT3DE color Doppler is complementary to 2D color Doppler adding superior 3D visualization of the size, geometry, and exact location of the regurgitant jet before and after mitral valve repair (■ Fig. 12.22).

Depending on the results of the mitral valve clipping procedure, a second clip or even more clips might be necessary if satisfactory reduction of mitral regurgitation was not achieved by the first clip. RT3DE has been demonstrated to be extremely useful for guiding deployment of additional clips accurately to the site of remaining mitral regurgitation and for visualizing the location of the clips as well as the resulting multiple orifice mitral valve (■ Fig. 12.23) [71][72][73][74]. In this context, RT3D TEE has been shown to be valuable in the detection and understanding of complications that can occur during the procedure as well as guiding the decision-making process [75].

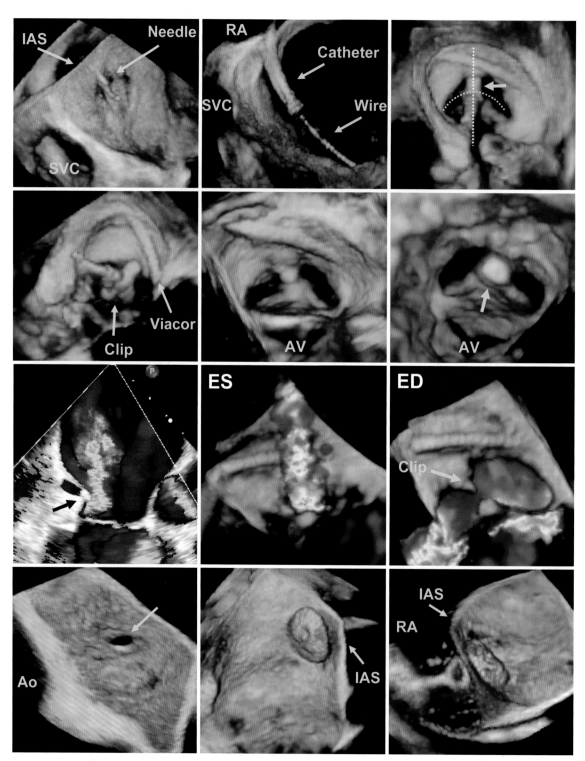

■ **Fig. 12.19** Periinterventional monitoring and guiding of percutaneous edge-to-edge mitral valve repair using RT3DE in the same patient shown in ■ Fig. 12.15 after ineffective percutaneous annulopasty. *Top left* RT3DE en face view of the interatrial septum (*IAS*) from a left atrial perspective showing the transseptal puncture using a Brockenbrough needle. *Top middle* Visualization of the 22-French guide catheter passing through the IAS over a thin guide wire. *Top right* En face view of the left atrium and mitral valve showing the guide catheter and the opened MitraClip™ (*arrow*) as well as the Viacor™ device in the coronary sinus (*CS*). The opened MitraClip™ is guided by RT3DE to be oriented perpendicular to the mitral valve coaptation line (*dotted lines*). *2nd row left* Side view to the guide catheter and opened MitraClip™. *2nd row middle* En face view of the mitral valve from the left atrial perspective after clipping of the anterior and posterior mitral leaflet resulting in a double orifice mitral valve. *2nd row right* En face view of the mitral valve from the left ventricular perspective to the clipped mitral valve. Note the exact median position of the clip (*arrow*). *3rd row left* Final result by 2D color Doppler showing mild-to-moderate mitral regurgitation (*MR*). Note the Viacor™ device in the coronary sinus (*black arrow*). *3rd row middle* End-systolic (*ES*) RT3DE color Doppler image showing the exact location of MR in the anterolateral orifice. *3rd row right* End-diastolic (*ED*) RT3DE color Doppler image representing the typical dual orifice mitral valve. *Bottom left* Remaining hole in the IAS (*arrow*) after transseptal puncture. *Bottom middle* RT3DE guiding of occluder implantation showing the left atrial occluder disk pulled towards the IAS (8 mm Amplatzer™ ASD occluder). *Bottom right* RT3DE side view of the IAS and occluder device showing unfolding of the right atrial occluder disk. *SVC* superior vena cava, *RA* right atrium, *AV* aortic valve, *Ao* aorta. [→Videos 12.19A–K]

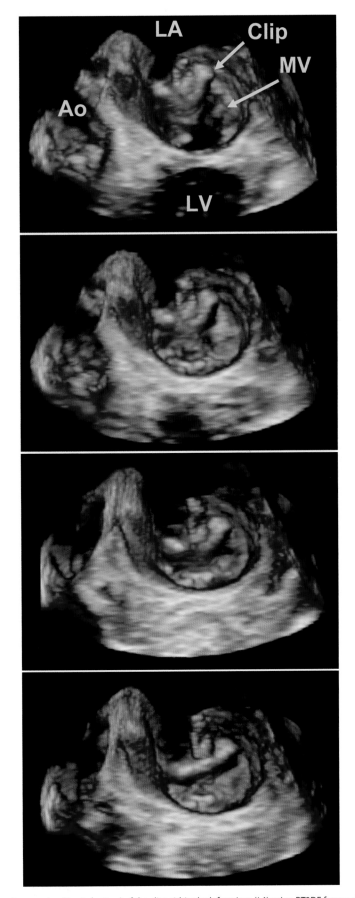

◻ **Fig. 12.20** Monitoring of progressive opening (*top to bottom*) of the clip within the left atrium (*LA*) using RT3DE from a side perspective to the clip and the mitral valve (*MV*). *Ao* aorta, *LV* left ventricle. [→Video 12.20]

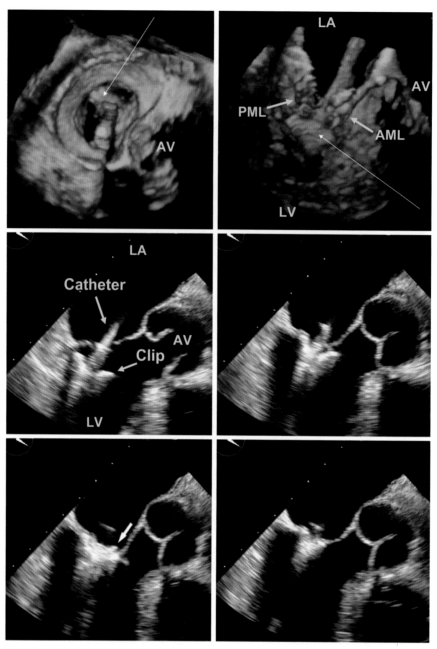

☐ **Fig. 12.21** Monitoring of grasping mitral leaflets and clip closure. *Top* RT3D TEE view from the left atrium (*LA*) toward the mitral valve (*left*) and oblique view from the left ventricle (*LV*) to the mitral valve (*right*). The opened clip (*white arrows*) is advanced through the mitral valve into the left ventricle and oriented perpendicular to the line of coaptation. *Bottom* The dynamic process of grasping the two mitral leaflets by the clip and closure of the clip can be best monitored by 2D imaging as shown in this sequence of images. *AV* aortic valve, *PML* posterior mitral leaflet, *AML* anterior mitral leaflet. [→Video 12.21]

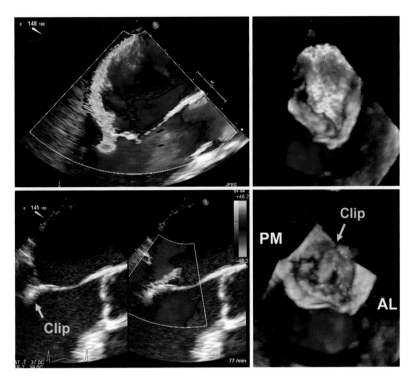

Fig. 12.22 The 2D and RT3D echocardiographic presentations of the result after successful edge-to-edge mitral valve repair. *Top* The 2D and RT3D echocardiographic demonstration of severe eccentric mitral regurgitation. RT3DE shows the broad jet origin along the commissure due to incomplete leaflet closure. *Bottom* After repair, 2D and RT3D echocardiography show only trace-to-mild mitral regurgitation. RT3DE clearly identifies the remaining jet in the antero-lateral location. *PM* postero-medial, *AL* antero-lateral. [→Videos 12.22A–D]

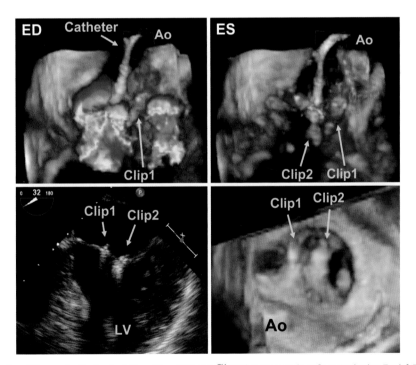

Fig. 12.23 RT3DE monitoring of the result after implantation of two MitraClips™ resulting in a triple orifice mitral valve. *Top left* End-diastolic (*ED*) RT3DE color Doppler oblique view from the left atrium of the mitral valve showing the three orifices while the second clip is placed. *Top right* End-systolic (*ES*) view showing the second clip attached to the delivery catheter, the first clip, and the remaining trace postero-medial mitral regurgitation. *Bottom left* The 2D echocardiographic representation of the two clips. *Bottom right* RT3DE en face view to the mitral valve showing the two clips and the triple orifice mitral valve. *Ao* aorta, *LV* left ventricle. [→Videos 12.23A–C]

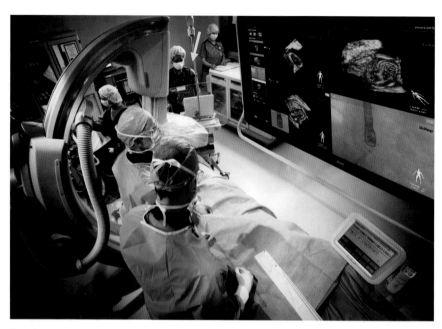

■ **Fig. 12.24** Illustration of a catheterization lab setting during transcatheter intervention of structural heart disease using EchoNavigator. In principle, in catheterization procedures not using the EchoNavigator x-ray imaging (*in front*) and 3D TEE imaging (*in back, yellow arrow*) are two total different modalities that are operated independently. In this example the echocardiographer and the interventionalists communicate based on the same synchronized view of x-ray and 3D image

12.3.5 EchoNavigator – integration of x-ray and RT3D TEE images during transcatheter interventions

The EchoNavigator is a novel application allowing for integration and synchronization of x-ray images and RT3D TEE images for improved navigation of wires and catheters and deploy implants like occluders, valves, and clips in the correct position in the heart. By merging the two, generally independently operated imaging modalities x-ray for imaging the catheters and devices and 3D echocardiography for imaging soft tissue heart structures which are required to guide catheter-based interventions, the EchoNavigator creates a single integrated and intuitive view.

Previously, the use of the two independent imaging modalities for guiding catheter-based interventions was difficult. Many of the challenges originate from the situation that x-ray imaging and 3D echocardiography are two completely separate techniques that have now been combined in the catheterization lab. Typically the interventionalist is familiar and comfortable with x-ray images, but his experience in interpreting the anatomy in 3D echocardiographic images is limited – and vice versa for echocardiographers interpreting x-ray images. In fact, the spatial relation between 3D echocardiographic and x-ray images is not trivial to understand because the x-ray image and 3D echocardiographic image orientation are not correlated. Left on the x-ray image might be right on the 3D echocardiographic image. Up on the 3D echocardiographic image might be down on the x-ray image. As a consequence, each time the interventionalist switches his view from x-ray to the 3D echocardiographic image, he needs to mentally re-register. Due to the fact that in critical moments both operators need to communicate information from two separate modalities, communication can be ambiguous. In

■ Fig. 12.24 the setting in a catheterization lab during intervention of structural heart disease (in this case with the use of the EchoNavigator) is illustrated.

The key characteristics of the work process of the EchoNavigator are briefly described. As a basic feature the EchoNavigator automatically finds and tracks the position of the head of the TEE probe in the x-ray image (■ Fig. 12.25). It also determines the direction of the head of the TEE probe based on the shape recognized in the x-ray image. Based on the position of the head of the TEE probe and directional information, the EchoNavigator displays the cone-shaped 3D echocardiographic volume in the x-ray image (*purple wire frame* in ■ Fig. 12.25) providing intuitive understanding of the spatial relationship between the 3D echo and x-ray image. Furthermore, the EchoNavigator provides automatic alignment between x-ray and 3D echocardiographic image orientation, making the device manipulation more straightforward as shown in cases of transseptal puncture (■ Fig. 12.25), MitraClip (■ Fig. 12.26), and ASD closure (■ Fig. 12.27). If the interventionalist moves the puncture device to the left in the x-ray image, the puncture device also moves to the left in the 3D echocardiographic image, thus, increasing the confidence in spatial orientation and anatomy and device orientation. With this synchronized view of x-ray and 3D echocardiographic image, the EchoNavigator will also automatically track and follow C-arm rotation. As another benefit of the synchronized x-ray and 3D echocardiographic image, the EchoNavigator allows specific anatomic structures or targets to be marked in the RT3D TEE image dataset and this ultrasound mark automatically appears in the x-ray image for improved guidance of device catheters, which is of crucial importance during the MitraClip procedure (■ Fig. 12.26). Finally, the EchoNavigator also allows the 3D echocardiographic image to be shown in different per-

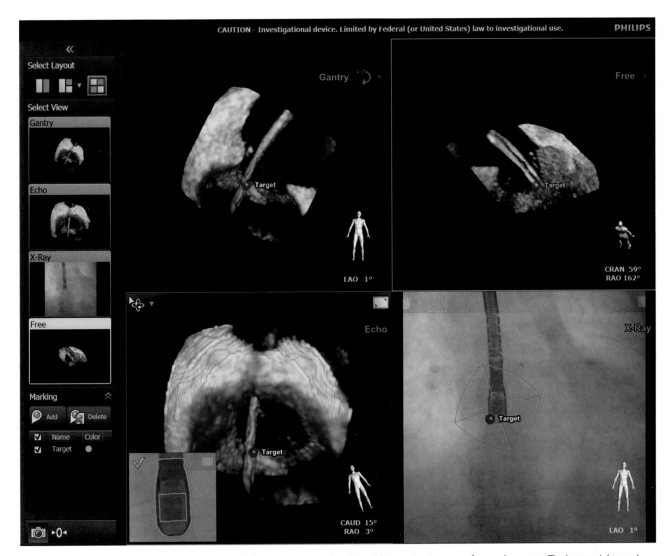

Fig. 12.25 Example of the EchoNavigator imaging displayed on the central multimodality monitor in a case of a septal puncture. The *bottom right panel* (x-ray) shows the typical x-ray image with the TEE probe, but with the characteristic display of the cone-shaped 3D echo volume (*purple wire frame*), the *blue tissue* marker at the target site on the inter atrial septum for transseptal puncture and the *silver man* for spatial orientation. The *upper left panel* (gantry) shows the 3D echocardiographic image perfectly aligned in space with the x-ray image (note the identical orientation of the guide catheter in the x-ray and 3D echocardiographic image as well as the identical orientation of the silver man). The *lower left panel* (echo) represents the 3D echocardiographic image as it is interrogated by the echocardiographer on the 3D echo machine providing also to visualize the anatomy simultaneously from different perspectives. In the *lower left panel* also automatic recognition and tracking of the head of the TEE probe is monitored. The *upper right panel* (free) allows the interventionalist to independently interrogate the 3D echocardiographic image from the table side

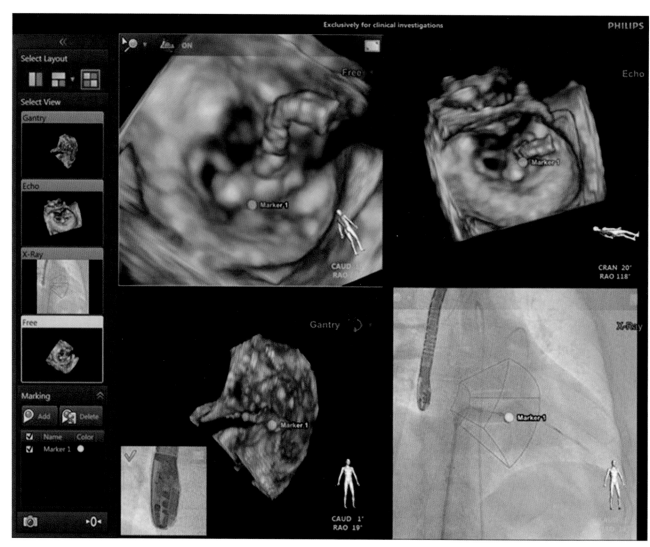

Fig. 12.26 Example of the use of the EchoNavigator in a MitraClip case at the point of steering the device catheter with the opened clip to the leaflets and orienting the clip perpendicular to the line of coaptation. Note that the four panels (x-ray, gantry, echo, free) are the same as in **Fig. 12.25** but are in a different order with the two synchronized and aligned x-ray and 3D echocardiographic images displayed side-by-side in the *bottom row*. The *yellow marker*, set in the 3D echocardiographic dataset, indicates the desired clip position at the level of the leaflets. As it automatically appears in the x-ray image, it gives the interventionalist a general idea of direction on where to steer the device to when looking at the x-ray image

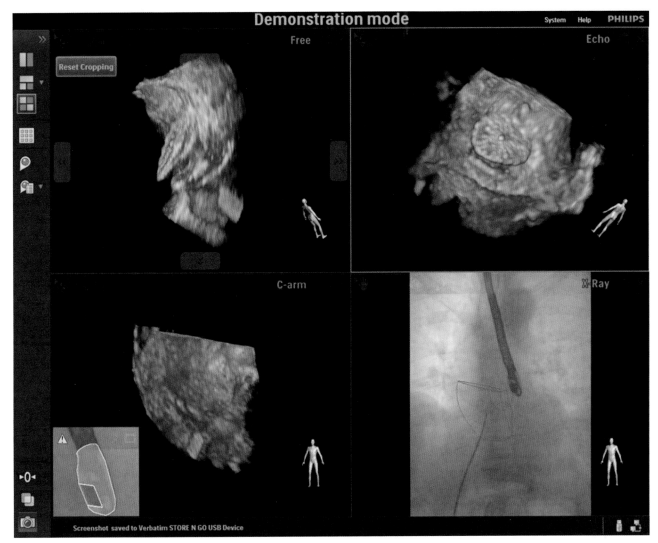

Fig. 12.27 Case of ASD closure with an Amplatzer occluder using the EchoNavigator. The display of the different views illustrates the feature of simultaneously showing the 3D echocardiographic image in different perspectives. In the 3D image in the *upper right panel* the ASD occluder device is shown en face from the left atrium with full deployment of the left-sided disk. In the *upper left panel,* the view is more along the device axis and also shows the deployment of the right-sided disk

spectives simultaneously (■ Fig. 12.25, ■ Fig. 12.26, ■ Fig. 12.27) and even enables the interventionalist who is experienced in RT3DE to interrogate (rotate and crop) the 3D echocardiographic image by himself from the table side. Thus, during critical moments of the procedure, for example just before deploying an ASD occluder or MitraClip, the interventionalist can be ensured of the good position of the device.

The novel EchoNavigator application not only provides synchronized x-ray and RT3D TEE imaging for improved understanding and guiding, but also introduces a whole new solution for ›synchronized‹ communication and work flow between echocardiographers and interventionalists in the cath lab, which potentially will also lead to reduced procedure and fluoroscopy time during catheter-based interventions for structural heart disease.

12.3.6 Left atrial appendage occluder implantation

Occluding the left atrial appendage (LAA) in nonvalvular atrial fibrillation is a potential alternative to long-term oral anticoagulation for stroke prevention as shown in the PROTECT AF study [76][77]. In the intervention group, the combined risk for ischemic and hemorrhagic stroke was lower compared to the control group (2.3 versus 3.2 events per 100 patient–years). In this study, the left atrial appendage was occluded by implantation of a self-expanding nitinol mesh device (Watchman™, Atritec Inc., Plymouth, MN, USA) placed under fluoroscopic and transesophageal echocardiographic guidance. A recently introduced device (Amplatzer™ Cardiac Plug, AGA Medical Cooperation, Plymouth, MN, USA), which is composed of a lobe being placed into the LAA with a connected disk that is placed to cover the orifice of the LAA, extends this concept [76].

Compared to ASD and PFO occluder implantation, echocardiographic monitoring and guiding is even more important during LAA occluder implantation. This is because transseptal puncture is required (see above) and accurate navigation of the device catheter into the complex shaped LAA can be difficult. RT3D TEE provides an anatomically realistic view of the left atrium and LAA as well as neighboring structures. Consequently, it has been demonstrated to be particularly useful in guiding transcatheter LAA occlusion as it provides accurate visualization and assessment of both the interatrial septum and the LAA [1] [68][78][79]. RT3D TEE has also been shown to provide accurate quantitative analysis of LAA anatomy including the number of lobes which is crucial for patient selection and appropriate occluder placement [80][81]. Device sizing requires careful measurement of the appendage dimensions. Since it rarely has a circular cross-section, RT3DE can be very helpful in this context. RT3D TEE has been demonstrated to provide more accurate assessment of the LAA orifice area compared to 2D TEE using cardiac computed tomography for reference [82]. Furthermore, RT3DE enables continuous monitoring and guiding of the all individual steps of the procedure (◘ Fig. 12.28) [83]. After the occluder disk has been released from the device catheter, the RT3DE en face view of the LAA gives greater confidence of sufficient occlusion by the occluder compared to 2D echocardiography. Beyond the procedure itself, RT3D TEE has recently been shown, because of its superior spatial information, to be valuable in the detection and monitoring of thrombus formation on Amplatzer occluder devices during routine follow-up examinations (► Chapter 11.1.1, ► Fig. 11.7) [84].

12.3.7 Percutaneous occluder implantation for paravalvular leaks

Percutaneous occluder implantation for paravalvular leaks of aortic or mitral valve prostheses has proved to be a valuable therapeutic option for patients with signs of hemolysis or progressive heart failure and with a risk for second cardiac surgery that is too high [1]. It has been particularly stimulated by the experiences made in percutaneous occluder implantations in cases of ASD,

PFO, LAA, and VSD. In addition to the procedure itself, selection of appropriate patients and criteria for understanding the pathology are of utmost importance for procedural success [1]. RT3D TEE has been validated to accurately provide determination of the locations and number of the leaks, as well as their shapes, lengths, widths, areas, and extent [85]. Particularly an en face view to the aortic or mitral valve prosthesis provides superior spatial information to accurately detect the location of the leaks by using a diagram of radians (► Fig. 7.25 in Chapter 7) [1]. Illustrative examples of paravalvular leaks and their quantification using RT3D TEE datasets are shown in ► Fig. 7.24, ► Fig. 7.25, ► Fig. 7.27, and ► Fig. 7.28 in Chapter 7. Accurate determination of size, shape and number of leaks is also of particular importance for decision-making on the number of closure devices needed [1, 86, 87].

In a recent study comparing 2D TEE and RT3D TEE, only RT3D TEE could accurately demonstrate the length of the paravalvular leak [88]. In principle, RT3D TEE en face visualization of aortic prostheses and paravalvular leaks is more difficult compared to mitral valve prostheses mainly because of the more confined anatomy. During the procedure after transseptal puncture, guiding navigation of the guide wire through the paravalvular leak can be extremely difficult using fluoroscopic or 2D echocardiographic imaging. RT3D TEE provides superior spatial visualization and orientation of the guide wire in relation to the paravalvular leak and is therefore ideally suited for guiding both the guide wire and the occluder device to the leak (◘ Fig. 12.29) [61][89][90].

Because of the spatial complexity of navigating the guide wire through the leak, this procedure is considered as an application, in which periinterventional RT3D TEE guiding is indispensable and was recently recommended as the preferred TEE imaging modality for this procedure [1]. The value of RT3D TEE during percutaneous implantation of one or multiple occluder devices to paravalvular leaks of the aortic or mitral valve has been demonstrated by several investigators (◘ Fig. 12.30) [61][87][89][91] [92][93][94]. More recently, as an alternative to antegrade transseptal access, a transapical or a retrograde transaortic approach to paravalvular leaks has been described where RT3D TEE was also demonstrated to be indispensable for guiding and monitoring the procedure [95][[96][97].

> RT3D TEE provides superior spatial visualization and orientation for navigating the guide wire through the paravalvular leak.

12.3.8 Percutaneous mitral valvuloplasty

Three-dimensional echocardiography and particular RT3D TEE has been shown to provide important image information in patients with mitral stenosis before, during, and after percutaneous mitral balloon valvuloplasty (PMV) [98]. Using RT3D TEE also allows assessment of the morphology of the MV considered for PMV, which is important for the evaluation of the mechanism, patient selection, and procedural success [99][100]. Examples of mitral stenosis of different pathomorphologies demonstrated by

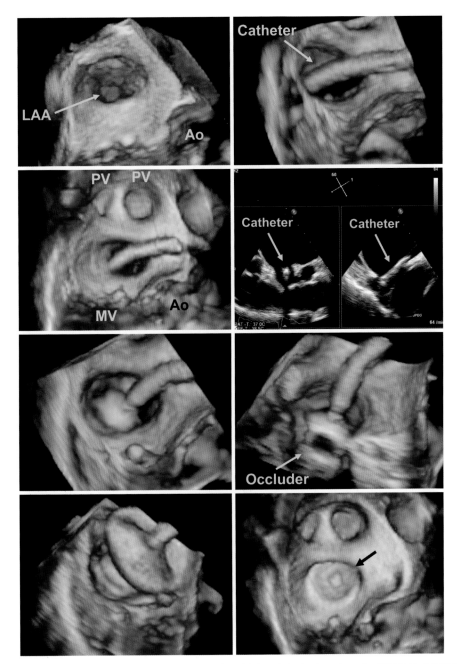

Fig. 12.28 Periinterventional monitoring and guiding of left atrial appendage (*LAA*) occluder implantation using RT3DE. *Top left* RT3DE aspect of the LAA before occluder implantation providing a view deep into the LAA. *Top right* Live 3D zoom image monitoring navigation of the delivery catheter into the LAA. *2nd row left* RT3DE full volume showing the delivery catheter placed into the LAA as well as neighboring structures like the mitral valve (*MV*), aortic valve, and the two left pulmonary veins (*PV*). *2nd row right* RT3DE xPlane image showing the delivery catheter with the LAA in two orthogonal views. *3rd row left* Monitoring of the opening of the distal part of the occluder (26 mm, Amplatzer™ Cardiac Plug) within the LAA. *3rd row right* Cross-section through the LAA and the occluder unfolded within. *Bottom left* Release of the proximal disk-shaped occluder to cover the LAA entrance. *Bottom right* RT3DE full volume en face view to the LAA successfully plugged by the occluder (*arrow*). *Ao* aorta. [→Videos 12.28A–H]

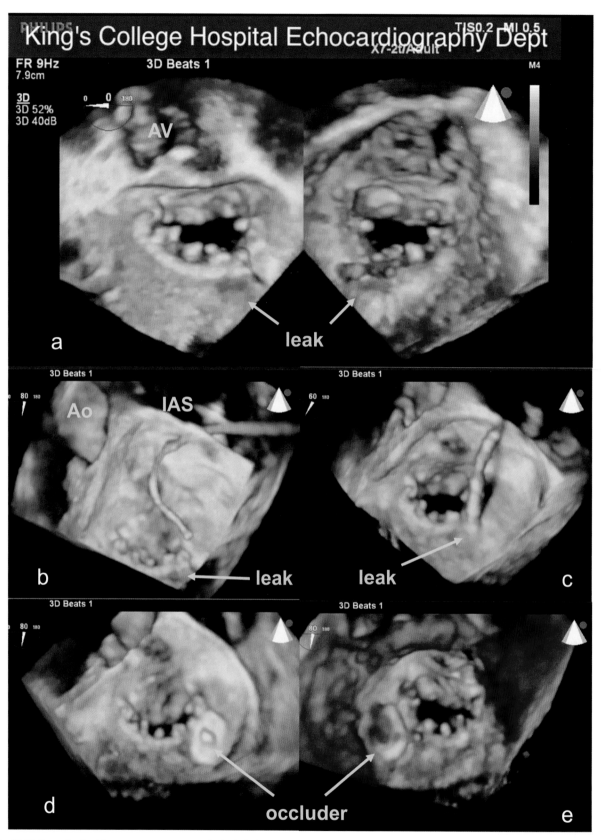

■ **Fig. 12.29** Example of guiding a percutaneous paravalvular leak closure in a case after surgical mitral annuloplasty using RT3D TEE. *Top* The 3D dual-view mode representation of a mitral valve repaired by annuloplasty with a paravalvular leak in the posterior location (*left image* shows view from the left atrium; *right image* shows view from the left ventricle). The paravalvular leak is more obvious in the ▶ Video. *Middle left* Guiding of the guide wire passing through the IAS and navigated towards the paravalvular leak. *Middle right* Demonstration of the guide catheter successfully positioned across the paravalvular leak. *Bottom left* Surgical view from the left atrium to the mitral valve showing the occluder device in final position. *Bottom right* Occluder device shown from left ventricle. *AV* aortic valve, *IAS* interatrial septum, *Ao* aorta. (Courtesy of M.J. Monaghan) [→Video 12.29a–e]

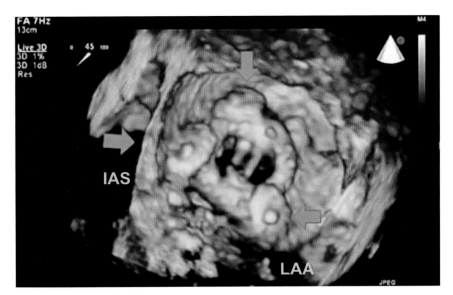

◘ Fig. 12.30 RT3D TEE en face view in an anatomic orientation from left atrium to a mechanical mitral valve prosthesis after percutaneous implantation of three occluder devices (*green arrows*) in paravalvular leaks. *IAS* interatrial septum, *LAA* left atrial appendage. (Courtesy of J. Zamorano)

RT3DE are shown in ▶ Chapter 8 (▶ Figs. 8.1–8.6). RT3DE provides an en face view of the mitral valve from either a left atrial or a left ventricular perspective, including detailed visualization of the commissures, leaflets, and subvalvular structures which often can not be clearly seen with 2D echocardiography [61] [101]. Like in other transcatheter mitral valve interventions described previously, RT3D TEE is of great value for guiding the different steps during the balloon valvuloplasty including transseptal puncture, guiding the balloon catheter into the mitral valve and appropriate positioning of the balloon within the mitral valve (◘ Fig. 12.31) [61][102].

> ❯ RT3D TEE is a suitable technique for monitoring percutaneous mitral valvuloplasty and provides accurate measurement of MVA immediately after PMV.

In the immediate post-PMV period, RT3D TEE provides accurate assessment of the mitral commissural splitting, stretching, or tearing after PMV by a direct en face view to the mitral valve either from a left atrial or a left ventricular perspective (◘ Fig. 12.31). RT3D TEE also provides immediate accurate determination of the commissure opening after PMV. Earlier studies have demonstrated large discrepancies between mitral valve area (MVA) measurements obtained using the Doppler-based PHT method and those derived invasively in the catheterization laboratory [103]. Following PMV, the mitral orifice becomes irregular and is technically difficult to trace, particularly in heavily calcified areas. In addition, due to the variable geometry of the stenotic MV orifice, correct plane orientation using conventional 2D techniques frequently becomes difficult [61]. Recent studies of RT3DE vs 2D planimetry and PHT for measurement of MVA immediately after PMV used the invasively derived MVA (Gorlin) for reference [101][104]. In this comparison, RT3DE proved to be the most accurate technique for measuring MVA, with better pre- and postprocedural agreement with the invasively derived MVA [104]. Thus, RT3DE is not only a very suitable technique for appropriate patient selection and

guiding the procedure, but also for monitoring the efficacy and potential complications of PMV.

12.3.9 Electrophysiological procedures

There is increasing need for imaging techniques to monitor and guide electrophysiological procedures. Navigation of diagnostic and therapeutic catheters in electrophysiology is normally performed using fluoroscopy. However, fluoroscopy can not be used to visualize myocardial tissue or the endocardial surface, which is of great importance especially during ablation procedures.

Electroanatomical mapping systems, using electromagnetic sensor localization, have become widely adopted for complex procedures. In addition, 2D intracardiac ultrasound systems have been used to guide electrophysiological interventions, thus, obtaining 2D images of cardiac structures during the procedure.

The potential added value of 3D anatomic information in electrophysiological procedures has been demonstrated by non-real-time 3D intracardiac ultrasound images reconstructed from a set of 2D image planes [105]. However, this method, besides its offline character, is limited by its invasive nature, using large sheaths with possible bleeding complications.

RT3D TEE has been validated to address these challenges by less invasively acquiring high-quality 3D images of the atria, pulmonary veins, and the mitral valve annulus (◘ Fig. 12.32) [22] [106][107][108]. As previously mentioned, the addition of the third dimension is also useful during transseptal puncture in patients receiving left atrial electrophysiological procedures, e.g., ablation of fibrillation (see also ◘ Fig. 12.16) [109][110][111]. Recently, RT3D TEE has been demonstrated in several clinical studies to provide superior 3D visualization of all pulmonary vein ostia and neighboring left atrial structures during ablation and to provide the operator successful guidance to position an ablation catheter or cryoballoon in the pulmonary veins [112] [113][114].

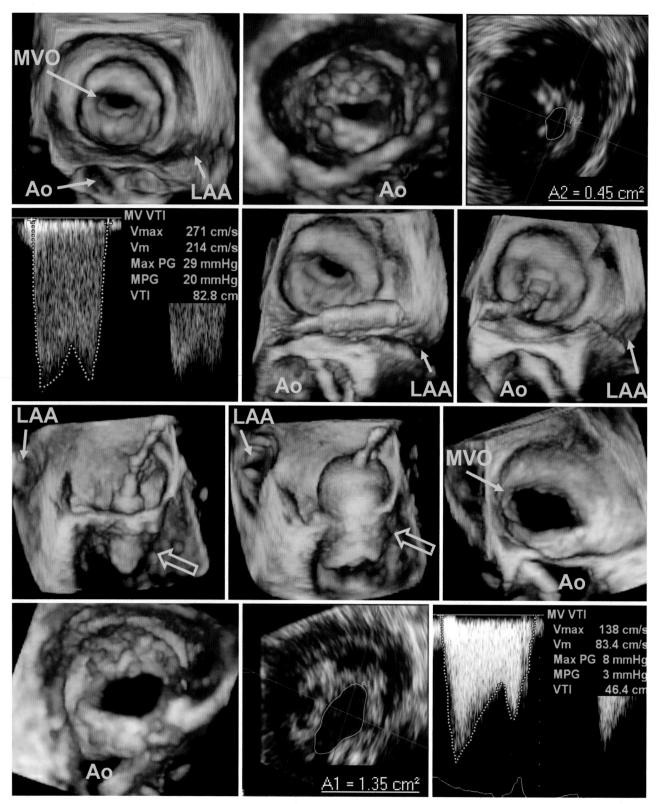

◘ **Fig. 12.31** Periinterventional monitoring and guiding of percutaneous mitral valvuloplasty (*PMV*). *Top left* RT3DE en face view of the stenotic mitral valve from the left atrial perspective. *Top middle* RT3DE en face view of the stenotic mitral valve from a left ventricular perspective. *Top right* RT3DE-based planimetry of a mitral valve orifice (*MVO*) area of 0.45 cm². *Second row left* CW Doppler measurement of a mean pressure gradient (*MPG*) of 20 mmHg. *Second row middle* RT3DE-guided navigation of the catheter with the deflated balloon; the balloon catheter is still malpositioned toward the left atrial appendage (*LAA*). Note the pigtail catheter through the aortic valve. *Second row right* Successful RT3D-guided navigation of the balloon catheter into the mitral valve. *Third row left* Positioning of the balloon (*contoured arrow*) within the mitral valve. *Third row middle* Monitoring of balloon inflation. *Third row right* Maximal opening of the mitral valve after valvuloplasty from a left atrial perspective. *Bottom left* Maximal opening of the mitral valve after valvuloplasty from a left ventricular perspective. *Bottom middle* RT3D-based planimetry of a mitral valve orifice area of 1.35 cm² after valvuloplasty. *Bottom left* CW Doppler measurement of a mean pressure gradient (*MPG*) of 3 mmHg after valvuloplasty. *Ao* aorta, *LAA* left atrial appendage. [→Videos 12.31A–H]

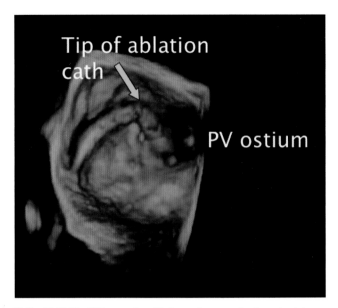

Fig. 12.32 The 3D image of an ablation catheter coming from the right atrium into the left atrium after transseptal puncture. View into the left upper pulmonary vein (*PV*); note the catheter crossing the interatrial septum and the location of the catheter tip near the PV ostium. The ablation catheter is rinsed with saline which forms small bubbles that can be seen in the PV ostium. [→Video 12.32]

References

1. Zamorano JL, Badano LP, Bruce C et al (2011) EAE/ASE recommendations for the use of echocardiography in new transcatheter interventions for valvular heart disease. Eur J Echocardiogr 12:557–584
2. Amitai ME, Schnittger I, Popp RL et al (2007) Comparison of three-dimensional echocardiography to two-dimensional echocardiography and fluoroscopy for monitoring of endomyocardial biopsy. Am J Cardiol 99:864–866
3. Roman KS, Nii M, Golding F et al (2004) Images in cardiovascular medicine. Real-time subcostal 3-dimensional echocardiography for guided percutaneous atrial septal defect closure. Circulation 109:e320–e321
4. Bartel T, Konorza T, Arjumand J et al (2003) Intracardiac echocardiography is superior to conventional monitoring for guiding device closure of interatrial communications. Circulation 107:795–797
5. Knackstedt C, Mischke K, Frechen D et al (2007) The role of intracardiac echocardiography in interventional electrophysiology. Minerva Cardioangiol 55:755–770
6. Kim SS, Hijazi ZM, Lang RM, Knight BP (2009) The use of intracardiac echocardiography and other intracardiac imaging tools to guide non-coronary cardiac interventions. J Am Coll Cardiol 53:2117–2128
7. Szili-Torok T, Bosch JG (2011) Transnasal transoesophageal ultrasound: the end of the intracardiac echocardiography age? Europace 13:7–8
8. Lang RM, Badano LP, Tsang W et al (2012) EAE/ASE recommendations for image acquisition and display using three-dimensional echocardiography. Eur Heart J Cardiovasc Imaging 13:1–46
9. Grewal J, Mankad S, Freeman WK et al (2009) Real-time three-dimensional transesophageal echocardiography in the intraoperative assessment of mitral valve disease. J Am Soc Echocardiogr 22:34–41
10. Sugeng L, Shernan SK, Weinert L et al (2008) Real-time three-dimensional transesophageal echocardiography in valve disease: comparison with surgical findings and evaluation of prosthetic valves. J Am Soc Echocardiogr 21:1347–1354
11. Hien MD, Rauch H, Lichtenberg A et al (2013) Real-time three-dimensional transesophageal echocardiography: improvements in intraoperative mitral valve imaging. Anesth Analg 2013; 116:287–295

12. Chikwe J, Adams DH, Su KN et al (2012) Can three-dimensional echocardiography accurately predict complexity of mitral valve repair? Eur J Cardiothorac Surg 41:518–524
13. Vegas A, Meineri M (2010) Core review: three-dimensional transesophageal echocardiography is a major advance for intraoperative clinical management of patients undergoing cardiac surgery: a core review. Anesth Analg 110:1548–1573
14. Shernan SK (2009) Intraoperative three-dimensional echocardiography: ready for primetime? J Am Soc Echocardiogr 22:27A–28A
15. Gripari P, Tamborini G, Barbier P et al (2010) Real-time three-dimensional transoesophageal echocardiography: a new intraoperative feasible and useful technology in cardiac surgery. Int J Cardiovasc Imaging 26:651–660
16. Fischer GW, Adams DH (2008) Real-time three-dimensional TEE-guided repair of a paravalvular leak after mitral valve replacement. Eur J Echocardiogr 9:868–869
17. Ender J, Koncar-Zeh J, Mukherjee C et al (2008) Value of augmented reality-enhanced transesophageal echocardiography (TEE) for determining optimal annuloplasty ring size during mitral valve repair. Ann Thorac Surg 86:1473–1478
18. Seo JS, Song JM, Kim YH et al (2012) Effect of atrial septal defect shape evaluated using three-dimensional transesophageal echocardiography on size measurements for percutaneous closure. J Am Soc Echocardiogr 25:1031–1140
19. Chen FL, Hsiung MC, Hsieh KS et al (2006) Real time three-dimensional transthoracic echocardiography for guiding Amplatzer septal occluder device deployment in patients with atrial septal defect. Echocardiography 23:763–770
20. Acar P, Massabuau P, Elbaz M (2008) Real-time 3D transoesophageal echocardiography for guiding Amplatzer septal occluder device deployment in an adult patient with atrial septal defect. Eur J Echocardiogr 9:822–823
21. Perk G, Lang RM, Garcia-Fernandez MA et al (2009) Use of real time three-dimensional transesophageal echocardiography in intracardiac catheter based interventions. J Am Soc Echocardiogr 22:865–882
22. Balzer J, Kuhl H, Rassaf T et al (2008) Real-time transesophageal three-dimensional echocardiography for guidance of percutaneous cardiac interventions: first experience. Clin Res Cardiol 97:565–574
23. Balzer J, Kuhl H, Franke A (2008) Real-time three-dimensional transoesophageal echocardiography for guidance of atrial septal defect closures. Eur Heart J 29:2226
24. Balzer J, Kelm M, Kuhl HP (2009) Real-time three-dimensional transoesophageal echocardiography for guidance of non-coronary interventions in the catheter laboratory. Eur J Echocardiogr 10:341–349
25. Martin-Reyes R, Lopez-Fernandez T, Moreno-Yanguela M et al (2009) Role of real-time three-dimensional transoesophageal echocardiography for guiding transcatheter patent foramen ovale closure. Eur J Echocardiogr 10:148–150
26. Lodato JA, Cao QL, Weinert L et al (2009) Feasibility of real-time three-dimensional transoesophageal echocardiography for guidance of percutaneous atrial septal defect closure. Eur J Echocardiogr 10:543–548
27. Taniguchi M, Akagi T, Watanabe N et al (2009) Application of real-time three-dimensional transesophageal echocardiography using a matrix array probe for transcatheter closure of atrial septal defect. J Am Soc Echocardiogr 22:1114–1120
28. Taniguchi M, Akagi T, Kijima Y, Sano S (2013) Clinical advantage of real-time three-dimensional transesophageal echo-cardiography for transcatheter closure of multiple atrial septal defects. Int J Cardiovasc Imaging 29:1273–1280
29. Lopez AL, Palomas JL, Rubio DM, Ortiz MR (2011) Three-dimensional echocardiography-guided repair of residual shunt after percutaneous atrial septal defect closure. Echocardiography 28:E64-E67
30. Balzer J, van Hall S, Rassaf T et al (2010) Feasibility, safety, and efficacy of real-time three-dimensional transoesophageal echocardiography for guiding device closure of interatrial communications: initial clinical experience and impact on radiation exposure. Eur J Echocardiogr 11:1–8
31. Acar P, Abdel-Massih T, Douste-Blazy MY et al (2002) Assessment of muscular ventricular septal defect closure by transcatheter or surgical approach: a three-dimensional echocardiographic study. Eur J Echocardiogr 3:185–191

32. Acar P, Abadir S, Aggoun Y (2007) Transcatheter closure of perimembranous ventricular septal defects with Amplatzer occluder assessed by real-time three-dimensional echocardiography. Eur J Echocardiogr 8:110–115

33. Tighe DA, Paul JJ, Maniet AR et al (1997) Survival in infarct related intramyocardial dissection importance of early echocardiography and prompt surgery. Echocardiography 14:403–408

34. Kakouros N, Brecker SJD (2009) Device closure for ventricular septal defect after myocardial infarction. Cardiac Interventions Today 43–49

35. Halpern DG, Perk G, Ruiz C et al (2009) Percutaneous closure of a postmyocardial infarction ventricular septal defect guided by real-time three-dimensional echocardiography. Eur J Echocardiogr 10:569–571

36. Charakida M, Qureshi S, Simpson JM (2013) 3D echocardiography for planning and guidance of interventional closure of VSD. JACC Cardiovasc Imaging 6:120–123

37. Grube E, Schuler G, Buellesfeld L et al (2007) Percutaneous aortic valve replacement for severe aortic stenosis in high-risk patients using the second- and current third-generation self-expanding CoreValve prosthesis: device success and 30-day clinical outcome. J Am Coll Cardiol 50:69–76

38. Leon MB, Smith CR, Mack M et al (2010) Transcatheter aortic-valve implantation for aortic stenosis in patients who cannot undergo surgery. N Engl J Med 363:1597–1607

39. Makkar RR, Fontana GP, Jilaihawi H et al (2012) Transcatheter aortic-valve replacement for inoperable severe aortic stenosis. N Engl J Med 366: 1696–1704

40. Smith LA, Monaghan MJ (2013) Monitoring of procedures: peri-interventional echo assessment for transcatheter aortic valve implantation. Eur Heart J Cardiovasc Imaging 14:840–850

41. Chin D (2009) Echocardiography for transcatheter aortic valve implantation. Eur J Echocardiogr 10:i21–i29

42. Moss RR, Ivens E, Pasupati S et al (2008) Role of echocardiography in percutaneous aortic valve implantation. JACC Cardiovasc Imaging 1:15–24.

43. Janosi RA, Kahlert P, Plicht B et al (2009) Guidance of percutaneous transcatheter aortic valve implantation by real-time three-dimensional transesophageal echocardiography - A single-center experience. Minim Invasive Ther Allied Technol 142–148

44. Janosi RA, Kahlert P, Plicht B et al (2011) Measurement of the aortic annulus size by real-time three-dimensional transesophageal echocardiography. Minim Invasive Ther Allied Technol 20:85–94

45. Ng AC, Delgado V, van der KF et al (2010) Comparison of aortic root dimensions and geometries before and after transcatheter aortic valve implantation by 2- and 3-dimensional transesophageal echocardiography and multislice computed tomography. Circ Cardiovasc Imaging 3:94–102

46. Santos N, de Agustin JA, Almeria C et al (2012) Prosthesis/annulus discongruence assessed by three-dimensional transoesophageal echocardiography: a predictor of significant paravalvular aortic regurgitation after transcatheter aortic valve implantation. Eur Heart J Cardiovasc Imaging 13:931–937

47. Jilaihawi H, Doctor N, Kashif M et al (2013) Aortic annular sizing for transcatheter aortic valve replacement using cross-sectional 3-dimensional transesophageal echocardiography. J Am Coll Cardiol 61:908–916

48. Husser O, Rauch S, Endemann DH et al (2012) Impact of three-dimensional transesophageal echocardiography on prosthesis sizing for transcatheter aortic valve implantation. Catheter Cardiovasc Interv 80:956–963

49. Smith LA, Dworakowski R, Bhan A et al (2013) Real-time three-dimensional transesophageal echocardiography adds value to transcatheter aortic valve implantation. J Am Soc Echocardiogr 26:359–369

50. Masson JB, Kovac J, Schuler G et al (2009) Transcatheter aortic valve implantation: review of the nature, management, and avoidance of procedural complications. JACC Cardiovasc Interv 2:811–820

51. Calleja A, Thavendiranathan P, Ionasec RI et al (2013) Automated quantitative 3-dimensional modeling of the aortic valve and root by 3-dimensional transesophageal echocardiography in normals, aortic regurgitation, and aortic stenosis: comparison to computed tomography in normals and clinical implications. Circ Cardiovasc Imaging 6:99–108

52. Goncalves A, Almeria C, Marcos-Alberca P et al (2012) Three-dimensional echocardiography in paravalvular aortic regurgitation assessment after transcatheter aortic valve implantation. J Am Soc Echocardiogr 25:47–55

53. Gripari P, Ewe SH, Fusini L et al (2012) Intraoperative 2D and 3D transoesophageal echocardiographic predictors of aortic regurgitation after transcatheter aortic valve implantation. Heart 98:1229–1236

54. Cubeddu RJ, Palacios IF (2010) Percutaneous techniques for mitral valve disease. Cardiol Clin 28:139–153

55. Feldman T, Cilingiroglu M (2011) Percutaneous leaflet repair and annuloplasty for mitral regurgitation. J Am Coll Cardiol 57:529–537

56. Daimon M, Shiota T, Gillinov AM et al (2005) Percutaneous mitral valve repair for chronic ischemic mitral regurgitation: a real-time three-dimensional echocardiographic study in an ovine model. Circulation 111:2183–2189

57. Kahlert P, Plicht B, Janosi RA et al (2009) The role of imaging in percutaneous mitral valve repair. Herz 34:458–467

58. Alfieri O, Maisano F, De Bonis M et al (2001) The double-orifice technique in mitral valve repair: a simple solution for complex problems. J Thorac Cardiovasc Surg 122:674–681

59. Feldman T, Kar S, Rinaldi M et al (2009) Percutaneous mitral repair with the MitraClip system: safety and midterm durability in the initial EVEREST (Endovascular Valve Edge-to-Edge REpair Study) cohort. J Am Coll Cardiol 54:686–694

60. Silvestry FE, Rodriguez LL, Herrmann HC et al (2007) Echocardiographic guidance and assessment of percutaneous repair for mitral regurgitation with the Evalve MitraClip: lessons learned from EVEREST I. J Am Soc Echocardiogr 20:1131–1140

61. Cavalcante JL, Rodriguez LL, Kapadia S et al (2012) Role of echocardiography in percutaneous mitral valve interventions. JACC Cardiovasc Imaging 5:733–746

62. Faletra FF, Pedrazzini G, Pasotti E, Moccetti T (2009) Real-time three-dimensional transoesophageal echocardiography showing sequential events of the percutaneous mitral clip procedure. Eur Heart J 30:2225

63. Altiok E, Becker M, Hamada S et al (2011) Optimized guidance of percutaneous edge-to edge repair of the mitral valve using real-time 3-D transoesphageal echocardiography. Clin Res Cardiol 100:675–681

64. Biner S, Perk G, Kar S et al (2011) Utility of combined two-dimensional and three-dimensional transesophageal imaging for catheter-based mitral valve clip repair of mitral regurgitation. J Am Soc Echocardiogr 24:611–617

65. Altiok E, Hamada S, Brehmer K et al (2012) Analysis of procedural effects of percutaneous edge-to-edge mitral valve repair by 2D and 3D echocardiography. Circ Cardiovasc Imaging 5:748–755

66. O'Gara P, Sugeng L, Lang R et al (2008) The role of imaging in chronic degenerative mitral regurgitation. JACC Cardiovasc Imaging 1:221–1237

67. Lang RM, Tsang W, Weinert L et al (2011) Valvular heart disease. The value of 3-dimensional echocar-diography. J Am Coll Cardiol 58:1933–1944

68. Faletra FF, Nucifora G, Ho SY (2011) Imaging the atrial septum using real-time three-dimensional transesophageal echo-cardiography: technical tips, normal anatomy, and its role in transseptal puncture. J Am Soc Echocardiogr 24:593–599

69. Swaans MJ, Post MC, Van den Branden BJ, Van der Heyden JA (2011) A complicated transseptal puncture during Mitraclip procedure: saved by 3D-TEE. Eur J Echocardiogr 12:E45

70. Swaans MJ, Van den Branden BJ, Van der Heyden JA et al (2009) Three-dimensional transoesophageal echocardiography in a patient undergoing percutaneous mitral valve repair using the edge-to-edge clip technique. Eur J Echocardiogr 10:982–983

71. Ciobanu A, Bennett S, Azam M et al (2011) Incremental value of three-dimensional transoesophageal echocardiography for guiding double percutaneous MitraClip (R) implantation in a 'no option' patient. Eur J Echocardiogr 12:E11

72. Paranskaya L, Kische S, Bozdag-Turan I et al (2012) Mitral valve with three orifices after percutaneous repair with the MitraClip system: the triple-orifice technique. Clin Res Cardiol 101:847–849

73. Kische S, Nienaber C, Ince H (2012) Use of four MitraClip devices in a patient with ischemic cardiomyopathy and mitral regurgitation: »zipping by clipping«. Catheter Cardiovasc Interv 80:1007–1013

74. Faletra F, Grimaldi A, Pasotti E et al (2009) Real-time 3-dimensional transesophageal echocardiography during double percutaneous mitral edge-to-edge procedure. JACC Cardiovasc Imaging 2:1031–1033

75. Pedrazzini GB, Klimusina J, Pasotti E et al (2011) Complications of percutaneous edge-to-edge mitral valve repair: the role of real-time three-dimensional transesophageal echocardiography. J Am Soc Echocardiogr 24:706–707

76. Landmesser U, Holmes DR, Jr (2012) Left atrial appendage closure: a percutaneous transcatheter approach for stroke prevention in atrial fibrillation. Eur Heart J 33:698–704

77. Holmes DR, Reddy VY, Turi ZG et al (2009) Percutaneous closure of the left atrial appendage versus warfarin therapy for prevention of stroke in patients with atrial fibrillation: a randomised non-inferiority trial. Lancet 374:534–542

78. Perk G, Biner S, Kronzon I et al (2012) Catheter-based left atrial appendage occlusion procedure: role of echocardiography. Eur Heart J Cardiovasc Imaging 13:132–138

79. Shah SJ, Bardo DM, Sugeng L et al (2008) Real-time three-dimensional transesophageal echocardiography of the left atrial appendage: initial experience in the clinical setting. J Am Soc Echocardiogr 21:1362–1368

80. Nakajima H, Seo Y, Ishizu T et al (2010) Analysis of the left atrial appendage by three-dimensional transesophageal echocardiography. Am J Cardiol 106:885–892

81. Chue CD, de GJ, Steeds RP (2011) The role of echocardiography in percutaneous left atrial appendage occlusion. Eur J Echocardiogr 12:i3–10

82. Nucifora G, Faletra FF, Regoli F et al (2011) Evaluation of the left atrial appendage with real-time 3-dimensional transesophageal echocardiography: implications for catheter-based left atrial appendage closure. Circ Cardiovasc Imaging 4:514–523

83. Unsworth B, Sutaria N, Davies DW, Kanagaratnam P (2011) Successful placement of left atrial appendage closure device is heavily dependent on 3-dimensional transesophageal imaging. J Am Coll Cardiol 58:1283

84. Plicht B, Konorza TF, Kahlert P et al (2013) Risk factors for thrombus formation on the amplatzer cardiac plug after left atrial appendage occlusion. JACC Cardiovasc Interv 6:606–613

85. Garcia-Fernandez MA, Cortes M, Garcia-Robles JA et al (2010) Utility of real-time three-dimensional transesophageal echocardiography in evaluating the success of percutaneous transcatheter closure of mitral paravalvular leaks. J Am Soc Echocardiogr 23:26–32

86. Phillips SA, Thompson A, bu-Halimah A et al (2009) Percutaneous closure of aortic pros-thetic paravalvular regurgitation with two amplatzer septal occluders. Anesth Analg 108:437–438

87. Johri AM, Yared K, Durst R et al (2009) Three-dimensional echocardiography-guided repair of severe paravalvular regurgitation in a bioprosthetic and mechanical mitral valve. Eur J Echocardiogr 10:572–575

88. Biner S, Kar S, Siegel RJ et al (2010) Value of color Doppler three-dimensional transesophageal echocardi-ography in the percutaneous closure of mitral prosthesis paravalvular leak. Am J Cardiol 105:984–989

89. Hamilton-Craig C, Boga T, Platts D et al (2009) The role of 3D transesophageal echocardiog-raphy during percutaneous closure of paravalvular mitral regurgitation. JACC Cardiovasc Imaging 2:771–773

90. Becerra JM, Almeria C, de Isla LP, Zamorano J (2009) Usefulness of 3D transoesophageal echocardiography for guiding wires and closure devices in mitral perivalvular leaks. Eur J Echocardiogr 10:979–981

91. Kim MS, Casserly IP, Garcia JA et al (2009) Percutaneous transcatheter closure of prosthetic mitral paravalvular leaks: are we there yet? JACC Cardiovasc Interv 2:81–90

92. Biner S, Rafique AM, Kar S, Siegel RJ (2008) Live three-dimensional transesophageal echocardiography-guided transcatheter closure of a mitral paraprosthetic leak by Amplatzer occluder. J Am Soc Echocardiogr 21:1282–1289

93. Tarantini G, Mojoli M, Napodano M (2013) Mitral paravalvular leak closure by antegrade percutaneous approach: Three-dimensional transesophageal echocardiographic guided multiple amplatzer implantation by a modified sequential anchoring-based technique. Catheter Cardiovasc Interv 82:e626–629

94. Hagler DJ, Cabalka AK, Sorajja P et al (2010) Assessment of percutaneous catheter treatment of paravalvular prosthetic regurgitation. JACC Cardiovasc Imaging 3:88–91

95. Swaans MJ, Post MC, Ten Berg JM (2011) Transapical repair of mitral valve paravalvular leakage using 3-D transesophageal guidance. Catheter Cardiovasc Interv 77:121–123

96. Rihal CS, Sorajja P, Booker JD et al (2012) Principles of percutaneous paravalvular leak closure. JACC Cardiovasc Interv 5:121–130

97. Nietlispach F, Johnson M, Moss RR et al (2010) Transcatheter closure of paravalvular defects using a purpose-specific occluder. JACC Cardiovasc Interv 3:759–765

98. Applebaum RM, Kasliwal RR, Kanojia A et al (1998) Utility of three-dimensional echocardiography during balloon mitral valvuloplasty. J Am Coll Cardiol 32:1405–1409

99. Binder TM, Rosenhek R, Porenta G et al (2000) Improved assessment of mitral valve stenosis by volumetric real-time three-dimensional echocardiography. J Am Coll Cardiol 36:1355–1361

100. Langerveld J, Valocik G, Plokker HW et al (2003) Additional value of three-dimensional transesophageal echocardiography for patients with mitral valve stenosis undergoing balloon valvuloplasty. J Am Soc Echocardiogr 16:841–849

101. Zamorano J, Perez de Isla L, Sugeng L et al (2004) Non-invasive assessment of mitral valve area during percutaneous balloon mitral valvuloplasty: role of real-time 3D echocardiography. Eur Heart J 25:2086–2091

102. Dobarro D, Gomez-Rubin MC, Lopez-Fernandez T et al (2009) Real time three-dimensional transesophageal echocardiography for guiding percutaneous mitral valvuloplasty. Echocardiography 26:746–748

103. Rodriguez L, Thomas JD, Monterroso V et al (1993) Validation of the proximal flow convergence method - calculation of orifice area in patients with mitral-stenosis. Circulation 88:1157–1165

104. Sebag IA, Morgan JG, Handschumacher MD et al (2005) Usefulness of three-dimensionally guided assessment of mitral stenosis using matrix-array ultrasound. Am J Cardiol 96:1151–1156

105. Knackstedt C, Franke A, Mischke K et al (2006) Semi-automated 3-dimensional intracardiac echocardiography: development and initial clinical experience of a new system to guide ablation procedures. Heart Rhythm 3:1453–1459

106. Faletra FF, Nucifora G, Regoli F et al (2012) Anatomy of pulmonary veins by real-time 3D TEE: implications for catheter-based pulmonary vein ablation. JACC Cardiovasc Imaging 5:456–462

107. Pua EC, Idriss SF, Wolf PD, Smith SW (2007) Real-time three-dimensional transesophageal echocardiography for guiding interventional electrophysiology: feasibility study. Ultrason Imaging 29:182–194

108. Yang HS, Srivathsan K, Wissner E, Chandrasekaran K (2008) Images in cardiovascular medicine. Real-time 3-dimensional transesophageal echocardiography: novel utility in atrial fibrillation ablation with a prosthetic mitral valve. Circulation 117:e304–e305

109. Chierchia GB, Van Camp G, Sarkozy A et al (2008) Double transseptal puncture guided by real-time three-dimensional transoesophageal echocardiography during atrial fibrillation ablation. Europace 10:705–706

110. Chierchia GB, Capulzini L, de Asmundis C et al (2008) First experience with real-time three-dimensional transoesophageal echocardiography-guided transseptal puncture in patients undergoing atrial fibrillation ablation. Europace 10:1325–1328

111. Lim KK, Sugeng L, Lang R, Knight BP (2008) Double transseptal catheterization guided by real-time 3-dimensional transesophageal echocardiography. Heart Rhythm 5:324–325

112. Ottaviano L, Chierchia GB, Bregasi A et al (2013) Cryoballoon ablation for atrial fibrillation guided by real-time three-dimensional transoesophageal echocardiography: a feasibility study. Europace 15:944–950

113. Regoli F, Faletra FF, Scaglione M et al (2012) Pulmonary vein isolation guided by real-time three-dimensional transesophageal echocardiography. Pacing Clin Electrophysiol 35:e76–e79

114. Faletra FF, Regoli F, Acena M, Auricchio A (2012) Value of real-time transesophageal 3-dimensional echocardiography in guiding ablation of isthmus-dependent atrial flutter and pulmonary vein isolation. Circ J 76:5–14

Service Part

Index – 304

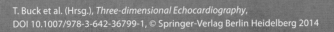

T. Buck et al. (Hrsg.), *Three-dimensional Echocardiography*,
DOI 10.1007/978-3-642-36799-1, © Springer-Verlag Berlin Heidelberg 2014

Index

Printing: Ten Brink, Meppel, The Netherlands
Binding: Stürtz, Würzburg, Germany